The Da Vinci Lupus Protocol

By Dr George J Georgiou

1

Dedication

First, I would like to deeply prostrate to the thousands of patients who have helped me understand the complexities of chronic diseases - for placing your trust in me, and allowing experimentation when things were not so clear.

All these patients over the years have been my "laboratory" for developing many treatment protocols through trial and error, backed by research.

I would also like to thank all the researcher scientists, lecturers and teachers who dedicate their life to helping others, and all the courageous health professionals who go against the grain of the establishment, while thinking outside the box.

A loving hug of gratitude to my wife and 4 children for their support and understanding during my professional endeavours throughout these years – they are all blessed.

In addition, I am deeply grateful to all the people and teams that have made it possible to produce the extensive series of health books that I have written and allow this information to spread across the globe to many other people in need.

Finally, I deeply embrace the Divine faith that I have been blessed with, that has helped me believe in the innate healing abilities of the body, through the power of Natural healing, without chemical intervention.

A profound blessing to you all, and may your healing journey be fruitful and fulfilling!

Published by
Inspired Publishing Ltd
27 Old Gloucester Street
London
WC1N 3AX

ISBN: 978-1-78555-043-0

Table of Contents

Chapter 1

The Da Vinci Lupus Treatment Protocol

Lupus is an autoimmune disease that causes swelling (inflammation) and a wide variety of symptoms. Lupus affects each individual uniquely. It causes high levels of persistent inflammation, which can negatively affect nearly every part of the body: the heart, joints, brain, kidneys, lungs and endocrine glands. Some people have only a few mild symptoms and others have more severe symptoms.

Lupus symptoms are very similar to many other health conditions, such as thyroid disorders, Lyme disease and fibromyalgia. Because of this, lupus can be very hard to diagnose.

Symptoms usually start in early adulthood, anywhere from the teen years into the 30s. As with some other autoimmune diseases, people with lupus generally experience flare-ups of symptoms followed by periods of remission. That's why early signs are easy to dismiss.

Common signs and symptoms of lupus include fatigue, headaches, joint pain, insomnia, GI issues and skin rashes. There are many others, so let's look at them in more detail below.

Common Lupus Symptoms
Symptoms of SLE may vary widely between individuals.

Brain: Persistent and unusual head-aches, memory loss, or confusion

Mouth and Nose: Sores inside the mouth and/or nose

Lungs/Heart: Shortness of breath and/or pain in the chest.

Eyes: Dry or puffy eyes, and increasing sensitivity to light

Skin: A "butterfly" rash on the face usually over the cheeks and bridge of the nose or other rashes that can worsen with sun exposure

Allow me to side-track a little and explain the premise of holistic medicine – I would strongly recommend that you read the chapter on holistic medicine in this book to understand the topic a little deeper. It is important because the label that is placed on the disease is not as important as trying to understand the underlying causative factors for the symptoms.

Whether you label all the symptoms I will describe below as lupus, rheumatoid arthritis, or Hashimoto's disease, or any other autoimmune disease, it does not really tell us what is triggering or causing all the symptoms to occur in the body. This is the $10 million question that every doctor needs to ask and answer for the benefit of the patient.

When a patient with lupus or any other chronic autoimmune disease walks into my office, the first thing that I will do is begin an investigation to discover the underlying causative factors.

At the Da Vinci Holistic Health Center where I work in Larnaca, Cyprus (www.naturaltherapycenter.com), I have developed the IDEL Diagnostic Programme which is a five-hour testing programme designed to bring many underlying causative factors to the fore. This is the only way to help such patients with such a complexity of symptoms. Indeed, IDEL stands for **ID**entify and **El**iminate. First, we identify the underlying causative factors and then we offload them and eliminate them so they cause no further problems in the body.

In the case of lupus, using a variety of drugs to suppress inflammation and symptoms does not really address many underlying causative factors that we will discuss below under holistic causes. Besides, many of these drugs have some very adverse side-effects and can damage other parts of the body causing further problems.

Let's examine some of the common symptoms that we often find in people suffering from lupus:

1. Fatigue

About 90% of people with lupus experience some level of fatigue, according to the Johns Hopkins Lupus Center. An afternoon nap does the trick for some people, but sleeping too much during the day can lead to insomnia at night. It may be hard to do, but if you can remain active and stick to a daily routine, you may be able to keep your energy levels up. If you are living with debilitating fatigue, speak to your doctor. Some causes of fatigue can be successfully treated.

2. Unexplained Fever

One of the early signs of lupus is a low-grade fever for no apparent reason. Because it may hover somewhere between 98.5 and 101 degrees Fahrenheit, you won't necessarily think to see a doctor. People with lupus may experience this type of fever on and off. Low-grade fever could be a sign of inflammation, infection, or imminent flare-up. If you have recurrent, low-grade fevers, make an appointment to see your doctor.

3. Hair Loss

Thinning hair is often one of the first signs of lupus. Hair loss is the result of inflammation of the skin and scalp. Some people with lupus lose hair by the clump, but more often, hair thins out slowly. Some people also have thinning of the beard, eyebrows, eyelashes, and other body hair. Lupus can cause hair to feel brittle, break easily, and look a bit ragged, earning it the name "lupus hair." Treating lupus successfully usually results in renewed hair growth. However, if you develop lesions on your scalp, hair loss in those areas may be permanent.

4. Skin Rash or Lesions

One of the most visible signs of lupus is the butterfly-shaped rash that appears over the bridge of the nose and both cheeks. About 50% of people with lupus have this rash, according to the Johns Hopkins Lupus Center. The rash can occur suddenly or appear after exposure to sunlight. Sometimes the rash appears just before a flare-up.

Signs And Symptoms Of Lupus

Lupus can also cause non-itchy lesions in other areas of the body. Rarely, lupus can cause hives. Many lupus patients are sensitive to the sun, or even to artificial lighting. Some experience discoloration of the fingers and toes.

5. Pulmonary Issues

Inflammation of the pulmonary system is another possible marker of lupus. Not only can the lungs themselves become inflamed, but the swelling can also extend to lung blood vessels. Even the diaphragm may be affected. These can all lead to chest pain when you try to breathe in, a condition often referred to as pleuritic chest pain.

Over time, breathing issues from lupus can literally shrink the lung size. Also called vanishing (or shrinking) lung syndrome, this condition is characterized by on-going chest pain and shortness of breath. The diaphragmatic muscles are so weak that they appear to move up in CAT scan imagery, according to the Lupus Foundation of America.

6. Kidney Inflammation

People with lupus can develop a kidney inflammation called nephritis. Inflammation makes it harder for the kidneys to filter toxins and waste from the blood. According to the Lupus Foundation of America, nephritis usually begins within five years of the start of lupus.

Symptoms include swelling in the lower legs and feet and high blood pressure. You may notice blood in your urine, or have to go more frequently at night. Also, you may have a pain in your side and your urine may be a bit darker than usual. Early signs may go unnoticed. Once diagnosed, monitoring of kidney function is recommended. Untreated lupus nephritis can lead to end-stage renal disease (ESRD).

7. Painful, Swollen Joints

Inflammation can cause pain, stiffness, and visible swelling in your joints, particularly in the morning. It may be mild at first, gradually becoming more obvious. Like other symptoms of lupus, joint problems can come and go.

If over-the-counter pain medications don't help, see your healthcare professional. There may be better treatment options, but your doctor must determine if your joint problems are caused by lupus or another condition, such as arthritis.

8. Gastrointestinal Problems

Some people with lupus experience occasional heartburn, acid reflux, or other gastrointestinal problems. Mild symptoms can be successfully treated with over-the-counter antacids. If you have frequent bouts of acid reflux or heartburn, try cutting down on the size of your meals, avoid beverages containing caffeine and don't lie down right after a meal. If symptoms continue, see your doctor so other conditions can be ruled out.

9. Thyroid Problems

It's not uncommon for people with lupus to develop autoimmune thyroid disease. The thyroid helps control your body's metabolism. A poorly functioning thyroid can affect vital organs like your brain, heart, kidneys, and liver. It can result in weight gain or weight loss. Other symptoms include dry skin and hair, as well as moodiness.

An underactive thyroid is known as hypothyroidism and an overactive one is called hyperthyroidism. Various treatments to get your metabolism back on track are available.

10. Dry Mouth, Dry Eyes

If you have lupus, you may have dry mouth. Your eyes may feel gritty and dry, too. That's because some lupus patients develop Sjogren's syndrome, another autoimmune disorder. Sjogren's syndrome causes malfunctioning of the glands responsible for tears and saliva. In some cases, women with lupus may also experience dryness of the vagina.

11. Other Symptoms

The list of potential symptoms of lupus is lengthy. Other symptoms include muscle pain, chest   pain, osteoporosis,   and depression.   Rare   symptoms include anaemia, dizziness, and seizures.

11

Fortunately, not everyone gets every symptom. While new symptoms can appear on the scene, old ones often disappear.

It takes many lupus patients years to be accurately diagnosed, sometimes leaving patients being prescribed various prescriptions over and over again that don't seem to fix the problem. Today, conventional medications for lupus include corticosteroid drugs, NSAID pain relievers, thyroid medications and even synthetic hormone replacement drugs - which help lower inflammation but can cause many unwanted side effects and even long-term health problems.

Although many patients with lupus aren't thrilled about the effects of the prescriptions they take, most feel they have no other choice and are desperate to find relief from their symptoms. Fortunately, natural remedies for lupus, including supplements, exercise and a healthy diet high in anti-inflammatory foods can all help manage symptoms and improve overall immune function, without raising the risk for complications.

Risk factors for lupus

Risk factors for developing lupus include:

- Having genetic susceptibility and a family history of lupus or other autoimmune disorders.
- Family history - first-degree or second-degree relatives of a person with lupus have a 4-8% risk of developing lupus. One study suggests that sisters of lupus patients have as high as a 10% chance of developing lupus. In another 10-year prospective study, researchers observed a 7% incidence of lupus in first-degree relatives of lupus patients. However, a genetic predisposition does not mean that you will develop lupus – the environment can also change the expression of genes, meaning that lifestyle changes can change the expression of the genes and the direction of the disease.
- Being a woman (90 percent of all lupus patients are women).
- Being between the ages of 15 - 45; women of "childbearing age" are by far the most likely to develop lupus.
- Being of African-American, Asian or Native American decent; these ethnicities develop lupus two to three times more often than Caucaisans do.
- Eating a poor diet and having nutrient deficiencies.
- GI troubles including leaky gut syndrome.

- Food allergies and sensitivities.
- Toxicity exposure.

- A history of infections and other autoimmune disorders.

It is uncommon for children under the age of 15 to have lupus. One exception is babies born to women with lupus. These children may have heart, liver or skin problems caused by lupus.

Pregnancy

Although pregnancy in women with lupus is considered high risk, most women with lupus carry their babies safely to the end of their pregnancy. Overall, women with lupus have a higher rate of miscarriage and premature births compared with the general population. In addition, women who have anti-phospholipid antibodies are at a greater risk of miscarriage in the second trimester because of their increased risk of blood clotting in the placenta.

Lupus patients with a history of kidney disease have a higher risk of preeclampsia (hypertension with a build-up of excess watery fluid in cells or tissues of the body). Pregnancy counselling and planning before pregnancy are important. Ideally, a woman should have no signs or symptoms of lupus and be taking no medications for several months before becoming pregnant.

The pathogenesis of lupus

The principle cause of lupus-mediated tissue injury is inflammation triggered by *autoantibody complexes.*

B cells, so-called because these immune cells originate in the **B**one marrow, produce and secrete the antibodies, which are specialized proteins that bind to other molecules. The immune system generates millions of different antibodies that target an extremely large variety of molecules on the surface of microbes, such as bacteria and viruses.

The antibody binds its specific molecule on a microbe in similar fashion to a key in a certain lock. When the "key" (antibody) and "lock" (microbe) fit together, the antibody sticks tightly to the microbe and marks it to be removed from the body. In people with lupus, many of the B cells secrete *autoantibodies,* which means that these antibodies bind to molecules on otherwise healthy tissues instead of molecules on microbes.

T cells, which are generated in the **T**hymus, produce various proteins called cytokines that help B cells grow, become activated, and stimulate B cells to produce antibodies. Other immune cells, including macrophages and neutrophils, migrate to the site of inflammation and produce tissue damaging *reactive oxygen species* (ROS), otherwise known as free radicals, as well as engulf microbes and cells through a process called *phagocytosis*.

One of the ways macrophages know when to engulf a microbe is by sensing that antibodies are stuck to their surface. All of these cells collectively are called leukocytes or white blood cells because of their lack of colour. B and T cells are a subset of leukocytes called lymphocytes.

The types of self-molecules ("the lock") that stick to autoantibodies ("the key") vary in each case of lupus. Self-molecules common in lupus often are associated with the cell nucleus, which is the compartment within a cell that contains DNA and other proteins that make up genes.

Lupus-mediated tissue damage can be summarized as follows:

1. B cells become activated and produce autoantibodies that bind various self-molecules.
2. Activated T cells produce proteins called cytokines that help activate more B cells.
3. Large complexes of antibodies stuck to self-molecules are formed.
4. These complexes become lodged in various tissues throughout the body, such as the kidney and joints.
5. The complexes cause an influx of neutrophils, macrophages, and other B cells and T cells into the tissue.
6. Proinflammatory cells secrete damaging reactive oxygen species or free radicals and more proteins that cause tissue damage.
7. If the inflammation is not treated and persists over time, the tissue may become permanently damaged.

How is Lupus Diagnosed?

Your doctor will do a physical exam to check for typical signs and symptoms of lupus, including:

*   sun sensitivity rashes, such as a malar or butterfly rash
*   mucous membrane ulcers, which may occur in the mouth or nose
*   arthritis

14

- hair loss
- hair thinning
- signs of cardiac or lung involvement, such as murmurs, rubs, or irregular heartbeats.

No one single test is diagnostic for SLE, but screenings that can help your doctor come to an informed diagnosis include:

- a urinalysis
- blood tests, such as antibody tests and a complete blood count
- a chest X-ray

Your doctor might refer you to a rheumatologist, which is a doctor who specializes in treating joint and soft tissue disorders and autoimmune diseases.

To summarize

- Lupus is not contagious, not even through sexual contact. You cannot "catch" lupus from someone or "give" lupus to someone.

- Lupus is not like or related to cancer. Cancer is a condition of malignant, abnormal tissues that grow rapidly and spread into surrounding tissues. Lupus is an autoimmune disease, as described above. However, some treatments for lupus may include immunosuppressant drugs that are also used in chemotherapy.

- Lupus is not like or related to HIV (Human Immune Deficiency Virus) or AIDS (Acquired Immune Deficiency Syndrome). In HIV or AIDS the immune system is underactive; in lupus, the immune system is overactive.

- Lupus can range from mild to life-threatening and should always be treated by a doctor. With good medical care, most people with lupus can lead a full life.

- More than 16,000 new cases of lupus are reported in the USA every year.

- It is estimated that at least 1.5 million Americans have lupus. The actual number may be higher; however, there have been no large-scale studies to show the actual number of people in the U.S. living with lupus.

- It is believed that 5 million people throughout the world have a form of lupus.

15

- Lupus strikes mostly women of childbearing age. However, men, children, and teenagers develop lupus, too. Most people with lupus develop the disease between the ages of 15-44.

- Women of colour are two to three times more likely to develop lupus than Caucasians.

- People of all races and ethnic groups can develop lupus.

Lupus Symptoms & Warning Signs

Lupus causes symptoms both directly due to inflammation, and also indirectly due to worsening levels of stress. Many lupus patients suffer psychologically and deal with symptoms of anxiety, depression, memory loss and insomnia — partially because lupus can cause nerve damage to the spinal cord and inflammation of the brain, but also because battling lupus can be very hard.

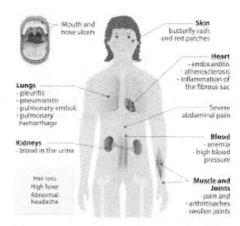

Systemic lupus erythematosus

Common Symptoms of Lupus Include:

- chronic fatigue
- joint pains
- muscle aches
- stiffness, swelling and oedema
- shortness of breath and chest pains
- headaches

- fever
- skin rashes and sunburns
- depression and anxiety
- insomnia
- blurred vision and dry eyes
- mouth and nose sores and ulcers
- anaemia and weakness
- memory loss and confusion
- complications including higher risk for high blood pressure and heart disease, kidney damage, lung damage, infections, seizures and stroke

The following systems in the body can also be affected by lupus:

- Kidneys: inflammation of the kidneys (nephritis) can impair their ability to get rid of waste products and other toxins from the body effectively

- Lungs: some people with lupus develop pleuritis, an inflammation of the lining of the chest cavity that causes chest pain, particularly with breathing. Patients with lupus may also get pneumonia

- Central nervous system: in some patients, lupus affects the brain or central nervous system. This can cause headaches, dizziness, depression, memory disturbances, vision problems, seizures, stroke or changes in behaviour

- Blood vessels: blood vessels may become inflamed (vasculitis), affecting the way blood circulates through the body

- Blood: people with lupus may develop anaemia, leukopenia (a decreased number of white blood cells) or thrombocytopenia (a decrease in the number of platelets in the blood, which assist in clotting)

- Heart: in some people with lupus, inflammation can occur in the heart itself (myocarditis and endocarditis) or the membrane that surrounds it (pericarditis), causing chest pain or other symptoms. Endocarditis can damage the heart valves, causing the valve surface to thicken and develop growths which can lead to heart murmurs.

Having lupus also increases your risk of:

- Infection: people with lupus are more vulnerable to infection because both the disease and its treatments weaken the immune system. Infections that most commonly affect people with lupus include urinary tract infections, respiratory infections, yeast infections, salmonella, herpes and shingles

- Bone tissue death (avascular necrosis): this occurs when the blood supply to a bone diminishes; often leading to tiny breaks in the bone and eventually to the bone's collapse. The hip joint is most commonly affected.

- Pregnancy complications: women with lupus have an increased risk of miscarriage. Lupus increases the risk of high blood pressure during pregnancy (preeclampsia) and preterm birth. To reduce the risk of these complications, doctors often recommend delaying pregnancy until your disease has been under control for at least six months.

Types of lupus

There are many different types of lupus, including the following five forms:

1) Systemic lupus erythematosus (SLE)

When most people talk about lupus, they are referring to SLE.

"Systemic" means that the disease can affect numerous parts of the body. The symptoms of SLE can be mild or severe, and although more common in people aged between 15 - 45, it can additionally occur during childhood or later in life.

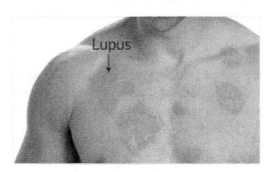

2) Discoid Lupus Erythematosus (DLE)

DLE is a chronic skin disorder in which a red, raised rash appears on the face, scalp or elsewhere on the body.

The raised areas may become thick and scaly and may cause scarring. The rash may last for days or years and may reoccur. Small percentages of people with DLE have or will develop SLE.

3) Subacute cutaneous lupus erythematosus

Subacute cutaneous lupus erythematosus refers to skin lesions that appear on parts of the body exposed to sun. The lesions do not cause scarring.

4) Drug-induced lupus

There are a number of medications that can cause drug-induced lupus such as some anti-seizure, high blood pressure, thyroid medications, antibiotics, antifungals and oral contraceptive pills. The symptoms usually completely disappear when you stop taking the drug.

Drug Induced Lupus
- Long term use of certain medications
- Symptoms of SLE
- Stopping medications reduces symptoms within weeks
- Some implicated medications
  - Chlorpromazine
  - Methyldopa
  - Hydralazine
  - Procainamide
  - Isoniazid
  - Dilantin
  - Penicillamine
  - Quinidine
  - Certain antibiotics
  - Allopurinol

5) Neonatal lupus

Neonatal lupus is a rare disease that can occur in new-born babies of women with SLE, Sjögren's syndrome, or with no disease at all. Most babies of mothers with SLE are healthy.

Scientists suspect that neonatal lupus is caused in part by autoantibodies in the mother's blood called anti-Ro (SSA) and anti-La (SSB).

At birth, babies with neonatal lupus have a skin rash, liver problems and low blood counts. These symptoms usually resolve by the time the child is 6 months old, but the most serious manifestation - congenital heart block - requires a pacemaker and has a mortality rate of around 20%.

It is important for women with SLE or other related autoimmune disorders to be under a doctor's care during pregnancy.

Conditions with Similar Symptoms

A number of conditions overlap with SLE:

- Scleroderma: Hardening of the skin caused by overproduction of collagen
- Rheumatoid arthritis: Inflammation of the lining of the joints
- Sojourn's syndrome: Characterized by dry eyes and dry mouth
- Mixed connective tissue disorder: Similar to SLE, but milder
- Myositis: Inflammation and degeneration of muscle tissues
- Rosacea: Flushed face with pus-filled blisters
- Seborrheic dermatitis: Sores on lips and nose

20

- Lichen planus: Swollen rash that itches, typically on scalp, arms, legs, or in the mouth
- Dermatomyositis: Bluish-red skin eruptions on face and upper body
- Lyme disease: Bulls-eye rash, joint inflammation, and flu-like symptoms

If lupus is not treated or controlled, these complications can result:

- Inflamed kidneys, which may cause no pain but can be detected with urine and blood tests.

-

- Central nervous system problems, such as headaches, dizziness, difficulty concentrating, mood swings or seizures.
- Blood and blood vessel problems. These include anaemia, increased risk of bleeding, increased risk of blood clots or inflamed blood vessels.

- Inflammation of the lungs and the linings of the chest cavity. This can make breathing painful and increase the risk of a form of pneumonia.

- Chest pain resulting from inflammation of the heart muscle, arteries or heart membrane. The leading cause of death for people with lupus today is cardiovascular disease, which can lead to heart attacks. It is not clear whether this is because people with lupus are living longer or whether it is a complication of treatment.
- Exercising, not smoking, controlling high blood pressure and reducing cholesterol levels all help reduce the risk of cardiovascular disease.

- Infection, from having the disease and from treatment.

- Tissue death, caused when the blood supply to certain areas is reduced. The hip joint is commonly affected and may result in pain when walking.

For women who are of the age to bear children, lupus creates special risks, including:

- Difficulty conceiving. Flare-ups of the disease and medications used to treat it can contribute to infertility.

-

- Greater risk for miscarriage. The risk is highest early or late in the pregnancy. The risk can be reduced by careful planning and medical care.

21

- More risk of complications during pregnancy. Flare-ups are more likely. The risk for high blood pressure, diabetes and kidney problems during pregnancy is also higher.

- Limited birth control options. Women may not tolerate birth control pills well, and they should not use intrauterine devices because of the risk of infection.

Causes of Lupus: The Medical Perspective

The exact cause of lupus is unknown by modern medicine. Some experts indicate that lupus develops in response to a combination of factors from both inside and outside of the body, including hormones, genetics and the environment. Let's look at some of these factors in a little more detail below.

1. Hormones

Hormones are chemical substances produced in the body that control and regulate the activity of certain cells or organs.

As 9 in every 10 occurrences of lupus are in females, researchers have looked at the possible relationship between oestrogen and lupus. Although both men and women produce oestrogen, the production of the hormone is greater in women.

Studies have shown that women have lupus symptom flare-ups just before menstrual periods and during pregnancy when oestrogen production is higher.

Oestrogen is known to be an "immune-enhancing" hormone, which means that women have stronger immune systems than men. For this reason, the incidence of autoimmune diseases is generally higher in women than in men.

Research has found that women have lupus symptom flare-ups just before menstrual periods and during pregnancy when oestrogen production is increased. This may suggest that oestrogen could regulate the severity of lupus. However, no causal effect has been proven, and studies including women taking oestrogen in the form of birth control pills or as postmenopausal therapy have shown no increase in disease activity.

Oestrogen actions tend to be proinflammatory, while the actions of progesterone, androgens, and glucocorticoids are anti-inflammatory (Cutolo 2004). Studies have documented low progesterone levels in women with lupus, suggesting that a relative imbalance in favour of oestrogen may contribute to immune reactivity in some female patients (Shabanova 2008).

Accordingly, studies in women with lupus revealed an increased rate of mild to moderate intensity disease flares associated with oestrogen-containing hormone replacement therapy (Buyon 2005). Experimental studies have suggested that testosterone may suppress immune reactivity in lupus animal models and in cells from patients with lupus (Walker 1994; Kanda 1997).

Based on the available data, Life Extension suggests that women with lupus evaluate their sex hormone levels and ensure that progesterone and testosterone levels are sufficient. If progesterone or testosterone levels are found to be low, women should consider using bioidentical progesterone or and/or testosterone creams to restore levels to a normal range (Gompel 2007).

2. Genetics

No specific gene or group of genes has been proven to cause lupus. Lupus is more prevalent among some families and certain genes have been identified as contributing to the development of lupus. However, these genetic associations alone are not conclusive for causing the disease, as highlighted by twins where only one of the twins develops lupus.

Identical twins may be raised in the exact same way in the same environment and feature the same inherited attributes, but only one of them may develop lupus. There is a 25% chance that an identical twin could develop the disease and a 2-3% chance for fraternal twins.

The risk for development of lupus in siblings of individuals with the disease is about 20 times higher than that of the general population.

Although there are occurrences of lupus developing in people with no family history of the disease, there are likely to be other autoimmune diseases such as thyroiditis, haemolytic anaemia and idiopathic thrombocytopenia purpura in some family members.

Ethnic groups such as people of African, Asian, Hispanic, Native American, Native Hawaiian, or Pacific Island descent have a greater risk of developing lupus, which may be related to genes they have in common.

3. Biomarkers

Biomarkers are another significant area of lupus research. Biomarkers are defined as molecules that reflect a specific biological or pathological process, a consequence of a process or a response to a therapeutic intervention. Simply put, they can let the doctor know what is happening in the body - or predict what is going to happen - based on something reliably measurable in tissues, cells or fluids.

Researchers have identified the following as potential biomarkers:

- Anti-double-stranded DNA antibodies and complement C3a - both of which can be found in blood tests - as biomarkers for flares

- Proteins in the urine of people with renal disease caused by lupus. These biomarkers can be used to indicate the type and severity of renal disease in these patients, as well as the extent of damage to the kidney

- C-reactive protein (CRP), a protein made by the liver, which correlates with disease activity and cardiovascular disease risk factors, and C4d, a protein in the blood that may indicate lupus disease activity or kidney involvement

4. Environment

According to the Lupus Foundation of America, researchers consider that environmental agents such as chemicals or viruses may contribute to triggering lupus in genetically susceptible individuals.

Environmental elements that may trigger lupus include:

- Ultraviolet rays from the sun - UVB in particular

- Ultraviolet rays from fluorescent light bulbs used in tanning

- Exposure to silica dust in agricultural or industrial settings

- Sulpha drugs, which make a person more sensitive to the sun

- Sun-sensitizing tetracycline drugs

- Penicillin or other antibiotic drugs

- Infections - including the effects of Epstein-Barr virus

- Cold or a viral illness

- Exhaustion

- Injury

- Emotional stress, such as divorce, illness, death in the family or other life complications

- Anything else that causes stress to the body such as surgery, physical harm, pregnancy or giving birth

- Smoking

According to the medical profession, there is presently no cure for lupus. However, lupus can be treated effectively and most people with the disease can lead active, healthy lives.

We will see that this statement is not absolutely true, as when many of the underlying causative factors are removed from the body, then it is possible to cure lupus, as it is many other autoimmune diseases.

Let's now take a look at what some of these other causative factors are – these factors are often overlooked by medical doctors, this is why it is titled the "holistic perspective" as it goes beyond what a normal doctor would look for.

Causes of lupus: The Holistic Perspective

Potential lupus causes include allergic reactions, viruses, emotional stress, oestrogen disruption due to pregnancy or birth control, hormonal imbalances, poor digestion, and heavy metal toxicity.

Let's examine some of these factors in a little more detail…

Vaccinations

Studies have found that lupus can be triggered by the hepatitis B-vaccination (HBV). These are cases reported in the scientific literature and to the Vaccine Adverse Event Reporting System (VAERS) (Geier et al, 2005; Older et al, 1999). There is also recent evidence that BCG vaccinations can also be a trigger (Spadaro et al, 2016).

The researchers conclude (Santoro et al, 2010):

> *"Hepatitis B vaccine can potentially trigger both the onset or the exacerbations of several autoimmune disorders, including systemic lupus erythematosus, by reduced immune complex clearance or molecular mimicry."*

Another study has found that some of the oil adjuvants placed in vaccinations can also trigger an auto-immune response in lupus. One study concluded (Satoh et al, 2003):

> *"The ability to induce lupus autoantibodies is shared by several hydrocarbons and is not unique to pristane. It correlates with stimulation of the production of IL-12 and other cytokines, suggesting a relationship with a hydrocarbon's adjuvanticity. The potential to induce autoimmunity may complicate the use of oil adjuvants in human and veterinary vaccines."*

Dr. John Bergman blames vaccines for this 'autoimmune' epidemic. He says:
"With 69 different vaccines injected into children... well, we now see a response in our bodies and a massive rise in inflammatory brain disorders like encephalitis and autism, or inflammatory lung disorders, like Asthma; inflammatory sinus issues like sinusitis; inflammatory gut reactions like colitis and Irritable Bowel Syndrome, etc.".

Toxic metals and Other Toxins

Lead and mercury have been implicated in causing lupus with the proper genotype or genetics – there are 4 predisposing loci that have been identified on the 1st, 4th and 7th chromosomes.

According to Dr. John Bergman, the body is responding appropriately to environmental stimuli, such as:

> ➢ *69 highly toxic vaccines injected into children (containing mercury, aluminium, etc.).*
> ➢ *Thousands of toxic pharmaceutical drugs, with deadly side-effects.*
> ➢ *Highly toxic Genetically Modified Foods (GMO) in our food supply.*
> ➢ *Thousands of toxic pesticides are used on our crops.*
> ➢ *Thousands of toxic additives and chemicals are present in processed foods.*
> ➢ *Antibiotics, sex hormones, growth hormones, etc. are found in meat products.*

> ➢ *Thousands of toxic chemicals are found in makeup and personal care products.*

Mercury from amalgam fillings in our teeth, as well as eating mercury-toxic fish is another reason for autoimmune diseases.

According to Amalgam.org:

"Mercury is a common cause of chronic conditions related to intestinal dysfunction, such as ulcerative colitis, Irritable Bowel Syndrome, Crohn's, psoriasis and lupus. When intestinal permeability is increased, food and nutrient absorption is impaired. Dysfunction in intestinal permeability can result in leaky gut syndrome, where larger molecules and toxins in the intestines can pass through the membranes and into the blood, triggering immune response. Progressive damage can occur to the intestinal lining, eventually allowing disease-causing bacteria, undigested food particles, and toxins to pass directly into the blood stream."

"Other common causes or factors in leaky gut and the related conditions include food allergies and intolerances; drugs (NSAIDs, aspirin, stomach h2 blockers, steroids, etc.); dysbiosis (overgrowth of organisms due to antibiotic use and/or low probiotic levels); alcohol consumption; synergistic toxic exposures and chemical sensitivity; chronic infections; and inadequate digestive enzymes. [...] food additives or processed foods that contain glutamate (MSG), aspartame, high-fructose corn syrup, dyes, etc. are common causes of leaky gut syndrome.
[...] In addition to improvements in many patients after amalgam replacement and detoxification, diet and nutritional measures are usually effective at improving lupus. The 4-R program has seen good success in many patients. The program removes all foods where there is suspicion of allergy that might produce inflammation. Common allergens include wheat/gluten, dairy, eggs, peanuts, tomatoes, corn, and red meat."

"Additionally, elimination of gastrointestinal parasites, undesirable bacteria, fungus, and yeasts are carried out. Sometimes a treatment such as nystantin is used to eliminate yeast. Then vital nutrients are replaced by dietary measures and supplementation of a good multivitamin and mineral, minerals found deficient such as iron, magnesium, calcium, selenium, zinc, iodine and vitamins, such as B-complex, B6, B12, and folic acid. Next the intestines are re-inoculated with friendly bacteria (Lactobacillus acidophilus and Lactobacilus bulgaricus.) Finally, measures are taken to repair the intestine to correct for the increased permeability. This is done by adding nutrients such as glutamine, pathothenic acid (B5), zinc, FOS, and vitamin C. DHEA and Butyrate have also been found effective in many patients at reducing inflammation."

It is certainly worth using a gentle, natural chelator of heavy metals in order to detoxify these lupus-triggering toxic metals. It is worth reading the chapter on toxicity to see more details of HMD™, the natural, scientifically-researched natural chelator.

However, lupus patients must detoxify very slowly, beginning with only one drop x three times daily, and increase by one drop every day until the adult dosage of 45 drops x 3 times daily is reached.

In addition, it is important to take drainage remedies in order to help these toxic metals eliminate from the body, such as LAVAGE (25 drops x 3 times daily) as well as CHLORELLA (2 caps x 2 times daily). The SUPER ULTIMATE DETOX PACK is what we recommend at the Da Vinci Center and contains all these products in one pack.

Oestrogens

There is evidence that oestrogens play a role in the aetiology of systemic lupus erythematosus (SLE) (Meier et al, 1998).

These findings suggest that longer term use of postmenopausal oestrogens plays a role in the aetiology of both SLE and discoid lupus. There is a suggestion that progestogen may reduce the effect of oestrogens on these autoimmune disorders, given that it is antagonistic to oestrogen.

Apart from the endogenous oestrogens that the body produces, there are also exogenous oestrogen-mimicking molecules that come from chemicals such as those found in plastics. The more well-known of these chemicals is PCB's or Phthalates and Bisphenyl A – these will create a condition of oestrogen-dominance in the body, in both males and females and can trigger lupus as well as other serious chronic diseases (Protera C, 2005; Ghosh et al, 2003).

Phthalates are found in adhesives, cosmetics, fragrances, vinyl flooring, polyvinyl chloride pipe, and certain toys and medical supplies.

Statins – Cholesterol-lowering Drugs

Several case reports of lupus-like syndrome suggest that statins could have triggered the development of this rare autoimmune disease (Hilda et al, 2011).

Vitamin D Deficiency

Vitamin D deficiency is highly prevalent in patients with SLE (Gao et al, 2016; Thudi et al, 2008; Kamen et al, 2006). This may also explain winter flare-ups in lupus patients who see little sun because of their photosensitivity. The body makes vitamin D when the skin is exposed to the sun. Severe deficiency increases the risk of moderate to severe disease activity, but not organ damage.

Moreover, mounting evidence suggests that vitamin D may be a critical missing link in virtually all autoimmune diseases, including lupus. Vitamin D is capable of modulating the activity of immune cells, and studies have identified widespread vitamin D deficiency in lupus patients (Toloza 2010; Lemire 1992). For example, one study found that a mere **1.2%** of lupus patients had adequate vitamin D levels, compared to 45% of healthy controls (Damanhouri 2009); another found that lower vitamin D levels were linked with more aggressive lupus autoimmunity (Ritterhouse 2011).

The Da Vinci strategy is centred upon easing inflammation and combines several scientifically studied nutrients to complement the *immunomodulatory* role of vitamin D. Additionally, avoiding inflammatory foods high in omega-6 fatty acids in favour of healthy omega-3's provides a nutritional foundation ideal for balancing an inappropriately reactive immune system. We will discuss these strategies in more detail below.

Vitamin D intervenes in the process of autoimmunity by tilting the properties of T- and B-cells towards "***tolerance***" of self -tissues. Tolerance is a phenomenon orchestrated by a variety of highly specialized cytokines and other cell-signalling molecules.

Early in the developmental process of immune cells, they are directed to become either "*effector*" or "*regulatory*" immune cells. In other words, to become immune cells that promote tissue destruction, or those that suppress tissue destruction respectively.

Patients with lupus have elevated numbers of effector cells (promoting tissue destruction) and lower numbers of regulatory cells (suppressing tissue destruction) (Bonelli 2010). Moreover, the regulatory cells of lupus patients malfunction (Bonelli 2010).

Vitamin D exerts multiple actions at the cellular level to balance the population of effector cells and regulatory cells (Bruce 2011). In a 2012 study, 20 lupus patients with initially low vitamin D blood levels received 100,000 IU of vitamin D weekly for 4 weeks, followed by 100,000 IU monthly for 6 months.

The treatment resulted in significantly increased vitamin D blood levels (from 18 ng/mL at baseline to 51 ng/mL at 2- and 6-month follow-ups), decreased effector T-cell counts and anti-DNA antibodies, and increased regulatory T-cells.

Over the 6-month follow-up period, no disease flares were noted (Terrier 2012). These lines of evidence establish a very strong case for the importance of maintaining sufficient vitamin D blood levels to combat lupus disease activity. The Da Vinci Center suggests an optimal vitamin D blood level of 50 – 80 ng/mL (measured as 25-hydroxyvitamin).

To get to these blood levels we recommend VITAMIN D3 – 5,000 I.U.

Antioxidant Deficiency

A study (Bae et al, 2002) compared plasma antioxidant/oxidant status and the dietary nutrient intake of patients with systemic lupus erythematosus (SLE) to those of healthy controls. Results showed that plasma antioxidant status is impaired and dietary antioxidant intake is decreased in patients with SLE.

Antioxidant deficiency can also lead to greater free radical damage which can damage mitochondria in cells, leading to autoimmune diseases such as lupus.

Mitochondria could provoke the inflammation characteristic of lupus. By-products of cells' power stations goad certain white blood cells into making mesh traps as a precursor to cell death. Mitochondrial DNA is spewed out, triggering a warning and a response that can damage various organ tissues (Lood et al, 2016).

In lab studies, the researchers noted that this extracellular release of oxygenated mitochondrial DNA promotes an inflammatory reaction. When this DNA is injected into mice, its unwelcome presence is detected by DNA sensors and leads to activation of a protein called STING. A chemical warning goes off. The resulting type 1 interferon signalling calls up antimicrobial defences and other immune responses that will result in inflammation.

At the Da Vinci Center we use a high-potency multivitamin that contains good quantities of antioxidants such as HMD MULTIS (one cap x 3 daily), as well as ALPHA-LIPOIC ACID (one cap x 2 daily).

Lupus low-density granulocytes spontaneously undergo NETosis - a process in which the immune cell throws out genetic material (DNA, blue) and antimicrobial molecules such as elastase (green) in a web-like structure.
Credit: Luz Blanco/NIAMS

Food Intolerances and Lupus

When the body is exposed to environmental allergens the immune system begins to produce IgE immunoglobulins as a response. This triggers the body to produce inflammatory chemicals through the mast cells, such as proteases and pro-inflammatory cytokines. This inflammation can persist even after the exposure of the environmental allergen. We know from other research that chronic inflammation is one of the precursors for autoimmune disease, so allergies causing inflammation have a direct relationship with autoimmune diseases such as lupus (Valenta et al, 2009).

Non-allergy Non-celiac Wheat Sensitivity (NCWS)

There is another syndrome that may also be related to lupus known as non-allergy non-celiac wheat sensitivity (NCWS).

Recent studies (Schuppan et al, 2015) and experimental data strongly indicate that NCWS exists in a substantial proportion of the population, that it is an innate immune reaction to wheat and that patients often present with extraintestinal

31

symptoms, such as worsening of an underlying inflammatory disease in clear association with wheat consumption, such as lupus.

A protein in wheat called Amylase-Trypsin Inhibitors (ATIs) have been identified as the most likely triggers of NCWS. They are highly resistant to protease enzymes that would normally digest them. They also trigger monocytes, which are types of white blood cells that produce inflammatory antibodies – this is known as the Toll-Like Receptor 4 (TLR4) complex in monocytes, macrophages and dendritic cells of the intestinal mucosa. Non-gluten containing cereals or staples display no or little TLR4 stimulating activity.

So, in summary, there is mounting research that has identified a group of proteins in wheat that may be responsible for triggering inflammation in chronic conditions such as lupus, rheumatoid arthritis, and multiple sclerosis. Indeed, many of the lupus patients that I have tested for food intolerances are intolerant to all gluten grains, so it is easy to advise that they keep away from these grains religiously, including wheat, barley, rye, oats, zea, kamut, and spelt.

Why is Gluten So Bad For Us?

There are a number of recent studies that support the following findings:

1. Gluten grains contain "protease inhibitors" which block the body's own digestive enzymes. In addition, our bodies simply aren't capable of breaking gluten down into single amino acids. The proteins remain as amino acid chains (peptides) which will ultimately impede proper digestion, destroy our intestinal flora, and can damage the gut lining itself.

2. Some gluten proteins mimic those present in various bacteria and viruses. If those proteins enter the bloodstream through a damaged gut lining, the body mistakenly mounts an attack against them, thinking they are pathogens. This can result in systemic inflammation, joint pain, and chronic fatigue – common symptoms in lupus patients.

GLUTEN (GLIADIN + GLUTENIN)

3. Gluten proteins can also be very similar in molecular structure to human tissue and result in an autoimmune response. The molecular structure of the gluten protein called *gliadin* is very similar to that of thyroid tissue. When the immune system sees gliadin, it creates antibodies to attack it and those same antibodies incorrectly attack thyroid tissue as well, causing another autoimmune disease known as Hashimoto's disease.

Wheat: An Exceptionally Unwholesome Grain

Wheat presents a special case as wild and selective breeding has produced variations which include up to 6 sets of chromosomes (3x the human genome worth!) capable of generating a massive number of proteins each with a potential of causing inflammation.

Common bread wheat (Triticum aestivum), for instance, has over 23,788 proteins catalogued thus far. In fact, the genome for common bread wheat is actually 6.5 times larger than that of the human genome! Maybe the human body was not designed to digest so many proteins, as almost inevitably the more ancient and purer forms of wheat had far fewer proteins.

Another big change in the wheat that we are eating today compared to the past, is that the new wheat has up to a 50% increase in gluten content in some varieties. If we had a glass of gluten and you stick your hands in it, they would get stuck in the glue-like substance. Imagine drinking this "glue" and what this might do to the body.

To add insult to injury, research has also found other nasty proteins in wheat that are not good for the body. There are other protein components of wheat known as gliadin, the sugar-binding protein known as lectin (Wheat Germ Agglutinin), the exorphin known as gliadomorphin, and the excitotoxic potentials of high levels of aspartic and glutamic acid found in wheat. Add to these the anti-nutrients found in grains such as phytates, enzyme inhibitors, etc. and you have a substance that is far from healthy!

At the Da Vinci Center, we try to persuade all patients with lupus to give up all the gluten grains religiously! Their health usually begins improving only from this one restriction, even though we will also advise that they cut out all the food intolerances that we identify during testing.

Let's look at some of the components in wheat that we have mentioned above in a little more detail so that you can really understand WHY you should avoid it. I generally find that explaining things to patients results in greater compliance and understanding.

Wheat Germ Agglutinin (WGA)

There is a powerful little chemical in wheat known as 'wheat germ agglutinin' (WGA) which is largely responsible for many of the health issues seen in celiac disease. What is unique about WGA is that it can cause **direct** damage to the majority of tissues in the human body. This may explain why chronic inflammatory and other degenerative conditions are endemic to wheat-consuming populations, even when overt allergies or intolerances to wheat gluten appear exceedingly rare.

Wheat Germ Agglutinin is capable of creating many symptoms and degenerative conditions in the body. Let us examine some of these mechanisms below:

1. WGA may be pro-inflammatory

At exceedingly small concentrations, WGA stimulates the synthesis of pro-inflammatory chemical messengers (cytokines) in intestinal and immune cells (Pellegrian et al, 2009). WGA has been shown to trigger the release of inflammatory free radicals (Karlsson, A, 1999). WGA has been shown to play a causative role in patients with chronic gut inflammation (Guzyeyeva G, 2008).

2. WGA may be immunotoxic

WGA induces thymus atrophy in rats and may directly bind to, and activate, leukocytes. Anti-WGA antibodies have been shown to cross-react with other proteins, indicating that they may contribute to autoimmunity (Tchernychev et al, 1996). Indeed, WGA appears to play a role in the pathogenesis of celiac disease (CD) that is entirely distinct from that of gluten, due to significantly higher levels of the immunoglobulins IgG and IgA antibodies against WGA found in patients with CD, when compared with patients with other intestinal disorders. These antibodies have also shown not to cross-react with gluten antigens.

3.   WGA may be neurotoxic

WGA can pass through the blood brain barrier (BBB) and is able to travel freely among the tissues of the brain. WGA may attach to the protective coating on the nerves known as the myelin sheath and is capable of inhibiting nerve growth factor which is important for the growth, maintenance, and survival of certain target neurons.

4.   WGA may be cytotoxic

WGA has been demonstrated to be cytotoxic to both normal and cancerous cell lines, capable of inducing either cell cycle arrest or programmed cell death (apoptosis).

5.   WGA may interfere with gene expression

WGA may prevent DNA replication and it may influence both genetic and epigenetic factors.

6.   WGA may disrupt endocrine function

WGA has also been shown to have an insulin-mimetic action, potentially contributing to weight gain and insulin resistance. WGA has been implicated in obesity and "leptin resistance" by blocking the receptor in the hypothalamus for the appetite satiating hormone leptin.

7.   WGA may be cardiotoxic

WGA induces platelet activation and aggregation, leading to thrombosis.

8.   WGA may adversely affect gastrointestinal function

WGA causes increased shedding of the intestinal brush border membrane, reduction in surface area, acceleration of cell losses and shortening of villi, via binding to the surface of the villi.

So, the message is clear! You need to avoid all gluten grains in any quantities, <u>forever</u>. This is not only going to help your lupus disease, but it will prevent any further autoimmune disease from developing.

We need to return back to nature and choose foods that are completely natural, such as fruit and vegetables, and avoid all packaged foods that come in wrappers, bags, boxes and so on, even though they may be gluten-free. Gluten-free does not mean gliadin-free.

Once these foods are eliminated, then you can begin to heal a wounded gut that now requires the proper nutrients in order to rebuild and regenerate.

Once unnatural chemicals and gut-destroying foods are eliminated, the focus should be on healing the gut. Given enough time and the right nutrients, the body will accomplish this on its own.

Amylase-Trypsin Inhibitors (ATI's)

In new research, presented at the United European Gastroenterology (UEG) Week 2016 in Vienna, Professor Detlef Schuppan with Johannes Gutenberg University in Germany and colleagues looked at a different family of wheat proteins, called amylase-trypsin inhibitors (ATIs). ATIs are proteins derived from plants that inhibit enzymes of common parasites in wheat, and play a role in metabolic processes that occur during seed development.

ATIs only make up about 4 percent of wheat proteins, but their consumption can lead to inflammation in the lymph nodes, kidneys, spleen, and brain - as well as in the gut, the researchers reported. For this reason, ATIs can aggravate symptoms of autoimmune diseases like lupus, rheumatoid arthritis, multiple sclerosis, asthma, inflammatory bowel disease, and non-alcoholic fatty liver disease.

In a news release, Professor Schuppan said:

> *"As well as contributing to the development of bowel-related inflammatory conditions, we believe that ATIs can promote inflammation of other immune-related chronic conditions outside of the bowel. The type of gut inflammation seen in non-coeliac gluten sensitivity differs from that caused by coeliac disease, and we do not believe that this is triggered by gluten proteins. Instead, we demonstrated that ATIs from wheat, that are also contaminating commercial gluten, activate specific types of immune cells in the gut and other tissues, thereby potentially worsening the symptoms of pre-existing inflammatory illnesses."*

The research team is now focused on gaining a better understanding of the role of ATIs in chronic conditions.

"We are hoping that this research can lead us towards being able to recommend an ATI-free diet to help treat a variety of potentially serious immunological disorders," Schuppan said.

Besides causing inflammation outside the bowel, ATIs may also contribute to the development of non-coeliac gluten sensitivity (NCGS) as we have already mentioned, which is now a recognized medical condition.

Its symptoms, which can begin up to 48 hours after ingesting gluten and continue for a long period, include abdominal pain and irregular bowel movements, as well as headaches, joint pain, and eczema. To diagnose NCGS, it is first necessary to rule out celiac disease, wheat allergy or other possible causes of symptoms. Gluten sensitivity may be diagnosed if improvement is seen when following a gluten-free diet.

Schuppan hopes that the findings could be used to redefine non-coeliac gluten sensitivity. *"Rather than non-coeliac gluten sensitivity, which implies that gluten solitarily causes the inflammation, a more precise name for the disease should be considered,"* he said.

The Role of Autophagy in Lupus

Recent research (Pullen, LC, 2016) has shown that lupus patients have difficulty clearing the dead cells that die in our body's daily. Every day, in each person, millions of cells die and generate cell debris that must be efficiently and effectively removed via the process known as autophagy. This process is important and genome-wide association studies have suggested that defects in autophagy are associated with inflammatory diseases, such as systemic lupus erythematosus (SLE) and Crohn's disease.

Further support of the role of autophagy in the pathogenesis of lupus comes from the fact that patients with lupus often have dead cells in their tissues. Scientists believe these dead cells trigger danger signals that can break tolerance and result in the generation of autoantibodies, such as the antibodies that are the hallmark of lupus. Likewise, researchers believe that if these dead cells could be cleared, then the danger signals would decrease, as would the inflammation and pathology.

Detoxification on many different levels, beginning with the Alkaline detoxification diet, the liver and gallbladder cleanse, heavy metals detox and perhaps taking systemic enzymes to digest a lot of these dead cells, can greatly facilitate the healing of lupus.

This is what we implement routinely at the Da Vinci Center – it would be worth reading the chapter on Detoxification in this book to see the details of these protocols.

Candida and Lupus

From my personal experience, having treated a number of patients with lupus over the years, the vast majority of them have Candida. When the Candida is treated, along with the avoidance of food intolerances that are also an important part of the inflammatory cycle, then lupus symptoms abate.

A study has discussed some of the ways in which Candida mycotoxins (79 of them) can irritate the gut. Specifically, Santelmann et al. (2005) discussed several theories as to why this might be:

- Candida acts to stimulate mast cells, leading them to release substances that contribute to inflammation within the intestines, as well as possibly triggering autoimmune   diseases.

- Candida produces "proteases", substances that can interfere with the function of immuglobin. This "Ig" effect can also contribute to gut inflammation.

In addition, Candida overgrowth can lead to candida yeast infection and Leaky gut syndrome which is medically referred to as intestinal permeability.

Leaky gut is a major gastrointestinal disorder that occurs when openings develop in the gut wall. These tiny holes can be created when candida overgrowth moves to a more serious stage of candida yeast infection and the candida yeast grows roots or hypha (plural hyphae) which is a long, branching filamentous cell of a fungus (read the chapter on Candida for more details).

This fungal growth is a more advanced stage of development in the candida albicans yeast infection. The hyphae spreads the bowel wall cells apart so that acidic, harmful microorganisms and macromolecules are able to pass through (leak into) these openings and enter the circulatory system.

This is where the name "Leaky Gut" came from. The body is alerted to the invader and creates antibodies for protection, activates the immune system, and thus a food allergy or intolerance is born. Food allergies are directly linked to leaky gut and candida yeast infection overgrowth.

As a result, leaky gut syndrome and candida yeast infection can directly lead to many other systemic inflammatory and immune-related symptoms beyond food allergies, including lupus, rheumatoid arthritis, ankylosing spondylitis, multiple sclerosis, eczema, fibromyalgia, Crohn's disease, Raynaud's phenomenon, chronic urticaria (hives), and inflammatory bowel disease.

These are all generally referred to as autoimmune diseases. Thus, candida yeast infection and candida overgrowth is related to lupus. Major signs and symptoms of leaky gut syndrome include:

- Facial swelling upon exposure to strong smells
- Bloating, gas, and cramps immediately after eating
- Alternating bouts of constipation and diarrhea
- Headaches, poor concentration, and irritability
- Food Allergies/intolerances

Inflammation of the gut lining, often involving candida yeast overgrowth, is the primary symptom of leaky gut syndrome. The originating cause may be prescription drug use and antibiotics which kill off healthy probiotic flora. Gut inflammation from candida yeast infection is usually instigated by one or several of the following factors:

- Prescription hormones (e.g. birth control pills and/or hormone replacement therapy) and prescription corticosteroids (e.g. hydrocortisone).
- Excessive use of antibiotics which kills off health bacteria, causing dysbiosis, candida overgrowth and candida yeast infection.
- Processed foods, as well as foods and beverages contaminated by parasites, fungus, and/or mould which promote the growth of candida yeast infection.
- Increased amounts of refined carbohydrates (e.g. candy bars, cookies, cake, soft drinks, and white bread) which also promote the growth of candida yeast overgrowth and dysbiosis.
- Increased alcohol and caffeine consumption. Remember that alcohol is a natural result of yeast overgrowth and sugar.

It is highly advisable to read the chapter on Candida and get yourself checked out. There is a Candida questionnaire that you can complete at the end of the chapter which will give you a good idea of how many symptoms you may have that would lead to a diagnosis of systemic Candidiasis.

Again, I repeat, from my own clinical experience, candida is almost always found in cases of lupus. There are, off course, other underlying causative factors that are also important in curing your lupus and other autoimmune diseases.

What other causative factors may be playing a role in lupus?

The Microbiome and Lupus

The gut plays a major role in the health of the immune system because it supports nutrient absorption and detoxification. More than 1,000 unique species of bacteria make up the gut microbiome. An overgrowth and depletion of certain bacteria is evident in individuals with lupus.

Researchers have found that low levels of beneficial *Lactobacilli* and *Bifidobacterium* and increased levels of the butyrate producing *Lachnospiraceae* were present in the early onset of lupus development (Zhang et al, 2014).

Individuals with lupus are recommended to take a daily probiotic and consume probiotic rich foods. Adding healthy probiotics rich in *Lactobacillaceae* bacteria can exhibit anti-inflammatory effects by suppressing pro-inflammatory T cells and interleukins and stimulating Treg cells to regulate immune cell homeostasis (Zhang et al, 2014).

Raw and organic vegetables are also an excellent choice to heal gut issues. Avoiding unnecessary toxins is required to balance gut flora, improve digestive motility, remove toxins and reduce inflammation. Raw vegetables improve homeostasis by promoting an alkaline environment that is not susceptible to disease.

A study (Cuervo et al, 2015) has recently shown the existence of a gut microbial dysbiosis (imbalance of good and bad bacteria) in systemic lupus erythematosus (SLE), supporting previous evidence involving intestinal bacteria in the initiation and amplification of autoimmune diseases.

Biofilms and Lupus

For years, the scientific community has been unsure of the reasons why conditions like lupus and multiple sclerosis (MS) misdirect the immune system to attack one's own body. Now, a team at Temple University School of Medicine (TUSM) may have gotten closer to finding an answer. The researchers discovered that bacterial biofilms (groups of bacteria) found in the gut might be partly responsible for why lupus develops. Other researchers have confirmed similar findings (Gallo et al, 2015).

Have you ever picked up a rock from a nearby stream and wondered why it's slimy on the surface? That slimy layer is actually a group of microorganisms, collectively called a biofilm.

A biofilm is a community of bacteria that attach to a surface by excreting a sticky, sugary substance that encompasses the bacteria in a matrix. This might be the first time you've heard the term biofilm, but they're all around us; in streams, drains, fish tanks, even on our teeth.

A biofilm can be composed of a single species or a conglomerate of species. In many cases, biofilms are only bacteria, but they can also include other living things such as fungi and algae, creating a microbial stew of sorts. Biofilms are complex systems that are sometimes compared to multicellular organisms.

Small intestine bacterial overgrowth (SIBO)

SIBO is a condition characterized by abnormal overgrowth of bacteria in the small intestine. One study reported that up to 84 percent of IBS patients have SIBO and that patients with IBS were 26 times more likely to have SIBO than controls (Pimentel et al, 2000). Eradication of the overgrowth eliminated irritable bowel syndrome in 48% of subjects. Other autoimmune diseases can also be related to SIBO, such as lupus.

Most bacteria are in your large intestine, but sometimes they can move up into the small intestine. Given that the small intestines should not contain unhealthy bacteria, only the good acidophilus species, this is not a healthy environment. If the bad bacteria populate the small intestine, they will begin fermenting food that you digest, particularly sugar or starchy foods.

So, when you eat starchy foods such as bread, cereals, pasta, rice and sugary foods, the bacteria in your gut ferment the sugars in the food. This fermentation process and its gases expand and you begin to feel pain and discomfort.

Traditionally, SIBO is treated by medical doctors using specific antibiotics, sometimes giving these in multiple serial dosages over quite some time. The disadvantage of this is that long-term use of antibiotics is likely to lead to a yeast overgrowth in the gut, or candida, which is another major factor underlying Lupus.

It is probably wiser, if you have or suspect that you have SIBO, to use antibiotic herbs and supplements to help bring back some balance into the gut. Some of these will include grapefruit seed extract, oregano oil, colloidal silver, Echinacea herb, vitamin C, as well as repopulating the gut with friendly bacteria while eradicating any yeasts. We will talk more about these later in this chapter.

This is more likely to lead to an alleviation of lupus symptoms, given that you're working on all of these factors concomitantly. It does not make sense to work with only one factor at a time, such as SIBO for example, without addressing nutritional deficiencies, candida, parasites, digestive disorders, optimising nutrition and so forth.

Treating SIBO

Generally, I do not focus on treating SIBO alone, but try to incorporate a more eclectic programme to cover all the other causative factors that may be accompanying SIBO. Many practitioners are using the low-FODMAP diet to treat SIBO.

What Are FODMAPs?

A low FODMAP diet, or FODMAP elimination diet, refers to a temporary eating pattern that has a very low amount of food compounds called FODMAPs.

The acronym stands for:

- **Fermentable** – meaning they are broken down (fermented) by bacteria in the large bowel
- **Oligosaccharides** – "oligo" means "few" and "saccharide" means sugar. These molecules are made up of individual sugars joined together in a chain
- **Disaccharides** – "di" means two. This is a double sugar molecule
- **Monosaccharides** – "mono" means single. This is a single sugar molecule
- **And Polyols** – these are sugar alcohols

The saccharides and polyols are short-chain carbohydrates that, if poorly digested, ferment in the lower part of your large intestine (bowel). This fermentation process draws in water and produces carbon dioxide, hydrogen, and/or methane gas that causes the intestine to stretch and expand.

The result is strong pain, bloating, visible abdominal distension and other related symptoms (Clausen et al, 1998; Rumessen et al, 1998; Barrett et al, 2009; Ong et al, 2008; Ladas et al, 2000).

The FODMAP diet basically involves cutting out the food indicated in Figure 4 for at least a couple of months to see how you go.

The FODMAPS Diet

excess fructose	lactose	fructans	galactans	polyols
fruit apple, mango, nashi, pear, tinned fruit in natural juice, watermelon **sweetners** fructose, high fructose corn syrup, concentrated fruit sources, large servings of fruit, dried fruit, fruit juice **honey** corn syrup, fruisana	**milk** milk from cows, goats or sheep, custard, ice cream, yogurt **cheeses** soft unripened cheeses, such as cottage cheese, cream, mascarpone, ricotta	**vegetables** asparagus, beetroot, broccoli, brussel sprouts, cabbage, eggplant, fennel, garlic, leek, okra, onion, shallots, spring onion **cereals** wheat and rye **fruit** custard apple, persimmon, watermelon **misc.** chicory, dandelion, inulin	**legumes** baked beans, chickpeas, kidney beans, lentils	**fruit** apple, apricot, avocado, blackberry, cherry, lychee, nashi, nectarine, peach, pear, plum, prune, watermelon **vegetables** cauliflower, bell pepper, mushroom, sweet corn **sweetners** sorbitol, mannitol, isomalt, maltitol, xylitol

Fig 4. FODMAPS Diet

A low-FODMAP (or low-carbohydrate) diet will keep symptoms under control simply by starving the bacteria in your small intestine. When these bacteria don't have food to eat, they aren't able to metabolize that food and produce gas as a result. This gas is what causes the common symptoms of SIBO - bloating, abdominal pain, diarrhoea (in the case of hydrogen gas), and constipation (in the case of methane gas).

But starving the bacteria over the short term does not eradicate the bacteria, which is what we're trying to accomplish, as the small intestine is not supposed to contain much bacteria. If you continue this restriction for a long period of time in an effort to kill the bacteria, you're also starving the bacteria in your large intestine that should be there and that play a vital role in your health.

Simply put, a low-FODMAP or low-carb diet does not eradicate an overgrowth in the small intestine in a short period of time, and continuing on a long-term low-

FODMAP/carbohydrate diet in an effort to starve the bacteria to death has potential detrimental effects on the bacteria in the large intestine.

There are many clients who have been on long-term low-FODMAP diets who still have positive breath tests for SIBO, despite their restricted diet. There is a difference between controlling symptoms and actually clearing the bacteria. We want to do the latter, which has the added benefit of improving symptoms as well.

FODMAPs are fermentable carbohydrates that help to feed the beneficial bacteria in the large intestine. When you begin to think about them this way, it becomes a lot easier to understand why adhering to a diet low in the substrates that our healthy gut bacteria thrive on may not be the best of ideas.

In one study (Halmos et al, 2015) it was shown that being on a FODMAP restriction diet decreased overall bacteria by 47%, along with a decline in bacteria that produce butyrate (a beneficial substance made when probiotics feed on fermentable fibres). There are studies that have shown a decrease in the probiotic strain bifidobacteria, too.

While these bacteria would likely thrive once again with the addition of prebiotic substances, staying in a chronically diet-induced altered microbiological state is likely not a healthy choice when you start to think about the importance of our microbiome and its effect on our health.

Hopefully, when you have understood the Da Vinci Lupus Treatment Protocol in full, you will not need to be on a long-term low-FODMAP diet to keep your symptoms under control.

Other Ways of Treating SIBO

So, if you're not treating your SIBO only with diet, what else is used to treat it?

Rifaximin is the most commonly used antibiotic prescribed by medical doctors for the treatment of SIBO and has been shown to be safe and well-tolerated. On average, it is about 50% effective (Peralta et al, 2009). As I have already mentioned, I am not in favour of using antibiotics that kill off the friendly bacteria in the gut, worsening any possible dysbiosis, or causing Candida.

The good news is that recent research (Chedid et al, 2014) has shown that herbal antimicrobials are at least as effective as rifaximin, and about 57% of those who fail on rifaximin will succeed on herbal antimicrobials.

Herbs that have been found to be beneficial include: Red thyme oil (thymus vulgaris), oregano oil (origanum vulgare), horsetail, pau'd arco, wormwood (Artemisia absinthium), yarrow leaf (achillea millefolium), berberine, licorice root, Chinese rhubarb root (rheum officinale), ginger (zingiber officinale) and olive leaf (Olea europaea).

At the Da Vinci Center we would normally give our NATURAL ANTIBIOTIC PACK which contains a variety of these herbs, grapefruit seed extract, colloidal silver and vitamin C, as well as possibly other herbs as and when required.

	HIGH FODMAP FOODS	LOW FODMAP FOODS
VEGETABLES	Asparagus, artichokes, onions(all), leek, garlic, sugar snap peas, beetroot, Savoy cabbage, cauliflower, celery, sweet corn, mushrooms	Alfalfa, bean sprouts, green beans, bok choy, capsicum, carrot, fresh herbs, choy sum, cucumber, lettuce, rocket, tomato, zucchini.
FRUIT	Apples, apricots, figs, pears, mango, pears, watermelon, nectarines, peaches, plums	Banana, blueberries, strawberries, cherries, kiwi, orange, mandarin, grapes, melon
GRAINS	Rye, wheat-containing breads, wheat-based cereals with dried fruit, wheat pasta, barley	Gluten-free bread and sourdough spelt bread, rice bubbles, oats, gluten-free pasta, rice, quinoa
MEAT & ALTERNATIVES	Legumes/pulses, cashews, pistachios	Meats, fish, chicken, Tofu, tempeh, almonds (<10 nuts), pumpkin seeds
DAIRY	Cow's milk, yoghurt, soft cheese cream, custard, ice cream	Lactose-free milk, lactose-free yoghurts, hard cheese

Fig 2. High and Low FODMAP diet

45

By adding these natural antibiotics, you will be eradicating the bad bacteria causing the fermentation, while you starve them with the low-FODMAPS diet.

After being on a low-FODMAP diet for 7-8 weeks, begin adding these foods back into the diet in moderation (Fig. 2). I normally tell my patients to eat as many FODMAP foods as they can tolerate. You may experience some uncomfortable symptoms like bloating or gas during this time, but as long as it is not interrupting their life or causing pain, the more FODMAPs or carbohydrates they can eat, the better.

Leaky Gut and Lupus

When different areas of the intestinal tract become irritated, inflamed or breached, we can suffer from an array of symptoms such as: constipation, diarrhoea, heartburn, nausea, indigestion, gas, bloating and cramps, and these are usually caused by a leaky gut which further causes allergies, autoimmune diseases such as lupus, psoriasis, anaemia, fatigue, weight loss, arthritis, eczema, muscle pain and more.

Symptoms can persist for years with people bouncing from doctor to doctor without ever being properly diagnosed. While these diseases have different names, they have one thing in common - a leaky gut.

In the era of classic Greece, Hippocrates - known as the Father of the Modern Medicine -made the famous proclamation that 'all diseases start in the gut'.

Hippocrates may not have known the science behind leaky gut syndrome, nor did he use the term, but he was spot on.

Leaky Gut: The Consequences

A leaky gut is a condition in which the small intestine wall becomes inflamed and breached with tiny pinholes that leak putrid food particles into the blood stream. Your immune system builds antibodies to the proteins in this faecal matter and your body attacks these proteins as if they were foreign germs.

That is why it is called an auto-immune disease, because your immune system becomes confused between its own protein and foreign protein. It goes on to attack protein in other parts of the body such as between the joints, causing rheumatoid arthritis, lupus and more.

These poisons infiltrate the blood and lymph and overload the liver's ability to detoxify them.

Leaky Gut Progression

What causes leaky gut?

Several important factors should be considered to answer this question. First and foremost, understand that it is the role of various probiotic bacteria to maintain the integrity of the gut lining – they are ultimately the first line of defence.

Let's look at some of the most common causes of leaky gut that need to be dealt with before the gut can heal:

- Food intolerances
- Abuse of antibiotics, cortisone, hormone drugs and others
- Candida
- Dysbiosis - a microbial imbalance in the gut
- Poor microbiota of the gut

- Deficient digestive or pancreatic enzymes
- Low stomach acid (hypochlorhydria)
- Poor digestion – eating on the run, not chewing food properly, eating under stress
- Small Intestine Bacterial Overgrowth (SIBO)
- Exposure to toxins – heavy metals, PCB's and many more
- Parasites in the gut
- Lectins from food
- Chronic stress
- Gluten grains
- GMO corn and other foods
- Soy
- Commercial dairy
- Processed foods, preservatives, dyes, and additives
- Refined sugars
- Refined oils

When the balance of bacteria within the gut is threatened by such things, the ability of the good bacteria to maintain the gut wall lining is challenged. In addition, it is known that *gliadin*, a protein found in gluten, may also threaten the integrity of the gut lining.

Chronic stress can also weaken your immune system over time, which cripples your ability to fight off foreign invaders like bad bacteria and viruses, leading to inflammation and leaky gut.

We come into contact with over 80,000 chemicals and toxins every single year, but the worst offenders for causing leaky gut include antibiotics, pesticides, tap water, aspirin and NSAIDS (anti-inflammatories).

The most common components of food that can damage your intestinal lining are the proteins found in un-sprouted grains, sugar, Genetically modified foods (GMO's) and conventional dairy.

The anti-inflammatory diet

Considering the inflammatory nature of lupus disease, it is not surprising that anti-inflammatory diets are gaining in popularity among lupus sufferers looking to find relief from their symptoms through dietary modification rather than drugs.

The anti-inflammatory diet that we recommend at the Da Vinci Center looks something like this:

- Eat plenty of fruits and vegetables that are rich in antioxidants
- Reduce the amount of saturated and trans fats in your diet
- Watch your intake of sugar and refined carbohydrates
- Get plenty of omega-3 fatty acids from foods (or supplements)
- Eat lean protein sources, such as fish and organic chicken, and cut back on red meat
- Avoid refined and processed foods

Keeping calories in check is also important as fat cells can release a lot of inflammatory molecules into your bloodstream, so the higher your body fat percentage, the more inflammation you are likely to have.

Vegetarian diets have been associated with improved lupus symptoms in some studies. Although meat is not typically completely forbidden on anti-inflammatory diets, they do suggest that vegetables and fruits should play a key role in your diet if your goal is to reduce chronic inflammation in your body.

After reading about the potential anti-lupus effects of a high vegetable intake above, you might be tempted to embrace a strict vegetarian diet. However, going pescetarian rather than vegetarian might make more sense (a pescetarian diet includes fish and other seafood, but not the flesh of land-based animals). Regular consumption of oily fish that are rich in anti-inflammatory omega-3 fatty acids – such as mackerel, sardines, salmon, pilchard, kipper or herrings – is useful in the treatment of lupus as a balanced immune system does require good-quality protein.

A number of studies have found that people with lupus have an increased risk of certain other health problems, and many of these conditions have an inflammatory basis, suggesting that an anti-inflammatory diet might also help prevent or fight these conditions.

Examples of conditions that occur more often in lupus sufferers than the general population and that have been linked to inflammation include:

- Type 2 diabetes
- Rheumatoid arthritis and psoriatic arthritis
- Asthma

Here are a few more details about the Da Vinci anti-inflammatory diet that we recommend that you follow:

- Eat a wide variety of fruits and vegetables which are rich in antioxidants. A high intake of fruit and vegetables has been associated with plasma concentrations of C-reactive protein (CRP), a key marker of inflammation (Esmaillzadeh et al, 2006).

- Reduce the amount of trans fats in your diet. A high intake of trans fats has been associated with high plasma concentrations of biomarkers of systemic inflammation (Mozaffarian et al, 2004). Foods that contain high amounts of saturated fat are usually restricted on anti-inflammatory diets.

- Get plenty of omega-3 fatty acids from foods (or supplements). These essential fatty acids have been shown to disrupt inflammation cell signalling pathways by binding to the GPR120 receptor (Oh et al, 2012).

- Minimize your intake of sugar and refined carbohydrates which have high glycaemic loads (GL), and focus on low-GI foods instead. Research suggests that low-GI diets are inversely associated with inflammation (Neuhouser et al, 2012).

- Avoid refined and processed foods. These foods often have high glycaemic loads, plus they often contain food additives, some of which have been shown to promote inflammation in animal studies (Nakanishi et al, 2015; Chassaing et al, 2006).

Ginger as a Natural Anti-inflammatory Herb

Ginger (*Zingiber officinale*) has a long history of use as a medicine. Among practitioners of herbal medicine, remedies derived from ginger root – such as ginger tea or ginger juice – are well known for their ability to alleviate digestive problems, but they may also help fight a range of other health problems, especially conditions linked to chronic inflammation.

Anecdotal reports suggest that ginger may help ease lupus symptoms in some people — not surprising considering that lupus is classified as an inflammatory condition.

A study published in the journal *Medical Hypotheses* found that more than three-quarters of study participants with rheumatoid arthritis or osteoarthritis (common in lupus) experienced relief in pain and swelling after treatment with powdered ginger root. The researchers who conducted this study believe the observed anti-arthritic effects of ginger might be linked, at least part, to its ability to inhibit the biosynthesis of pro-inflammatory compounds called prostaglandins and leukotrienes.

You can use fresh ginger root in so many sweet and savoury recipes, way beyond the typical stir-fries and ginger root tea.

Incorporating ginger into homemade fruit juices or smoothies is also one of the best ways to reap the wonderful health benefits of fresh ginger root. Fruits and vegetables that pair well with ginger in juices include carrots, oranges, mandarins, apples, and grapefruit.

Fruit and vegetable smoothies

We have already looked at some of the studies that have shown that eating fruit and vegetables is helpful for lupus. There is another good way to get the antioxidant nutrients that these fruits and vegetables contain, and that is by drinking smoothies. Let's look at a few examples that you can add to your daily diet…

Green smoothie with ginger, spinach and flaxseed

This smoothie pairs nutrient-rich baby spinach with mango and banana to create a tasty and nutritious green smoothie. Ground flaxseed and fresh ginger, both of which contain anti-inflammatory compounds, are added to the mix to further boost its health-giving properties.

Ingredients

- About 1 ⅔ cups water and/or non-dairy milk of your choice (rice, almond, coconut)
- 1 small banana
- 1 small mango
- 2 cups baby spinach
- 1 tsp. grated fresh ginger
- 1 Tbsp. ground flaxseed
- 8 ice cubes

Directions

- Peel, rinse, pit and cut the ingredients as needed, and put them in a high-powered blender in the order listed above.
- Secure the lid and process in short bursts until the ice cubes have been thoroughly crushed. Then, slowly increase the speed, and blend at full speed for about 1 minute, or until the smoothie is very smooth and consistent in colour. Add water if needed to adjust the consistency. Makes 2 servings.

Gingery carrot juice

The potential inflammatory-fighting effects of carrot juice can be attributed, at least in part, to the high concentration of beta-carotene in carrots.

As you may already know, beta-carotene is a strong antioxidant that helps neutralize free radicals. Free radicals are unstable molecules that can damage DNA and cell membranes, thereby contributing the development of a wide range of health problems, including inflammation in people with lupus.

The following juicing recipe for lupus sufferers combines fresh carrots with ginger, another food you should definitely look into if you suffer from lupus. Practitioners of herbal medicine believe that ginger is good for lupus sufferers due to its strong anti-inflammatory properties, and anecdotal reports seem to support the use of ginger as a natural remedy for lupus.

Ingredients

- 8 organic carrots
- 1 ½ inch slice fresh ginger

Directions

- Scrub the carrots under cold running water and trim their tops. Peel the ginger.
- Pass the carrots and ginger through a juicer. Clean the juicer right after use. Serves 1.

Turmeric as an Anti-inflammatory Herb

Turmeric (known by its scientific name *Curcuma longa)*, has a long history of use in traditional Indian medicine as a treatment for inflammatory conditions such as Lupus.

Intrigued by this, Nita Chainani-Wu from the University of California, in 2003, decided to systematically review animal and human studies investigating the anti-inflammatory activity and safety of curcumin, the main active compound of turmeric.

She found that not only does curcumin appear to be safe, it also appears to be an effective anti-inflammatory agent. According to this review, laboratory studies suggest that the anti-inflammatory properties of curcumin are linked to its ability to inhibit a number of pro-inflammatory molecules, including phospholipase, leukotrienes, thromboxane, prostaglandins, lipooxygenase, cyclooxygenase 2, nitric oxide, collagenase, elastase, hyaluronidase, monocyte chemoattractant protein-1, interferon-inducible protein, tumour necrosis factor, and interleukin-12.

You can add curcumin to your fruit and vegetable smoothies.

Carrot, mango and turmeric smoothie

This recipe pairs fresh mango with carrot juice to create a luscious, brightly-coloured smoothie. The frozen banana this recipe calls for is added to give this vegan blend a creamy texture, while the turmeric powder ensures your body will get a generous dose of anti-inflammatory compounds.

Ingredients

- 1 ⅔ cups carrot juice
- 1 ripe mango, peeled and pitted
- 1 ½ tsp. pure turmeric powder
- 1 Tbsp. chia seeds
- 1 banana, peeled, sliced and frozen
- Water, as needed

Directions

- Add the carrot juice to a blender, followed by the remaining ingredients.
- Blend until thoroughly combined, stopping to scrape down sides and to check the consistency.
- If the smoothie seems too thick, add some water.
- Pour into tall glasses, and serve right away; serves 2.

Consume Foods that Contain Quercetin

Quercetin, a bioflavonoid that is found in high concentrations in yellow and red onions, has strong anti-inflammatory properties and therefore help alleviate lupus symptoms. Quercetin inhibits the action of phospholipase, an enzyme that generates free arachidonic acid. Arachidonic acid increases the levels of prostaglandins and leukotrienes, which are potent pro-inflammatory chemicals that our bodies do not need.

In addition to onions, good dietary sources of quercetin include capers, apples, lovage, broccoli, red grapes, cherries, citrus fruits, tea, and many berries, including raspberry, lingonberry, and cranberry.

Limit High Glycaemic and Sugary Foods

There is some evidence that a diet high in sugary and high-glycaemic foods (which rapidly raise blood sugar levels) can increase inflammation. One study revealed that women, particularly overweight women, eating large amounts of high glycaemic foods such as potatoes and white rice had elevated levels of C-reactive protein (CRP). CRP is a substance that the body releases in response to inflammation, and therefore CRP levels act as a measurement of inflammation in the body.

Furthermore, sugary foods are thought to promote the overgrowth of the Candida yeast in the body, which has been linked to lupus.

Conventional Lupus Treatment: Risks and Side Effects

As we have already mentioned, the medical profession believes that there is no known cure for lupus, but there are treatments used for managing symptoms. So, these treatments are really only geared to your symptoms; it is a symptom-suppression model of managing disease. The goals of treatment are to:

- Prevent flares

- Treat symptoms when they occur

- Reduce organ damage and other problems

Your treatment might include using medicines to:

- Reduce swelling and pain

- Prevent or reduce flares

- Calm the immune system

- Reduce or prevent damage to the joints

- Reduce or prevent organ damage

There are many medical and pharmaceutical drugs that are used to control symptoms of lupus without actually curing the disease. Many of these are simply fighting the chronic inflammation that is causing the symptoms.

Let's briefly examine some of the more common ones that are used by medical doctors – please note, that as part of the Da Vinci Treatment Protocol we do not recommend these drugs, but if the patient is already taking them upon prescription from their medical doctor, then we can often work with them.

Nonsteroidal anti-inflammatory drugs (NSAIDs)

NSAIDs are used to treat pain, inflammation, and stiffness due to lupus. These medications are available as over-the-counter (OTC) and prescription drugs. If you have kidney disease from lupus, talk to your doctor before taking an NSAID. You may need a lower dosage or your doctor may want you to avoid these medications.

OTC NSAIDs include:

- aspirin
- ibuprofen (Motrin)
- naproxen

Prescription NSAIDs include:

The most common side effects of these NSAIDs include:

- nausea
- heartburn
- ulcers in your stomach or intestines
- bleeding in your stomach or intestines

Taking a high dosage of an NSAID or using these drugs for a long time increases your risk of bleeding or stomach ulcers. Some NSAIDs are gentler on the stomach than others. Always take NSAIDs with food and never take them right before lying down or going to sleep. These precautions can reduce your risk of stomach problems.

Corticosteroids

Corticosteroids, also called glucocorticoids or steroids, can help treat symptoms of lupus. These drugs mimic how cortisol works. Cortisol is a hormone that your body makes. It helps fight inflammation and controls your immune system. Regulating your immune system can ease symptoms of lupus.

Steroids include:

- prednisone
- cortisone
- hydrocortisone

In general, steroids are effective. But like all drugs, they may cause side effects. These can include:

- weight gain
- fluid retention or swelling
- acne
- irritability
- trouble sleeping
- infections
- osteoporosis

Steroids often work quickly. Your doctor may give you a short steroid treatment until your longer-term drugs start working. Doctors try to prescribe the lowest possible dosage of a steroid for the shortest length of time to avoid side effects. When you need to stop taking steroids, your doctor will slowly reduce your dosage over time to reduce your risk of side effects.

Corticosteriods can have many side effects, so your doctor will give you the lowest dose possible. Short-term side effects can include: a round or puffy face, acne, heartburn, increased appetite, weight gain, and mood swings. These side effects typically stop when the drug is stopped. However, the weight gain will not reverse on its own, so be careful not to overeat while on steroids.

Long-term side effects can include: easy bruising, thinning skin and hair, weakened or damaged bones, high blood pressure, damage to the arteries, high blood sugar, infections, muscle weakness, and cataracts. Some people may have ulcers, depression, or even congestive heart failure. Your doctor can prescribe medicines to take with corticosteroids to prevent some side effects. Corticosteroids can be used during pregnancy with your doctor's supervision.

Antimalarial drugs: Medicines used to prevent or treat malaria are used to treat joint pain, skin rashes, fatigue, and inflammation of the lungs. Side effects of antimalarials can include stomach upset, nausea, vomiting, diarrhoea, headache, dizziness, blurred vision, trouble sleeping, and itching. People treated with antimalarials should see an eye doctor every year because of the low risk of eye problems. Studies have found that taking antimalarials can stop flares and some help people with lupus live longer.

BLyS-specific inhibitors: These drugs limit the number of autoantibodies found in people with lupus. The drug blocks the action of a specific protein in the body that is important in immune response. Clinical studies have reported more deaths and serious infections in those on the drugs than those not taking the drug. The most common side effects included nausea, diarrhoea, and fever.

Immunosuppressive agents/chemotherapy: These agents are used in severe cases of lupus when major organs are affected and other treatments do not work. These drugs suppress the immune system to limit the damage to the organ. These drugs can cause serious side effects including nausea, vomiting, hair loss, bladder problems, decreased fertility, and a risk of cancer and infection. These drugs can also cause birth defects. If you take these medicines, your doctor may tell you to avoid pregnancy.

Natural Treatments for Lupus

In addition to medications and other medical care from doctors, a growing number of people are turning to other healing practices to try to improve their health. There are many natural therapies that can be used, but what we have found at the Da Vinci Center is that when a number of these are combined, patients often get the maximum benefits.

This combination requires diagnostics in order to understand the underlying causative factors that need to be offloaded. Whether these be toxins, heavy metals, chronic inflammation, food intolerances, allergies, digestive disorders, SIBO, leaky gut, Candida, other microorganisms – we have developed protocols to offload all these factors to see how a person suffering from lupus can work towards helping themselves and not be reliant on symptom-suppressing drugs.

Let's begin with one of the most important underlying causative factors: Chronic inflammation.

Think about your body being a barrel with a number of hose pipes feeding it at the top, pouring inflammatory chemicals into it. Over the years, this barrel is bound to fill up and overflow, triggering an autoimmune response as the body becomes overwhelmed with the overflow.

What we need to do is cut off the source of the inflammation – this could be toxins, food intolerances, gluten grains, high acidic foods, preservatives and colouring agents in foods, vaccinations, and more.

Concomitantly, we need to open the tap at the bottom of this barrel and allow some of this inflammation to begin draining out. It is only when the barrel begins to empty that your autoimmune response will reset and symptoms will simply melt away.

Obviously, it is much better to be supervised during this process, which at the Da Vinci Center does not take longer than 90 days after the initial diagnostics are found from the IDEL Diagnostic Programme – see www.naturaltherapycenter.com

So, let's begin by looking at how we can get rid of inflammation first and foremost…

Omega-3 Fatty Acids

Omega-3 fats are required for many biological processes. Multiple studies have shown that their anti-inflammatory properties are significantly beneficial in managing lupus. Oily fish such as salmon, mackerel, herring, sardines and tuna are great sources of omega-3 fats-aim for at least two servings per week. Walnuts, flaxseeds, soy products, and green, leafy vegetables are also great sources of omega-3 fats.

Garlic

Garlic possesses a whole host of great health benefits. It not only boasts anti-Inflammatory properties, but it also has anti-thrombotic and vasodilating properties to help improve cholesterol levels, lower blood pressure, and decrease clot formation. In addition, garlic contains antioxidants to help prevent cancer.

To active the beneficial compounds in garlic, let it sit for at least 60 seconds after being chopped/crushed. Incorporate garlic into meals where it can be the last ingredient added in order to avoid overcooking it. Adding it to salads and rice dishes is a great way to add flavour without the extra calories. Try combining it with ginger and add to grilled chicken and seafood.

Note: Some lupus patients report garlic as a trigger for flare ups. If you think that fresh garlic is related to flares, talk to your doctor or try eliminating it from your diet.

Turmeric

For over 4000 years, turmeric has been used in dishes in order to alleviate a wide variety of ailments including inflammation, digestive problems, infections, and even cancers. Turmeric is best known for its use in curry dishes and gives them the mustard yellow colour. The yellowish pigment in curry is called curcumin. Numerous studies have found that curcumin's anti-inflammatory effects are comparable to the drugs hydrocortisone and phenylbutazone.

There are many benefits of Turmeric for lupus patients. Let's examine 10 SUPER POWERFUL benefits for lupus patients, along with the research to back it:

1. Turmeric inhibits the activity of autoantibodies in lupus

Bright JJ, in his paper *'Curcumin and autoimmune disease'* comments that curcumin ameliorates conditions like multiple sclerosis, rheumatoid arthritis, psoriasis, inflammatory bowel disease, lupus etc. It does so by regulating the activity of inflammatory agents and pathways activated in immune cells.

In their paper *'Heat-solubilized curry spice curcumin inhibits antibody-antigen interaction in in vitro studies: a possible therapy to alleviate autoimmune disorders'*, Kurien et. al (2010) demonstrated that heat solubilised curcumin and turmeric attenuated binding of autoantibodies in serum samples of SLE patients by 52% and 70% respectively.

In other words, this experimental study shows that curcumin inhibits autoantibodies produced in lupus from binding to target cells and these findings, if proven in humans, pretty much solves the issue of 'there is no cure for lupus'.

One interesting point the scientists mentioned is that the main issue that hinders us from making the most of curcumin is its bioavailability issue. So, what they boiled both curcumin and turmeric in water for 10 minutes before using it in the study.

Curcumin's solubility was increased by 12 folds and turmeric's solubility was increased by 3 folds!

Kurien et. al recently published a study in Lupus Science & Medicine (2015) where they used ultrasoluble curcumin and turmeric in animal model of lupus. Here the solubility of curcumin in water was increased by 35 folds using heat and pressure.

Curcumin reduced lesions, production of autoantibodies, prevented increase in lymphocytes (type of white blood cells), reduced kidney damage and protected salivary glands. <u>Curcumin and turmeric increased the survival rate.</u>

2. Curcumin as an immunomodulatory agent

Curcumin as an immunomodulatory agent regulates the activity of various immune cells like T cells, B cells, macrophages, neutrophils, natural killer cells, and dendritic cells. It also reduces production of inflammatory cytokines.

Srivastava et.al comment that this immune modulating property has been found to be useful in many inflammatory and metabolic diseases.

A very interesting point they put forth: *'During inflammation the functional influence of lymphocytes and the related cross-talk can be modulated by curcumin to achieve the desired immune status against diseases.'*

Curcumin and turmeric are immunomodulatory agents - they regulate immune responses. Dose dependently they may stimulate immune response as defence against infection and regulate inappropriate immune responses in case of autoimmune diseases such as lupus.

So, it is a myth that turmeric is an immune booster and hence you cannot take it to treat lupus or any autoimmune disease.

3.   Curcumin can restore immune function in SLE patients

A very recent concept that is being researched in the field of SLE is the balance between T helper cell 17 (Th17) and regulatory T cells. These are different types of immune cells, but in lupus there is an imbalance in their populations. If these could be balanced, then the immune system would begin regulating immune response – currently there is no drug that can do this.

A study published in Central European Journal of Immunology (Handono et al, 2015) examined whether this immunomodulatory property of curcumin can actually help in achieving balance in immune cell populations in SLE. The results were very encouraging!

It was found that curcumin reduced the numbers of Th17 and increased the levels of Treg cells, thereby helping regulate immune responses.

And curcumin did not reproduce these effects in T cells from healthy individuals. Handono et. al commented that curcumin can be used as a novel therapeutic agent for SLE by alleviating immune response and balancing Th17 and Treg cell population.

Curcumin is proven to balance the population of immune cells in samples taken from SLE patients. These findings suggest that it can help in regulating immune responses and thereby prevent progression of lupus!

4.   Anti-inflammatory properties

Curcumin as well as curcumin-free turmeric, have anti-inflammatory properties. Unlike regular non-steroidal anti-inflammatory drugs which inhibit only the COX enzyme, curcumin inhibits both COX and LOX, two important enzymes that participate in inflammation (Chainani-Wu, I, 2003; Aggarwal et al, 2013).

These properties combined with curcumin's immunomodulatory properties can help control and prevent spread of inflammation to other organs in lupus. An edge curcumin and turmeric have over other NSAIDs is that they do not cause side effects like gastric erosion.

Turmeric's anti-inflammatory property can help in controlling as well as preventing spread of inflammation to other organs in lupus.

5. Skin protection

70-80% of the individuals suffering from lupus present with skin lesions or rashes. These can be painful, itchy and photosensitive (Kole et al, 2009; Cojocaru et al, 2011). Topical immunomodulators or steroids are prescribed to treat such rashes.

Turmeric is traditionally used to treat skin diseases including inflammation. Research suggests that curcumin can be a novel treatment in skin disorders.

Curcumin's anti-inflammatory, immunomodulatory and skin protective properties make it a potential therapeutic compound for skin related symptoms of lupus.

6. Can reduce pain

Curcumin works as a natural painkiller- it attenuates various kinds of pain. Curcumin's analgesic or pain killing effect has been proven in an experimental model of postoperative pain (Kapoor, 2012; Sahbaie et al, 2014).

2g of Meriva (400mg curcumin) is found to have analgesic activity comparable to 1g of paracetmol and it has lesser side effects than painkillers like nimesulide and paracetmol (Pierro et al, 2013).

In treatment of osteoarthritis, curcumin is found to be as effective as painkiller ibuprofen and also has reduced side effects on the stomach (Kuptniratsaikul et al, 2014).

In fact, recent research shows that turmeric could possibly be better than opioid painkillers and protect from their side effects.

Curcumin found in turmeric is proven to have natural pain killing properties and in many studies, it has been proven to outperform conventional painkillers. Also, it does not cause any side effects like gastric erosion like NSAIDs do.

7. Combats fatigue

Systemic inflammation, joint pain, blood and bone related abnormalities contribute to negative effects on health in lupus thus paving way for fatigue and sleep disturbances (Ahn et al, 2012).

Turmeric's anti-inflammatory and analgesic action help reduce pain in arthritis. Additionally, animal studies show that by virtue of its anti-inflammatory and antioxidant activity, curcumin reduces chronic fatigue (Gupta et al, 2009).

Curcumin may even protect from side effects of sleep deprivation and reduce sleep disturbances (Huang et al, 2015).

8. It treats kidney damage in lupus

Lee et al. (2013) demonstrated that curcumin treats lupus nephritis by interacting with T reg cells. In this animal study, it was observed that curcumin reduced proteinuria (excess of proteins in urine occurring as a result of damaged kidney function) and reduced inflammation in the kidney.

A very popular study (Khajehdehi et al, 2012) highlighted when talking about turmeric's utility in lupus, that *"Oral supplementation of turmeric decreases proteinuria, hematuria, and systolic blood pressure in patients suffering from relapsing or refractory lupus nephritis."*

In this study, 24 individuals with relapsing or treatment resistant lupus nephritis were enrolled. 12 were treated with 500mg turmeric (22.1mg curcumin) three times a day while 12 were treated with placebo.

A significant decrease in proteinuria (excess protein in urine) was seen and reduction in blood in urine and systolic blood pressure (minimum blood pressure your heart experiences when filling with blood) was observed.

Researchers stated that short term turmeric supplementation can attenuate symptoms of lupus nephritis and aid as a safe adjuvant therapy.

9. Acts at a genetic level

Lupus could manifest as a result of genetic errors and one such genetic error is DNA methylation. For simplicity sake, DNA methylation is a process that controls gene expression or activates your gene and error in that mechanism results in abnormalities.

Curcumin is found to have the ability to regulate such epigenetic processes. It can regulate the activity of enzymes involved in gene expression (Teiten et al, 2013).

Though not assessed in relation with lupus, this property of curcumin is found to be beneficial in cancer, neurodegenerative and inflammatory disorders (Boyanapalli et al, 2015).

At the Da Vinci Center we recommend lupus patients take a high-potency TUMERIC 10,000 mg – one tablet a couple of times daily.

Lifestyle Changes

Lifestyle, including diet, physical activity, and stress levels, can have a potent effect on many different chronic diseases, including lupus. A healthy lifestyle is an important factor in preventing flares, reducing disease severity, and improving overall quality-of-life.

The level of stress an individual with lupus experiences can significantly affect disease. Whether this stress comes from work, finances, relationships, or from managing this chronic disease, it can trigger flares or worsen lupus severity.

A recent study found that the people with lupus who had a greater ability to cope with stress reported a greater quality-of-life (Hyphantis 2011). Additional data suggests that people who participate in a short stress-management program have less pain (Greco 2004).

Ultra-violet (UV) light from the sun can cause or exacerbate the skin lesions often associated with lupus. Therefore avoiding or reducing exposure to the sun may be necessary for some people to avoid triggering these symptoms. One study found that photosensitivity was tightly linked with lupus disease, irrespective of the type of lupus, the level of serum autoantibodies, and use of anti-inflammatory medications (Sanders 2003).

Fortunately, avoiding sun exposure or applying sunscreen is quite effective in preventing the damaging effects of UV light (Kuhn 2011). Ironically, the need to avoid exposure to sunlight may exacerbate the widespread vitamin D deficiency in lupus patients.

Exercising regularly is important for everyone's health, but is especially important for individuals with lupus. Exercise helps prevent inflamed joints from becoming excessively stiff and keeps muscles, bones, and cartilage strong (Chilibeck 1995). Physical activity has also been shown to improve physical fitness in individuals with lupus, but can also help improve feelings of depression and overall quality-of-life (Carvalho 2005).

Exercise can be daunting to those who are already feeling ill because of lupus, but remaining active is an important part of remaining as healthy as possible, even during flares. Those feeling too ill for more vigorous exercise can participate in gentle range-of-motion exercises so that muscles and joints can remain as flexible as possible.

One small pilot study with individuals with lupus confirmed that both aerobic exercise and the gentler range-of-motion exercises are safe for people with lupus and did not worsen signs or symptoms (Ramsey-Goldman 2000).

Nutritional Supplements

Vitamin D

Vitamin D is an essential nutrient and the precursor to the active form is produced in the skin after absorbing ultra-violet light. Other sources of vitamin D include fatty fish like salmon and mackerel; organic milk products, and vitamin D supplements (Berdanier 2008).

Studies have shown that vitamin D is important in reducing the risk of lupus (Cantorna 2004). It has been shown that higher blood levels of vitamin D are associated with less severe lupus disease activity (Amital 2010).

Two observational studies found that women with systemic lupus erythematosus have significantly lower levels of 25-hydroxy vitamin D (Toloza 2010; Borba 2009).

Another study found that, while 22% of healthy control women had a deficiency in vitamin D, 69% of women with lupus exhibited a deficiency in this vitamin (Ritterhouse 2011).

Reduced levels of vitamin D in people with lupus may be due to one or both of two possible scenarios:

1. The deficiency is related to the disease itself
2. The deficiency is caused/exacerbated by avoiding sun exposure due to increased photosensitivity

As discussed above, lupus and some of its treatments can cause bone loss and lead to osteoporosis. Healthy levels of vitamin D are necessary to help the body absorb calcium and keep bones as strong as possible. This is especially important in individuals with lupus.

At the Da Vinci Center we recommend that 25-hydroxyvitamin D levels be kept between **50 and 80 ng/ml** for optimal health. This usually necessitates supplementation with 5,000 – 10,000 IU vitamin D daily for most individuals – we use <u>VITAMIN D3 5,000 IU</u>. However, supplemental doses should always be determined based upon blood test results that your doctor can run for you.

Fish oil

The oil from fatty fish, such as mackerel, wild salmon, and halibut, is especially rich in omega-3 fatty acids (Kris-Etherton 2000). Fish oil is rich in two types of omega-3 fatty acids: docosahexaenoic acid (DHA) and eicosapentaenoic acid (EPA).

Omega-3 fatty acids, also sometimes referred to as polyunsaturated fatty acids (PUFAs), promote health in a number of ways. EPA and DHA are of particular interest in lupus.

Similar to vitamins, the body needs EPA and DHA, but can only produce them in very limited quantities. Therefore, these fatty acids must be included in the diet in adequate amounts (Connor 2000).

Recent evidence has revealed a critical role for EPA and DHA in establishing balanced immunity in autoimmune disease. Experimental studies found that EPA was able to induce immune cells into a regulatory phenotype, thus countering the action of aggressive effector immune cells (Iwami 2011).

Two clinical studies found that taking fish oil reduced lupus severity (Duffy 2004; Walton 1991). Another study found that taking fish oil reduced the level of serum lipids in people with lupus (Clark 1993), which may be useful as they are at a greater risk of developing heart disease.

The ratio between inflammatory omega-6 fatty acids and anti-inflammatory omega-3 fatty acids in the blood is of critical importance in autoimmune diseases. If the ratio is too high, disease activity may increase (Simopoulos 2008).

At the Da Vinci Center, we recommend that everyone strive to maintain an <u>omega-6 to omega-3 ratio</u> of **4:1 or lower**. We also recommend <u>KRILL OIL</u> as this is "cleaner," given that it comes from small crustacean that do not accumulate as much mercury as larger fish.

Minerals and Vitamins

Vitamin E

There are several forms of <u>VITAMIN E</u>, tocopherols and tocotrienols, each of which has different levels of activity in the human body. Vitamin E has been shown to reduce several different markers of inflammation in the body, including inflammatory cytokines (Singh 2005).

Since inflammation is responsible for the widespread tissue damage in lupus, antioxidant vitamins may aid in prevention or delay of the disease.

Vitamin E helps stabilize membranes of lysosomes, or immune cells that contain destructive enzymes used to fight intruders. When membranes are unstable, these enzymes cause damage to surrounding healthy tissue. Vitamin E can help prevent the onset of autoimmune attacks by stabilizing membranes of lysosomes (Ayres 1978). The symptoms of mice with lupus that were treated with vitamin E greatly improved. The mice lived longer, immune cell activity was normalized, anti-DNA antibodies were reduced, and kidney function improved (Weimann 1999).

One study indicates that vitamin E can reduce the level of autoantibodies in lupus patients (Maeshima 2007). A case report of two patients indicates that a topical formula containing vitamin E improves the health of skin in people with discoid lupus erythematosus (Yildirim-Toruner 2011).

Vitamin A

The active form of VITAMIN A, called retinol, is important for healthy skin, bones, and soft tissues (Coates 2010), and supports healthy immune function (Harbige 1996). Since people with lupus have an abnormally functioning immune system and a higher risk of osteoporosis, healthy vitamin A levels are especially important for this population.

Interestingly, one study showed that people with lupus consumed less vitamin A in their diets than age-matched healthy controls, which may contribute to a vitamin A deficiency (Bae 2002).

Consumption of beta-carotene, a vitamin A precursor, is an ideal way to ensure that vitamin A levels are sufficient while simultaneously avoiding vitamin A toxicity. The body will convert beta-carotene into active vitamin A as necessary and excrete any excess.

Plants and Herbs

Ginkgo

Ginkgo biloba, or more simply "ginkgo", is an herb that has been used for thousands of years in traditional Chinese medicine. This nutrient is often prepared by making an extract from the dried leaves. These extracts contain high concentrations of molecules called flavonoids and terpenoids, which are antioxidants and improve blood flow, respectively (McKenna 2001).

A clinical study revealed that taking 120mg of *Ginkgo biloba* extract three times per day for 10 weeks significantly reduced the number of Raynaud's phenomenon attacks, a set of symptoms that often affect people with lupus (Muir 2002).

We use GINGKO BILOBA 120 mg extract at the Da Vinci Center.

Pine bark extract

There is evidence that extract from the bark of the pine tree (*Pinus pinaster*) helps improve lupus inflammation.

One study found that administration of pine bark extract reduced oxidative stress and improved lupus signs and symptoms in six patients that received the supplement in addition to prescription medications compared to a placebo group (Stefanescu 2001). Specifically, the patients who took pine bark extract exhibited a reduction in SLEDAI score, meaning that disease as a whole was decreased.

White peony extract

White peony (*Paeonia lactiflora*) root is a traditional Chinese medicinal herb that contains bioactive compounds called glucosides. A water and alcohol extract of the peony root, known as total glucosides of peony, has more than 15 identified compounds. The most active and abundant of these is paeoniflorin, which represents more than 90% of the total glucosides of peony (Feng 2016; He 2011).

A number of studies have shown paeoniflorin and total glucosides of peony have immunomodulatory, anti-inflammatory, and pain-relieving properties, and provide supportive evidence for peony's historical use in the treatment of autoimmune conditions, including lupus (He 2011; W Zhang 2012; Feng 2016).

One study that examined case histories of lupus patients treated with total glucosides of peony found that consistent treatment for five years or more was associated with lower medication dosages and lower disease activity compared with patients who had not used peony extract (Zhang 2011).

In a mouse model of lupus, levels of lupus antibodies decreased significantly and disease-associated kidney damage was reduced after 15 and 30 days of treatment with total glucosides of peony (Ding 2011).

Laboratory and animal investigations indicate in conditions of immune over-activation, total glucosides of peony strengthen immune regulation and quiet immune over-activity (He 2011).

Other Natural Therapies

Dehydroepiandrosterone (DHEA)

DHEA is a hormone naturally produced by the adrenal gland that is converted into sex hormones. In addition to being produced in the body, DHEA can be derived from the Mexican yam (Coates 2010).

Low levels of DHEA-s, a plentiful metabolite of DHEA in humans, have been observed in patients with lupus and other inflammatory diseases (Sawalha 2008). DHEA and its various metabolites exert considerable influence over immune system activity by regulating production of multiple cytokines (Sawalha 2008).

In a clinical trial, when individuals with lupus took 200mg of DHEA daily for 24 weeks, the number of patients who experienced lupus flares was significantly reduced (Chang 2002).

In another study, the same investigators showed that taking 200mg of DHEA daily for 24 weeks reduced blood levels of the cytokine IL-10, which enhances antibody production (Chang 2004). This reduction in IL-10 may have contributed to the reduced incidence of lupus flares seen in the first study.

Another double-blind, randomized, controlled trial involving 41 women found that six months' treatment with 20–30mg DHEA daily improved mental and emotional well-being in lupus patients (Nordmark 2005).

Also, at a dose of 200mg daily, DHEA improved bone mineral density in postmenopausal women with lupus (Hartkamp 2004).

Plants to Avoid

The seeds of the alfalfa plant have the potential to cause transient lupus-like symptoms, including autoimmune-related anaemia (Montanaro 1991; Bardana 1982). Alfalfa seeds are rich in the amino acid L-canavanine, which was shown to be the responsible triggering agent in humans and in certain types of mice (Montanaro 1991; Akaogi 2006). Due to these potential effects, people with lupus should avoid alfalfa seeds.

Where to begin

We have presented a large amount of information in this chapter that may take another reading to really assimilate it all. However, in summary, let's go through the basic steps that you need to take and you can fill in the details when you do a second reading.

The first thing that I do with a patient with lupus is to identify and eliminate food intolerances – this I do using Bioresonance diagnostics, so if you have access to a Bioresonance practitioner they may be able to help.

If it is an international client who has a complex of chronic health problems, usually we go through a 5-hour testing programme called the IDEL DIAGNOSTIC programme – you can see details at www.naturaltherapycenter.com

Once you have identified your food intolerances, remove these from your diet religiously – even small amounts are enough to create an inflammatory response.

Then follow the alkaline detoxification diet outlined in the chapter on detoxification. If there is a lot of inflammation and bloating, start gently by eating lots of vegetable soups and broths, stir fried vegetables, oven vegetables, drink fresh vegetable juices, hot herbal teas, soft fruit such as avocado and bananas (avoid fruit with skins), and maintain this for a couple of weeks.

Add some coconut oil to your vegetables as this also has a healing and anti-inflammatory effect. Obviously, you need to eliminate any fruit and vegetables that you may intolerant to.

Lupus is due in great part to the over-acidification of the body, where the acid accumulates and degenerates your intestinal mucosa, causing inflammation. It is important to neutralize this acidity with the alkaline detoxification diet.

Much of the inflammation should abate by the end of the two weeks, particularly if you have been taking some of the supplements recommended in this chapter.

During the alkaline detoxification diet, consider running a parasite detox too using the herbal formula PARAFORM PLUS ONE – one capsule x 3 times daily, with food, along with the PARAFORM TINCTURE – 2 teaspoons in some water away from food, preferably at night.

In addition, if there are problems with constipation, take the appropriate supplements and herbs recommended to overcome this problem.

An extremely important part of the detoxification is to undergo the liver and gallbladder cleanse, again as recommended in the appropriate chapter. It is critically important to keep the liver fully functional and optimize all its metabolic processes.

After the detoxification protocols mentioned, stay on the Anti-Inflammatory Diet mentioned in this chapter.

Amongst the many lupus cases that I have seen, I've never seen even one case that did not have an underlying candida problem.

This is why it's important to read the chapter on candida and determine whether this is a treatment protocol that you need to add onto the other protocols mentioned here. It does take three months to complete, but in my clinical experience, the therapeutic effects can be very profound within this short space of time.

I cannot emphasize enough how important this part of the therapy is. In addition, read what is required for healing leaky gut, and begin applying that too. A lot of what applies to healing candida will also apply to healing your leaky gut.

Take a look again at the supplements that are recommended for healing leaky gut.

71

Foods and Beverages to Eliminate

Cut out all the following, again religiously, as they are almost definitely going to be adding to the inflammation:

- all food intolerances that you have identified
- foods high in lectins and phytates
- genetically modified foods (GMOs)
- all foods contain gluten and gliadin
- sugar - in all its forms
- processed foods – replace with whole, organic foods
- alcohol
- smoking
- soft drinks
- bread and baked goods – anything that contains wheat, gluten, or baker's yeast
- commercial dairy products - no milk, no cheese, no ice cream, no yoghurts. Natural, organic butter is OK in small amounts.
- peanuts
- red meat - organic, 'clean' meat in small amounts is OK, but seafood is better
- aspartame, other artificial sweeteners, colourings, preservatives
- MSG
- tap water – always drink good quality, mineral water – 1.5 – 2 litres daily
- toothpaste with fluoride – use organic toothpastes

Supplements and natural remedies

There are a number of supplements and herbal remedies that have been found to be beneficial for lupus – we will summarize these below, but please refer back to the beginning of the chapter for more details regarding how these supplements can be beneficial. Most of the supplements that we use at the Da Vinci Center are available at www.worldwidehealthcenter.net

HMD MULTIS – a high-potency, multivitamin and mineral formula with no excipients or chemicals that is doctor-formulated and clinically tried and tested by myself with many Crohn's cases. Take 2 caps x 2 times daily, with food.

KRILL OIL extracted from small crustaceans, as these are likely to have less mercury than Omega 3 fatty acids extracted from large fish.

<u>TURMERIC (10,000 mg)</u> – take one cap x 2 or even 3 times daily.

<u>VITAMIN C</u> – a mixture of calcium and magnesium ascorbate which is an alkaline form that is much gentler on the stomach and gut than pure ascorbic acid. Take one capsule x 3 times daily.

<u>VITAMIN D3</u> – take one daily (5,000 I.U) for maintenance, but during the first couple of months of therapy you can take two daily, morning and evening, with food.

<u>VITAMIN E (200 I.U)</u> – take one cap x 2 times daily.

Alterations in the bacterial milieu of the gut are common in lupus patients, as already discussed. The use of various probiotic bacteria to promote a balance of appropriate intestinal flora is highly recommended. This will help to balance any dysbiosis, boosting the innate immune system of the gut to help it heal.

Personally, I have used a number of probiotics, but my two favourites are:

<u>ACIDOPHILUS AND BIFIDUS</u> – a high-potency mix of acidophilus and bifidobacteria, with each capsule containing 60 billion live bacteria.

<u>SUPER PROBIO</u> - a practitioner-strength, multi-strain probiotic supplement with 20 billion friendly bacteria per capsule – equivalent to 40 pots of probiotic yoghurt, but without the added sugar, dairy and fat. It provides 8 strains of friendly lactic bacteria which should inhabit a healthy gut, and offers full-spectrum support of the upper and lower bowel.

Glutamine supplementation (1,000 - 4,000 mg per day) is recommended for patients on the basis that it decreases the permeability of the intestinal wall and heals leaky gut. It also reduces bacterial translocation that occurs as a result of intestinal wall permeability. We recommend:

<u>GLUTAMINE PLUS</u> – this is a powder and is easy to take – one teaspoon per day will give 5,000mg which is ample, in a small amount of water.

Butyric Acid may reduce Inflammation in lupus patients. Butyrate decreases proinflammatory cytokine expression (decreases inflammation in the gut) – this is critically important if you want to heal your leaky gut.

We use <u>BUTYRIC ACID</u> – 1 cap x 3 times daily.

QUERCETIN has also been shown to improve gut barrier function by sealing the gut because it supports creation of tight junction proteins. It also stabilizes mast cells and reduces the release of histamine, which is common in food intolerance. New studies have also shown its effectiveness in healing ulcerative colitis. Take 500 milligrams three times daily with meals.

Supplemental Pancreatic Enzymes may be a useful treatment for lupus patients (many patients are deficient in Pancreatic Enzymes). We recommend:

DIGESTIZYME – these are pancreatic enzymes to help digest food in the intestine to prevent putrefaction and fermentation of foods.

GASTRIC AID – these are for the digestion of food in the stomach and contain hydrochloric acid and pepsin – many celiac patients have a deficiency of hydrochloric acid and pepsin that can lead to leaky gut syndrome.

GINGKO BILOBA 120 mg – take one tab daily for the first month, then increase to two tabs for the following 2-3 months.

Homeopathic Remedies for Crohn's Disease

Unlike other forms of alternative medicine, there are no predefined remedies in homeopathy. Rather than have a set of remedies for each disease, homeopathy treats each patient individually.

To individualize the treatment of each patient, a proper consultation with a homeopath is required. A homeopath investigates more than the symptoms. He/she needs to also determine the physical, psychological and emotional constitution of each patient in order to prescribe the right "cures".

The basic principle of homeopathy is "like cures like". This means that homeopathic remedies are really toxic, harmful compounds.

However, instead of using the large doses that harm the body, homeopaths extract and considerably dilute these toxins. The result are watered down solutions of these toxins. Such homeopathic remedies contain none of the toxicity of the raw materials and are, therefore, safe.

In addition, the diluted homeopathic remedy carries a minute dose of the active ingredients of the raw material and that small dose is healing rather than toxic.

Therefore, there is no harm in trying out homeopathy in the treatment of lupus disease. However, homeopathic remedies are not recommended as the primary therapy in the management of lupus disease.

The clinical support for the use of homeopathy in the treatment of lupus disease may be sparse but there are a number of positive results from patients who successfully kept the disease in remission with homeopathy.

When prescribing remedies for lupus, the homeopath seeks to relieve symptoms of the disease, prevent flare-ups, maintain remission and address the underlying problems perpetuating the disease.

Here are some of the homeopathic remedies that are likely to help lupus patients:

Constitutional Treatment

Individuals can be classified according to the characteristic reaction patterns of body. For example, somebody who has a phosphoric constitution will experience pain as a burning sensation. These individuals are very anxious and indeed may become overwhelmed and "burnt out" by their anxieties.

Thus, a Phosphorus patient who develops lupus will have a tremendous anxiety about their health, will be very fearful, especially when alone and is particularly frightened of thunderstorms. The pains in their joints and muscles will be described as "burning". Pain in other parts of the body (e.g. migrainous headaches) will also have a burning quality.

A patient with a Nux vomica constitution will experience the same disease in a very different way. This is usually a very driven ambitious person who may lie awake at night worrying about business affairs, and will become very angry and frustrated with their illness. Typically, relapses in the condition will follow periods of overworking and stress. Joint pains will be worse at night in bed, worse for cold and better for warmth.

A Pulsatilla patient will again present a different picture. They will be a soft, gentle person who weeps easily and may be particularly tearful during flare-ups. They will require lots of comforting and consolation. One of the main characteristics of Pulsatilla is "changeability" and the aches and pains of lupus may be experienced as throbbing one day and stabbing the next.

The constitutional approach is usually the most effective when treating a multisystem disease such as lupus.

Local remedies

Flare-ups of lupus may affect different parts and organs at different times, and homeopathic remedies may be very useful in alleviating symptoms.

<u>Joint pains</u>

A number of homeopathic remedies can help joint pains:

Aconite: sudden severe joint pains which may occur following exposure to a cold, dry wind; hot tender joints.

Apis: hot swollen red inflamed joints. Relieved by cold applications.

Bryonia: sharp stitching joint and muscle pain worse with even the slightest movement.

Dulcamara: joint pains occurring in cold damp weather, better with heat and motion.

Rhus tox: painful stiff joints, worse with initial movement (e.g. on rising from bed), better with continued motion.

Rhododendron: joint pain worse in wet weather, especially before a storm.

Ruta: stiff painful joints and tendons especially following overuse. Worse from cold and damp.

Skin

Homeopathic medicines can be used to treat the cutaneous manifestations of lupus:

Apis: red burning rashes, often associated with fluid retention and swelling (oedema). Better from cold applications.

Fluoric acid: hair loss, especially alopecia areata.

Sepia: yellow/brown "saddle" across the bridge of the nose.

Sulphur: red itchy rashes. Worse with heat, especially the heat of the bed at night. Worse at night. Worse for bathing.

Lungs

Pleurisy may develop during flare-ups of lupus. The following remedies may be useful in helping to control the pain.

Aconite: sudden onset of sharp pains, especially after fright or shock. Worse after exposure to cold dry wind.

Bryonia: stitching pains (such as found in pleurisy) worse from the slightest movement.

Migraine

Many homeopathic remedies are helpful in the treatment of these headaches:

Belladonna: intense throbbing head pains beginning in the right occiput and extending forwards to the right eye. Worse at 3.00pm. Worse with any jarring. Better lying still in a dark room.

Natrum muriaticum: bursting pain, sometimes described as a small hammer in one spot. Worse around 10.00am. Aggravated by sunlight.

Spigelia: stitching neuralgic pain on the left side in or above the left eye. Better with heat or hot bathing.

Putting it All Together

There are many things that you can do to take control of your lupus symptoms and slowly reverse the autoimmune response that the body has developed. It is highly recommended that you work with a naturopathic physician or an experienced holistic medicine practitioner who can guide you along, conduct some tests to determine some of the underlying causative factors, as well as design the supplement programme for you to follow, while monitoring you.

Let's summarize the most important steps, so you can begin somewhere. Let's put things into some sort of "To-Do" order, as follows:

1. Identify food intolerances and remove those completely – read the chapter on food intolerances to understand why this is so important.

2. Go organic as much as possible. Biotech companies genetically modify their crops to increase their natural pesticide (lectin) abilities. Lectins are known for causing leaky gut and aggravating Lupus symptoms. Aside from that, organic meats and produce have higher nutrient concentrations and are pesticide-free, antibiotic-free, and GMO-free.

3. Adopt a plant-based diet. Many of our best nutrient sources are dark, leafy-green and brightly coloured vegetables. Kale, spinach, broccoli, asparagus, collards etc. should be eaten daily. Eat plenty of fermented vegetables containing healthy bacteria such as sauerkraut and other fermented veg. Kombucha tea and coconut milk kefir are also good additions.

4. Follow the anti-inflammatory diet explained above to reduce general inflammation in the body as well as the gut.

5. Add ginger and turmeric juices, which are highly anti-inflammatory, into your daily diet – see instructions above.

6. Drink a minimum of 1.5 – 2 litres of clean mineral water (not tap water) daily – this is critically important if you really want to heal.

7. Follow the strategies for a gluten-free lifestyle. Prepare your kitchen and check out the foods that are safe in order to increase the variety of food that you can add to your diet.

8. It would be good to take a good quality multi-vitamin formula such as HMD MULTIS (1 cap x 3 daily), as well as HEPATO PLUS (1 cap x 3 daily), a

herbal formula to help clean and strengthen the liver and COENZYME Q10 (1 cap daily). Remember that research has shown that many patients with lupus are deficient in vitamins and minerals.

9. Take anti-parasite herbs throughout the 15 days of the detox – PARAFORM PLUS ONE (1 cap x 3 times daily) and PARAFORM TINCTURE (2 tsp. in morning in water, away from food).

10. Take anti-inflammatory herbs, OMEGA PLUS (1 cap x 2 daily) or KRILL OIL (1 cap x 2 daily) fatty acids as well as the herb TURMERIC (1 tab x 2 daily) and QUERCETIN (1 cap x 3 times daily).

11. Take digestive enzymes such as DIGESTIZYME (1 cap with each meal) and GASTRIC AID (1 cap with each meal) for stomach digestion.

12. Take supplements for a leaky gut such as L-GLUTAMINE and BUTYRIC ACID to heal the mucosa of the gut, along with VITAMIN D3.
    The healing process will never be complete until the healthy bacterial strains in the gut are replenished. Until then, digestion and immunity will remain impaired. This is one step lupus patients often miss and they never heal completely because of it. Drink some organic bone broth as this also helps to heal the gut due to its reinforcing amino acids.

13. Make certain that you are not constipated, otherwise take a herbal remedy such as CONSTFORM, OXYGUT and COLFORM to help clean the gut.

14. Strictly avoid all the foods mentioned in the chapter on nutrition, as well as this chapter, including alcohol, sugar, yeasts.

15. Take probiotics to help the dysbiosis such as SUPER PROBIO, but also oregano oil to help eradicate bad bacteria from the gut. There is also a number of other NATURAL ANTIBIOTICS that can be taken in case of SIBO.

16. Begin taking the heavy metals protocol mentioned – the HMD ULTIMATE DETOX PACK – and if you have any amalgam fillings you may begin removing only one per month while taking the HMD™ all the way through – read the chapter on heavy metals and toxicity.

17. Run a Hair Mineral Analysis which will show the level of minerals in circulation, as well as the level of toxic metals. Take minerals and the HMD

protocol mentioned above, then run the test again in a couple of months in order to see whether the mineral levels have increased (they may not due to a leaky gut). See if there is a higher level of toxic metals indicating that there are metals stored in tissues and organs. Take zinc if this is low on the hair test, as many Lupus patients have been found to be low in zinc, and this is critical for immunity and healing in the body.

18. If there are joint problems, then taking GLUCOSAMINE COMPLEX will be helpful for the inflammation and rebuilding these joints.

19. Use organic protein powders (gluten-free and lactose-free) a couple time per week to substitute protein without fat – HEMP PLUS, PEA PLUS, RICE PLUS

20. Use SUPER GREEN PLUS – this organic mixture of wheat and barley grass, plus a host of other green vegetables, is excellent in vegetable and fruit juices and smoothies.

21. You can purchase and use the Bioresonance devices mentioned in the Energy Medicine chapter – you will also require the DEINFO USB in order to programme the DEVITA AP and the DEVITA RITM devices.

22. Examine any psychological, emotional and spiritual issues that may be causing or maintaining your lupus – forgive and do not hold grudges – read the chapter on this topic.

23. If you suspect having Candida – read the Candida chapter and begin the Da Vinci Candida Protocol after you have completed the alkaline detox, the parasite detox and the liver and gallbladder cleanse, not before.

24. Revise any medications you may be taking such as birth control pills and other over the counter medications that may be maintaining the inflammation.

25. Avoid using pesticides, fly killers, air fresheners and any other chemicals that will aggravate symptoms.

26. Avoid overuse of mobile phones, Wi-Fi and do not sleep with electromagnetic devices and phones next to your bedside – electromagnetic radiation is another invisible cause of much inflammation in the body. Protect yourself with Tachyon products.

27. Get a good night's sleep.

28. Exercise when you can, even walking is fine. Get short bursts of intense, rigorous exercise. This is the best way to reverse the effects of stress. You have to go all-out for 10-15 minutes, as though you're trying to exhaust yourself. This is best accomplished with sprints, running stairs, or doing bodyweight exercise. You'll feel the difference in your body and mind within minutes afterward.

29. Do fun things. Stress is bad in more ways than you can imagine. It flips our entire hormonal, digestive, and immune systems upside down. The best way to flip it right-side-up again is to have fun, engage in your hobbies, and do things that make you happy.

30. Learn the art of Prayer.

Most of the supplements mentioned are available at www.worldwidehealthcenter.net There is a lot of information in this book that is often difficult to assimilate in one reading, so go back to the beginning and read it with more attention to detail, underlining whatever is important for you.

Personally, I have seen many patients with lupus get well using these protocols, so there is no reason why you should not also see these benefits.

If all else fails, then you are welcome to come to the Da Vinci Holistic Health Center (www.naturaltherapycenter.com) in Larnaca, Cyprus and undergo the IDEL Diagnostic programme that will help us understand the underlying causative factors in order to design a bespoke treatment programme just for you.

References

Adriana Cuervo, Arancha Hevia, Patricia López, Ana Suárez, Borja Sánchez, Abelardo Margolles, Sonia González. Association of polyphenols from oranges and apples with specific intestinal microorganisms in systemic lupus erythematosus patients. Nutrients. *2015 ;7(2):1301-17. Epub 2015 Feb 16.*

Aggarwal BB, Yuan W, Li S, Gupta SC. Curcumin-free turmeric exhibits anti-inflammatory and anticancer activities: Identification of novel components of turmeric. Mol Nutr Food Res. 2013 Sep;57(9):1529-42.

Akaogi, J., et al., Role of non-protein amino acid L-canavanine in autoimmunity. Autoimmunity reviews, 2006. 5(6): p. 429-35.

Amital, H., et al., Serum concentrations of 25-OH vitamin D in patients with systemic lupus erythematosus (SLE) are inversely related to disease activity: is it time to routinely supplement patients with SLE with vitamin D? Annals of the rheumatic diseases, 2010. 69(6): p. 1155-7.

Amitha Thudi, Su Yin, Amy E Wandstrat, Quan-Zhen Li, Nancy J Olsen. Vitamin D levels and disease status in Texas patients with systemic lupus erythematosus. Am J Med Sci. *2008 Feb;335(2):99-104.*

Armstrong, C. Harskamp and E. Armstrong (2012). The association between psoriasis and obesity: a systematic review and meta-analysis of observational studies. Nutrition and Diabetes (2012), 2, e54.

Bae, S.C., S.J. Kim, and M.K. Sung, Impaired antioxidant status and decreased dietary intake of antioxidants in patients with systemic lupus erythematosus. Rheumatology international, 2002. 22(6): p. 238-43.

Bardana, E.J., Jr., et al., Diet-induced systemic lupus erythematosus (SLE) in primates. American journal of kidney diseases: the official journal of the National Kidney Foundation, 1982. 1(6): p. 345-52

Barrett JS, Gearry RB, Irving PM et al. Dietary poorly absorbed short-chain carbohydrates (FODMAPs) increase the volume and fermentable substrate content of ileal output. Gastroenterology 2009; 136 (Suppl. 1): A876.

Barrett, B., Efficacy and safety of echinacea in treating upper respiratory tract infections in children: a randomized controlled trial. The Journal of pediatrics, 2004. 145(1): p. 135-6.

Berdanier, C.D., J.T. Dwyer, and E.B. Feldman, Handbook of nutrition and food. 2nd ed2008, Boca Raton: Taylor & Francis. 1265 p.

Bonelli M et al. Treg and lupus. Ann Rheum Dis. 2010 Jan;69Suppl1:i65-66.

82

Borba, V.Z., et al., Vitamin D deficiency in patients with active systemic lupus erythematosus. Osteoporosis international : a journal established as result of cooperation between the European Foundation for Osteoporosis and the National Osteoporosis Foundation of the USA, 2009. 20(3): p. 427-33.

Boyanapalli SS, Tony Kong AN. "Curcumin, the King of Spices": Epigenetic Regulatory Mechanisms in the Prevention of Cancer, Neurological, and Inflammatory Diseases. Curr Pharmacol Rep. 2015 Apr;1(2):129-139. Epub 2015 Jan 30

Bright, J.J., Curcumin and autoimmune disease. Advances in experimental medicine and biology, 2007. 595: p. 425-51.

Bruce D et al. Converging pathways lead to overproduction of IL-17 in the absence of vitamin D signaling. IntImmunol. 2011 Aug;23(8):519-28. Epub 2011 Jun 22.

Buyon JP, Petri MA, et al. The effect of combined estrogen and progesterone hormone replacement therapy on disease activity in systemic lupus erythematosus: a randomized trial. Ann Intern Med . 2005 Jun 21;142(pt 1):953-62.

Cantorna, M.T. and B.D. Mahon, Mounting evidence for vitamin D as an environmental factor affecting autoimmune disease prevalence. Experimental biology and medicine, 2004. 229(11): p. 1136-42.

Carvalho, M.R., et al., Effects of supervised cardiovascular training program on exercise tolerance, aerobic capacity, and quality of life in patients with systemic lupus erythematosus. Arthritis and rheumatism, 2005. 53(6): p. 838-44.

C-C Gao, S-Y Liu, Z-Z Wu, T-F Li, G-M Gao, Z-S Liu, Z-H Zheng. Severe vitamin D deficiency increases the risk for moderate to severe disease activity in Chinese patients with SLE. Lupus. 2016 Feb 25. Epub 2016 Feb 25.

Chainani-Wu N. Safety and anti-inflammatory activity of curcumin: a component of tumeric (Curcuma longa). J Altern Complement Med. 2003 Feb;9(1):161-8.

Chang, D.M., et al., Dehydroepiandrosterone suppresses interleukin 10 synthesis in women with systemic lupus erythematosus. Annals of the rheumatic diseases, 2004. 63(12): p. 1623-6.

Chang, D.M., et al., Dehydroepiandrosterone treatment of women with mild-to-moderate systemic lupus erythematosus: a multicenter randomized, double-blind, placebo-controlled trial. Arthritis and rheumatism, 2002. 46(11): p. 2924-7.

Chassaing, B, Koren O, Goodrich JK, Poole AC, Srinivasan S, Ley RE, Gewirtz AT. Dietary emulsifiers impact the mouse gut microbiota promoting colitis and metabolic syndrome. Nature. 2015 Mar 5;519 (7541):92-6.

Chen YZ et al. Meta-analysis of Tripterygiumwilfordii Hook F in the immunosuppressive treatment of IgA nephropathy. Intern Med. 2010;49(19):2049-55. Epub 2010 Oct 1.

Chilibeck, P.D., D.G. Sale, and C.E. Webber, Exercise and bone mineral density. Sports medicine, 1995. 19(2): p. 103-22.

Christian Lood, Luz P Blanco, Monica M Purmalek, Carmelo Carmona-Rivera, Suk S De Ravin, Carolyne K Smith, Harry L Malech, Jeffrey A Ledbetter, Keith B Elkon, Mariana J Kaplan. Neutrophil extracellular traps enriched in oxidized mitochondrial DNA are interferogenic and contribute to lupus-like disease. *Nature Medicine*, 2016.

Clark, W.F., et al., Fish oil in lupus nephritis: clinical findings and methodological implications. Kidney international, 1993. 44(1): p. 75-86.

Clausen MR, Jorgensen J, Mortensen PB. Comparison of diarrhea induced by ingestion of fructooligosaccharide Idolax and disaccharide lactulose: role of osmolarity versus fermentation of malabsorbed carbohydrate. Dig. Dis. Sci. 1998; 43: 2696–707.

Coates, P.M., Encyclopedia of dietary supplements, 2010, Informa Healthcare, New York. p. 1 online resource (xix, 898 p.).

Connor, W.E., Importance of n-3 fatty acids in health and disease. The American journal of clinical nutrition, 2000. 71(1 Suppl): p. 171S-5S.

Cutolo M et al. Sex hormones influence on the immune system: basic and clinical aspects in autoimmunity. Lupus. 2004;13(9):635-8.

D Santoro, G Vita, R Vita, A Mallamace, V Savica, G Bellinghieri, S Benvenga, S Gangemi. HLA haplotype in a patient with systemic lupus erythematosus triggered by hepatitis B vaccine. Clin Nephrol. *2010 Aug;74(2):150-3*. PMID: 20630136

Damanhouri LH. Vitamin D deficiency in Saudi patients with systemic lupus erythematosus. Saudi Med J. 2009. 30(10): p. 1291-5.

Detlef Schuppan, Geethanjali Pickert, Muhammad Ashfaq-Khan, Victor Zevallos. Non-celiac wheat sensitivity: Differential diagnosis, triggers and implications. Best Practice & Research Clinical Gastroenterology. Volume 29, Issue 3, June 2015, Pages 469–476

Di Pierro F, Rapacioli G, Di Maio EA, Appendino G, Franceschi F, Togni S. Comparative evaluation of the pain-relieving properties of a lecithinized formulation of curcumin (Meriva(®)), nimesulide, and acetaminophen. J Pain Res. 2013;6:201-5.

Diane L. Kamen, Glinda S. Cooper, Henda Bouali, Stephanie R. Shaftman, Bruce W. Hollis, Gary S. Gilkeson. Vitamin D deficiency in systemic lupus erythematosus. Autoimmunity Reviews. Volume 5, Issue 2, February 2006, Pages 114–117.

Ding ZX, Yang SF, Wu QF, et al. [Therapeutic effect of total glucosides of paeony on lupus nephritis in MRL/lpr mice]. Nan fang yi ke da xue xue bao = Journal of Southern Medical University. Apr 2011;31(4):656-660.

Duffy, E.M., et al., The clinical effect of dietary supplementation with omega-3 fish oils and/or copper in systemic lupus erythematosus. The Journal of rheumatology, 2004. 31(8): p. 1551-6.

Elaine Pace Spadarol, John Xuereb Dingli, Rainer Doffinger, Kumararatne Dinakantha, Alexandra Betts, David Pacel. BCG induced lupus vulgaris: an unexpected adverse event. BMJ. 2016.

Esmaillzadeh, A., Masoud Kimiagar, Yadollah Mehrabi, Leila Azadbakht, Frank B Hu, and Walter C Willett. Fruit and vegetable intakes, C-reactive protein, and the metabolic syndrome. Am J Clin Nutr 2006; 84:1489

Feng Z, Xu J, He G, Cao M, Duan L, Chen L, Wu Z. The Efficacy and Safety of the Combination of Total Glucosides of Peony and Leflunomide for the Treatment of Rheumatoid Arthritis: A Systemic Review and Meta-Analysis. Evidence-based complementary and alternative medicine: eCAM. 2016; 2016:9852793.

Gallo, P.M., Glenn J. Rapsinski, R. Paul Wilson, Gertrude O. Oppong, Uma Sriram, Mark Goulian, Bettina Buttaro, Roberto Caricchio, Stefania Gallucci, Çagla Tükel. Amyloid-DNA Composites of Bacterial Biofilms Stimulate Autoimmunity.

Gompel A et al. Systemic lupus erythematosus and hormone replacement therapy. Menopause Int. 2007 Jun;13(2):65-70.

Grace E Ahn, Rosalind Ramsey-Goldman. Fatigue in systemic lupus erythematosus. Int J Clin Rheumtol. 2012 Apr 1; 7(2): 217–227.

Greco, C.M., T.E. Rudy, and S. Manzi, Effects of a stress-reduction program on psychological function, pain, and physical function of systemic lupus erythematosus patients: a randomized controlled trial. Arthritis and rheumatism, 2004. 51(4): p. 625-34.

Greenberg, A.S., and Martin S Obin. Obesity and the role of adipose tissue in inflammation and metabolism. Am J Clin Nutr 2006;83(suppl):461S–5S

Gupta A, Vij G, Sharma S, Tirkey N, Rishi P, Chopra K. Curcumin, a polyphenolic antioxidant, attenuates chronic fatigue syndrome in murine water immersion stress model. mmunobiology. 2009;214(1):33-9.

Harbige, L.S., Nutrition and immunity with emphasis on infection and autoimmune disease. Nutrition and health, 1996. 10(4): p. 285-312.

Hartkamp A et al. The effect of dehydroepiandrosterone on lumbar spine bone mineral density in patients with quiescent systemic lupus erythematosus. Arthritis Rheum. 2004 Nov;50(11):3591-5.

He DY, Dai SM. Anti-inflammatory and immunomodulatory effects of paeonia lactiflora pall., a traditional chinese herbal medicine. Frontiers in pharmacology. 2011; 2:10.

Hilda J I de Jong, Jan Willem Cohen Tervaert, Siti R F Saldi, Rob J Vandebriel, Patrick C Souverein, Ronald H B Meyboom, Henk van Loveren, Olaf H Klungel. Association Between Statin Use and Lupus-Like Syndrome Using Spontaneous Reports. Semin Arthritis Rheum. 2011 Aug 23. Epub 2011 Aug 23.

Huang GZ et al. [Pathological study on autopsy died of Tripterygium intoxication--report of 4 cases]. ZhongguoZhong Xi Yi Jie He ZaZhi. 2009 Feb;29(2):165-8.

Huang L et al. Decreased bone mineral density in female patients with systemic lupus erythematosus after long-term administration of TripterygiumWilfordii Hook. F. Chin Med J (Engl). 2000 Feb;113(2):159-61.

Huang WC, Chiu WC, Chuang HL, Tang DW, Lee ZM, Wei L, Chen FA, Huang CC. Effect of curcumin supplementation on physiological fatigue and physical performance in mice. Nutrients. 2015 Jan 30;7(2):905-21.

Husen Zhang, Xiaofeng Liao, Joshua B. Sparks, Xin M. Luo. Dynamics of Gut Microbiota in Autoimmune Lupus. Appl Environ Microbiol. 2014 Dec; 80(24): 7551–7560.

Hyphantis, T., et al., Coping with health-stressors and defence styles associated with health-related quality of life in patients with systemic lupus erythematosus. Lupus, 2011. 20(9): p. 893-903.

Iwami D, Nonomura K, Shirasugi N, et al. Immunomodulatory effects of eicosapentaenoic acid through induction of regulatory T cells. Int Immunopharmacol. 2011. 11(3): p. 384-9.

Junker Y, Zeissig S, Kim S-J et al. Wheat amylase trypsin inhibitors drive intestinal inflammation via activation of toll-like receptor 4. J Exp Med 2012;209(13):2395-408.

Kanda N et al. Testosterone suppresses anti-DNA antibody production in peripheral blood mononuclear cells from patients with systemic lupus erythematosus. Arthritis Rheum. 1997 Sep;40(9):1703-11.

Khajehdehi P, Zanjaninejad B, Aflaki E, Nazarinia M, Azad F, Malekmakan L, Dehghanzadeh GR. Oral supplementation of turmeric decreases proteinuria, hematuria, and systolic blood pressure in patients suffering from relapsing or refractory lupus nephritis: a randomized and placebo-controlled study. J Ren Nutr. 2012 Jan;22(1):50-7.

Kris-Etherton, P.M., et al., Polyunsaturated fatty acids in the food chain in the United States. The American journal of clinical nutrition, 2000. 71(1 Suppl): p. 179S-88S.

Kuhn, A., et al., Photoprotective effects of a broad-spectrum sunscreen in ultraviolet-induced cutaneous lupus erythematosus: a randomized, vehicle-controlled, double-blind study. Journal of the American Academy of Dermatology, 2011. 64(1): p. 37-48.

Kumar Kole, Alakendu Ghosh. Cutaneous manifestations of systemic lupus erythematosus in a tertiary referral center. Indian J Dermatol. 2009 Apr-Jun; 54(2): 132–136.

Kuptniratsaikul V, Dajpratham P, Taechaarpornkul W, Buntragulpoontawee M, Lukkanapichonchut P, Chootip C, Saengsuwan J, Tantayakom K, Laongpech S. Efficacy and safety of Curcuma domestica extracts compared with ibuprofen in patients with knee osteoarthritis: a multicenter study. Clin Interv Aging. 2014 Mar 20;9:451-8.

Kurien BT, D'Souza A, Scofield RH. Heat-solubilized curry spice curcumin inhibits antibody-antigen interaction in in vitro studies: a possible therapy to alleviate autoimmune disorders. Mol Nutr Food Res. 2010 Aug;54(8):1202-9.

Kurien BT, Harris VM, Quadri SM, Coutinho-de Souza P, Cavett J, Moyer A, Ittiq B, Metcalf A, Ramji HF, Truong D, Kumar R, Koelsch KA, Centola M, Payne A. Danda D, Scofield RH. Significantly reduced lymphadenopathy, salivary gland infiltrates and proteinuria in MRL-lpr/lpr mice treated with ultrasoluble curcumin/turmeric: increased survival with curcumin treatment. Lupus Sci Med. 2015 Sep 8;2(1):e000114.

Kusworini Handono, Mirza Zaka Pratama, Agustina Tri Endharti, Handono Kalim. Treatment of low doses curcumin could modulate Th17/Treg balance specifically on CD4+ T cell cultures of systemic lupus erythematosus patients. Cent Eur J Immunol. 2015; 40(4): 461–469.

Ladas SD, Grammenos I, Tassios PS, Raptis SA. Coincidental malabsorption of lactose, fructose, and sorbitol ingested at low doses is not common in normal adults. Dig. Dis. Sci. 2000; 45: 2357–62.

Laura C. Pullen. Researchers Hone in on Defect in Autophagy that May Underlie Lupus. The Rheumatologist. June 13, 2016.

Lee H, Kim H, Lee G, Chung HS, Bae H. Curcumin attenuates lupus nephritis upon interaction with regulatory T cells in New Zealand Black/White mice. Br J Nutr. 2013 Jul 14;110(1):69-76.

Lee, A.N. and V.P. Werth, Activation of autoimmunity following use of immunostimulatory herbal supplements. Archives of dermatology, 2004. 140(6): p. 723-7.

Lemire, J.M., Immunomodulatory role of 1,25-dihydroxyvitaminD3. Journal of cellular biochemistry, 1992. 49(1): p. 26-31.

Lim SY, Ghosh SK (2003) Autoreactive responses to an environmental factor: 1. Phthalate induces antibodies exhibiting anti-DNA specificity. Immunology 110:482–492. PubMed

M R Geier, D A Geier. A case-series of adverse events, positive re-challenge of symptoms, and events in identical twins following hepatitis B vaccination: analysis of the Vaccine Adverse Event Reporting System (VAERS) database and literature review. Clin Chim Acta. *2006 Feb;364(1-2):196-204. Epub 2005 Aug 10.*

Maeshima, E., et al., The efficacy of vitamin E against oxidative damage and autoantibody production in systemic lupus erythematosus: a preliminary study. Clinical rheumatology, 2007. 26(3): p. 401-4.

Manole COJOCARU, Inimioara Mihaela COJOCARU, Isabela SILOSI, Camelia Doina VRABIE. Manifestations of Systemic Lupus Erythematosus. Maedica (Buchar). 2011 Oct; 6(4): 330–336.

McKenna, D.J., K. Jones, and K. Hughes, Efficacy, safety, and use of ginkgo biloba in clinical and preclinical applications. Alternative therapies in health and medicine, 2001. 7(5): p. 70-86, 88-90.

Meier, C. R., et al. Postmenopausal estrogen replacement therapy and the risk of developing systemic lupus erythematosus or discoid lupus. J Rheumatol. 25(8):1515-1519, 1998.

Minoru Satoh, Yoshiki Kuroda, Hideo Yoshida, Krista M Behney, Akiei Mizutani, Jun Akaogi, Dina C Nacionales, Thomas D Lorenson, Robert J Rosenbauer, Westley H Reeves. Induction of lupus autoantibodies by adjuvants. J Autoimmun. *2003 Aug;21(1):1-9.*

Montanaro, A. and E.J. Bardana, Jr., Dietary amino acid-induced systemic lupus erythematosus. Rheumatic diseases clinics of North America, 1991. 17(2): p. 323-32.

Mozaffarian, D, Pischon T, Hankinson SE, Rifai N, Joshipura K, Willett WC, Rimm EB. Dietary intake of trans fatty acids and systemic inflammation in women. Am J Clin Nutr. 2004 Apr;79(4):606-12.

Muir, A.H., et al., The use of Ginkgo biloba in Raynaud's disease: a double-blind placebo-controlled trial. Vascular medicine, 2002. 7(4): p. 265-7.

Nakanishi Y, Tsuneyama K, Fujimoto M, Salunga TL, Nomoto K, An JL, Takano Y, Iizuka S, Nagata M, Suzuki W, Shimada T, Aburada M, Nakano M, Selmi C, Gershwin ME. Monosodium glutamate (MSG): a villain and promoter of liver inflammation and dysplasia. J Autoimmun. 2008 Feb-Mar;30(1-2):42-50.

NCCAM. National Center for Complementary and Alternative Medicine. "Thunder God Vine". Available at: http://nccam.nih.gov/health/tgvine/ Accessed 10/18/2011.

Neuhouser, M.L. Yvonne Schwarz, Chiachi Wang, Kara Breymeyer, Gloria Coronado, Chin-Yun Wang, Karen Noar, Xiaoling Song, and Johanna W. Lampe. A Low-Glycemic Load Diet Reduces Serum C-Reactive Protein and Modestly Increases Adiponectin in Overweight and Obese Adults. J Nutr. 2012 Feb; 142(2): 369–374.

Nordmark G et al. Effects of dehydroepiandrosterone supplement on health-related quality of life in glucocorticoid treated female patients with systemic lupus erythematosus. Autoimmunity. 2005 Nov;38(7):531-40.

Oh DY, Talukdar S, Bae EJ, Imamura T, Morinaga H, Fan W, Li P, Lu WJ, Watkins SM, Olefsky JM. GPR120 is an omega-3 fatty acid receptor mediating potent anti-inflammatory and insulin-sensitizing effects. Cell. 2010 Sep 3;142(5):687-98.

Ong DK, Mitchell SB, Smith S et al. The intestinal fermentative response to dietary FODMAPs: failure to switch to methane production in patients with irritable bowel syndrome. J. Gastroenterol. Hepatol. 2008; 23 (Suppl. 4): A219.

Potera, C. Autoimmune Disease: Phthalate Linked to Lupus in Mice. Environ Health Perspect. 2005 December; 113(12): A809.

Ramsey-Goldman, R., et al., A pilot study on the effects of exercise in patients with systemic lupus erythematosus. Arthritis care and research : the official journal of the Arthritis Health Professions Association, 2000. 13(5): p. 262-9.

Ritterhouse, L.L., et al., Vitamin D deficiency is associated with an increased autoimmune response in healthy individuals and in patients with systemic lupus erythematosus. Annals of the rheumatic diseases, 2011. 70(9): p. 1569-74.

Rudolf Valenta, Irene Mittermann, Thomas Werfel, Holger Garn, Harald Renz. Linking allergy to autoimmune disease. Trends in Immunology. Volume 30, Issue 3, March 2009, Pages 109–116

Rumessen JJ, Gudmand-Hoyer E. Fructans of chicory: intestinal transport and fermentation of different chain lengths and relation to fructose and sorbitol malabsorption. Am. J. Clin. Nutr. 1998; 68: 357–64.

S. A. Older, D F Battafarano, R J Enzenauer, A M Krieg. Can immunization precipitate connective tissue disease? Report of five cases of systemic lupus erythematosus and review of the literature. Semin Arthritis Rheum. *1999 Dec;29(3):131-9.*

Sahbaie P, Sun Y, Liang DY, Shi XY, Clark JD. Curcumin treatment attenuates pain and enhances functional recovery after incision. Anesth Analg. 2014 Jun;118(6):1336-44.

Sanders, C.J., et al., Photosensitivity in patients with lupus erythematosus: a clinical and photobiological study of 100 patients using a prolonged phototest protocol. The British journal of dermatology, 2003. 149(1): p. 131-7.

Sang-Cheol Bae, Soo-Jin Kim, Mi-Kyung Sung. Impaired antioxidant status and decreased dietary intake of antioxidants in patients with systemic lupus erythematosus. Rheumatology International. November 2002, Volume 22, Issue 6, pp 238–243

Sawalha AH et al. Dehydroepiandrosterone in systemic lupus erythematosus. CurrRheumatol Rep. 2008 Aug;10(4):286-91.

Shabanova SS et al. Ovarian function and disease activity in patients with systemic lupus erythematosus. ClinExpRheumatol. 2008 May-Jun;26(3):436-41.

Shailendra Kapoor. Curcumin and Its Emerging Role in Pain Modulation and Pain Management. Korean J Pain. 2012 Jul; 25(3): 202–203.

Simopoulos AP. The importance if the omega-6/omega-3 fatty acid ratio in cardiovascular disease and other chronic diseases. Exp Biol Med (Maywood). 2008. 233(6): p. 674-88.

Singh, U., S. Devaraj, and I. Jialal, Vitamin E, oxidative stress, and inflammation. Annual review of nutrition, 2005. 25: p. 151-74.

Spelman, K., et al., Modulation of cytokine expression by traditional medicines: a review of herbal immunomodulators. Alternative medicine review: a journal of clinical therapeutic, 2006. 11(2): p. 128-50.

Srivastava RM, Singh S, Dubey SK, Misra K, Khar A. Immunomodulatory and therapeutic activity of curcumin. Int Immunopharmacol. 2011 Mar;11(3):331-41.

Stefanescu, M., et al., Pycnogenol efficacy in the treatment of systemic lupus erythematosus patients. Phytotherapy research : PTR, 2001. 15(8): p. 698-704.

Teiten MH, Dicato M, Diederich M. Curcumin as a regulator of epigenetic events. Mol Nutr Food Res. 2013 Sep;57(9):1619-29.

Terrier B, Derian N, Schoindre Y, et al. Costedoat-Chalumeau N. Restoration of regulatory and effector T cell balance and B cell homeostasis in systemic lupus erythematosus patients through vitamin D supplementation. Arthritis research & therapy. Oct 17 2012;14(5):R221.

Toloza, S.M., et al., Vitamin D insufficiency in a large female SLE cohort. Lupus, 2010. 19(1): p. 13-9.

Walker SE et al. Accelerated deaths from systemic lupus erythematosus in NZB x NZWF1 mice treated with the testosterone-blocking drug flutamide. J Lab Clin Med. 1994;124(3):401-7.

Walton, A.J., et al., Dietary fish oil and the severity of symptoms in patients with systemic lupus erythematosus. Annals of the rheumatic diseases, 1991. 50(7): p. 463-6.

Wang BX et al. [A tablet of Tripterygiumwilfordii in treating lupus erythematosus]. Zhong Xi Yi Jie He ZaZhi. 1989 Jul;9(7):407-8, 389.

Weimann BJ, Hermann D. Inhibition of autoimmune deterioration in MRL/lpr mice by vitamin E. Int J VitamNutr Res . 1999 Jul;69(4):255-61.

Yildirim-Toruner, C. and B. Diamond, Current and novel therapeutics in the treatment of systemic lupus erythematosus. The Journal of allergy and clinical immunology, 2011. 127(2): p. 303-12; quiz 313-4.

Zevallos V, Weinmann-Menke J, Meineck M et al. Alpha-amylase/trypsin inhibitors (ATIs) accelerate murine systemic lupus erythematosus. Poster presentation at the 16th International Coeliac Disease Symposium, 21-24 June 2015, Prague, Czech Republic. Poster P168.

Zevallos V, Yogev N, Nikolaev A et al. Consumption of wheat alpha-amylase/trypsin inhibitors (ATIs) enhances experimental autoimmune encephalomyelitis in mice. Oral presentation at the 16th International Coeliac Disease Symposium, 21-24 June 2015, Prague, Czech Republic.

Zhang W, Dai SM. Mechanisms involved in the therapeutic effects of Paeonia lactiflora Pallas in rheumatoid arthritis. International immunopharmacology. Sep 2012;14(1):27-31

Chapter 2

The Holistic Model of Health

I am certain that everybody reading this book will have come across the term "Holistic medicine" at some point in time. There is considerable confusion about the meaning of *holistic*. If you have ever entered into a discussion about Holistic medicine, you will see that everybody has their own opinion. This is not surprising, since there are no accepted standard definitions for Holistic medicine. Most people use the term as a synonym for alternative therapies; basically meaning that they are turning away from any conventional medical options and using alternative treatment exclusively. This is not exactly correct.

Holistic medicine means taking into consideration the complete person - physically, psychologically, socially, and spiritually - in the management and prevention of disease. It is underpinned by the concept that there is a link between our physical health and our more general 'well-being'. A Holistic approach means that the doctor is informed about a patient's *whole* life situation (Strandberg et al, 2007).

In the Holistic approach to medicine, there is the belief that our well-being relies not just on what is going on in our body physically in terms of illness or disease, but also on our psychological, emotional, social, spiritual and environmental state. These different states are equally important. They should be managed together so that a person is treated as a whole. In fact, some feel that the word holistic should really be spelt 'wholistic'.

Holistic medicine needs to look at the whole person; how they interact with their environment and the people around them. It needs diagnostic and therapeutic tools to examine and balance the physical, nutritional, environmental, psychological, emotional, social and spiritual levels of health. It therefore encompasses all modalities of diagnosis and treatment, including allopathic medicine using drugs and surgery if there are no other safer alternatives

The ultimate goal of Holistic medicine is to use all diagnostic and treatment modalities available to optimize the health of the person on all levels of well-being, <u>without doing harm to the person</u>. It is the optimization of all resources to bring about a cure in the person, no matter what school or modality they belong to. Holistic medicine treats symptoms, but also looks for underlying causes of these symptoms.

Holistic medicine =

Disease and symptoms

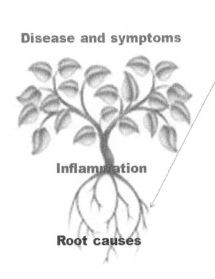

Inflammation

Root causes

Conventional treatments
+
Treating the whole person
+
Finding the root cause
+
Unconditional love
+
Utilize all the tools in our tool belt to heal the patient from inside out

Targeting the root cause can treat multiple conditions and symptoms simultaneously – promoting optimal health ☺

Research in Australia demonstrated that one of the reasons so many Australians seek out alternative and complementary medicine is because of the Holistic philosophy which guides their work. Conversely, it is also the reason why many Australians are becoming less enthusiastic about western or conventional medicine. They see it as non-holistic in nature (Hassed, 2004).

Holistic medicine is something that alternative medicine practitioners traditionally use as a basis for their treatments. However, it is a common misconception that holistic medicine is just 'alternative' or 'complementary' medicine. It is true though, that holistic medicine allows for a wider range of treatment approaches to be used together and encourages open-mindedness for these different approaches.

Some of these approaches may include the use of complementary and alternative medicine, but holistic medicine does not dismiss conventional medicine. It uses conventional medicine as part of the treatment approach. Nutrition, exercise, homeopathy, prayer, acupuncture and meditation are just a few other treatments that may be used together with conventional medicine as part of a Holistic approach.

There are a number of diagrams (Fig 1) that have tried to explain the multimodal approach of Holistic medicine. Perhaps one of the oldest was developed in the 1980's by Dr. Dietrich Klinghardt,[1] one of the leading proponents of Holistic medicine that has provided many tools for practitioners in this field.

The physical body is at the lowest level and is the foundation upon which everything else rests. This is the level that interests medical doctors as well as natural medicine practitioners such as herbal medicine, nutritionists and chiropractors.

On the second level is the electromagnetic body – it is the summation of all electric and magnetic events caused by the neuronal activity of the nervous system. This level is generally not examined by medical practitioners as it requires different tools to access this electromagnetic body. Acupuncturists tap into the meridians and chakras that are part of this second level.

The third-level body is called the "Mental body" and consists of our conscious and subconscious thoughts, attitudes and beliefs. This is where psychotherapists will work, but there are also other natural medicine healing modalities such as homeopathy, applied psychoneuro-biology and meditation that can access this level.

On the fourth level, the "Intuitive body", is the level beyond our level of consciousness; the level of the unconscious, meditative state and trance state. Hypnotherapy, regression therapy and Hellinger's Family Constellation therapy can access this level.

The fifth level, the "Soul", is perhaps the most profound level and the one that is least accessed by therapists of all kinds. It is the level where we are at one with a Higher Consciousness, a Higher Power, God. Prayer and the Spiritual aspects of religion can access this level.

It is generally believed that the first three levels belong to the personal realm, meaning the individual detached from others. The fourth and fifth levels belong to the transpersonal realm, meaning that these are levels that relate to our relationships with others. The lower levels generally supply energy to the higher levels, but the higher levels have an organizing influence on the lower levels.

---

1 http://www.klinghardtacademy.com

The premise of Holistic medicine is to attempt to treat the whole patient on all levels, as opposed to just the symptoms. Often a complaint such as migraines may have a myriad of different causes in each patient – so there is no standard therapy for migraines as the cause would be different in each person. This is why it is important to take into account all the causative factors for each person, and ultimately treating the *patient* and not the *disease* per se. It appears that this wise statement made by Hippocrates, the Father of medicine, has been forgotten by modern medicine! Instead of looking at the person and trying to understand WHY they have the bunch of symptoms that make up their diagnosis, we consume ourselves with LABELLING the disease and suppressing its symptoms, when we should clearly be looking for its root causes.

> *"It is more important to know what sort of PERSON has a disease than to know what sort of DISEASE a person has."*
>
> -   Hippocrates, about 2,500 years ago

We can extrapolate from this that Holistic medicine is based on a "health-care system" and not a "disease-care system". It encompasses preventative medicine by attempting to catch developing health issues early on, instead of waiting until they reach pathological parameters. **Optimizing health should be the ultimate goal of all Holistic medicine practitioners.**

Often Holistic medicine is not interested in labelling the disease itself because this rarely gives information regarding the causes of the symptoms the person is suffering with. Holistic medicine should first identify the causes of the symptoms, which are the body's way of "talking" to the practitioner, without necessarily being overly concerned with the "diagnosis."

This can be clearly illustrated when a person goes to their medical doctor with bowel distension and pain after eating, as well as bouts of intermittent diarrhoea and constipation. The doctor diagnoses Irritable Bowel Syndrome (IBS) and usually gives antispasmodic medication to alleviate the symptoms.

The 5 Levels of Healing – A Guide to Diagnosis and Treatment

Level Body/Sphere	Our Experience at this Level	Anatomical & Conceptual Designation	Related Science	"Diagnostic" Method	Related Medical Treatment & Healing Techniques
5th Level Spiritual Body	Bliss, Oneness with God, Satori	Spirit, Higher Consciousness	Religion & Spirituality	Knowing & Awareness	Self-Healing, Prayer, True Meditation, Chanting
4th Level Intuitive Body	Intuition, Symbols, Trance, Meditative States, Dreams, Magic Curses, Spirit Possession, Out of body & near-death experiences	Collective Unconscious, "No Mind"	Mathematics & Quantum - Physics	Intuition, Applied Psycho-Neurobiology APN II, Systemic Family - Constellation, Sound & Voice Analysis, Radiesthesia, Dream Analysis, Syntonic Optometry, Art Therapy	Applied Psycho-Neurobiology APN II, Systemic Family Constellation, Color and Sound Therapies, Shamanism, Hypnotherapy, Jungian Psychotherapy, Radionics, Rituals
3rd Level Mental Body	Thoughts, Beliefs, Attitudes, Long distance -healing, Consensus reality	Mind & Mental Field - [conscious & subconscious mind], Morphic field, The "Wall"	Psychology & Homeopathy	Autonomic Response Testing ART I & II, Applied Psycho-Neurobiology APN I & II, Psychological Interview - [MMPI], Homeopathic Repertorizing	Applied Psycho-Neurobiology APN I, Mental Field Therapy, Psychotherapy, TFT, EMDR, Homeopathy
2nd Level Energy Body	Feelings - [anger, joy, etc.], Chi [qigong energy], 6th sense & other "energy" perceptions	Nervous System, Meridians, Chakras, Aura, Bio-Electric System, GAGS, Microtubules	Physiology & Physics	Autonomic Response Testing ART I & II, Thermogram, EEG, EKG, EMG, VAS, EAV, Kinesiology, Chinese Pulses, Kirlian Photography, X-rays, MRI, CAT scan	Neural Therapy NTA & B*, Microcurrent Therapies, Acupuncture, Bodywork/Touch, Breath Therapy, Yoga, Qigong, Meditation, Radiation Therapy
1st Level Physical Body	Sensations - [touch, smell, etc.], Action, Movement	Structure & Biochemistry	Mechanics & Chemistry	Direct Resonance - Autonomic Response Testing ART II, Physical Exam, Lab Tests, BDORT	Diet Therapy - Exercise, Osteopathy & Chiropractic, Surgery, Physical Therapy, Drugs & Herbs, Orthomolecular Medicine, Aromatherapy

The Five "Bodies"

5 SB
4 IB
3 MB
2 EB
1 PB

Spheres Model

Objective Reality — Subjective Reality

5th Spiritual (5 SB)
4th Intuitive (4 IB)
3rd Mental (3 MB)
2nd Energy Body (2 EB)
1st Physical Body (1 PB)

Levels Model

The "Emotional Body" is a composite of Levels 1 through 3
The "Soul" is a composite of Levels 2 through 4

Fig. 1. The 5-levels of healing as postulated by Dr. Klinghardt[2]

A Holistic medicine practitioner, however, would begin to investigate the causes of these symptoms such as:

❖ Lack of hydrochloric acid production in the stomach and deficiency in pancreatic enzymes, leading to poor digestion of food with resulting fermentation and bloating.

---

[2] Klinghardt, D. Explore! Volume 14, November 4, 2005

❖ Food intolerances to wheat, lactose, caffeine and eggs, causing the production of inflammatory chemicals such as cytokinines and COX-2's.

❖ Dehydration - the person only drinks 2-3 glasses of water daily, so is severely dehydrated and digestive processes suffer as a result.

❖ Eating a lot of junk food which is nutritionally deficient, resulting in a downward spiral of nutritional deficiencies.

❖ The patient is constantly stressed at home due to marital discord, poor communication with his wife and an autistic child.

❖ The patient is holding a grudge against a family member that hurt them many years ago, and is simply not "letting go" by forgiving them.

Once all of these causes are rectified, then the IBS will disappear forever. The IBS is the result of these causative factors provoking the symptoms and discomfort, and not because the person is lacking in anti-spasmodic medication, or any other medication.

Based on the abovementioned example, it is clear to see that there are no limits to the range of diseases and disorders that can be treated in a Holistic way; simply find all the potential causative factors, remove them, then help the body to repair, rebuild and rebalance. But this needs to be done on all levels – physical body, energetic body, etheric body, mind, emotions, and spirit.

This is why when an individual seeks Holistic treatment for a particular illness or condition, other health problems automatically improve without direct intervention, as the same causative factors could also be responsible for a myriad of other symptoms.

Holistic health teaches the person to reach and maintain higher levels of wellness, optimizing health as well as preventing illness. People generally enjoy the vitality and well-being that results from their positive lifestyle changes, and this provides the motivation to continue this process throughout their lives.

In Holistic medicine the healthcare professional and the patient work as partners. This is really the only way of succeeding, since healing is not really related to the practitioner's skill but the willingness of the patient to work with the practitioner and implement their bespoke healing programme.

Rather than just eliminating or masking symptoms, the symptom is used as a guide to look below the surface for the *root cause*. Whenever possible, treatments are selected that support the body's natural healing system.

HOLISTIC MEDICINE

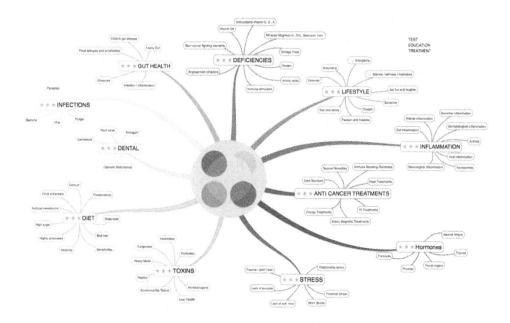

The Medical Model of Disease

Recently I have been discussing issues of Holistic medicine on national TV in Cyprus, where I work and live, in the presence of medical doctors. This has opened up some interesting observations into how allopathic or medical doctors perceive and tackle diseases in their patients. Generally, with few exceptions, allopathic doctors perceive the body as a physical and chemical entity, much like a mechanic would view a machine. Using this "mechanistic" approach, their concern is to examine these structures using a variety of technologies such as X-rays, MRI's, CT scans, gastroscopy, colonoscopy, biochemical lab tests and the like.

These technologies and testing techniques are all measuring the physical and chemical structure of different body parts; the "physical body" which is on the first level of the five levels of healing. They will examine the body's organs, the various tissues, down to the cellular level, to determine pathology (disease) of their structure and the biochemical constituents of the blood, plasma and other body fluids.

Allopathic doctors are extremely well-trained in looking at the physical and chemical composition of the body, and they spend many years in medical school doing just this. However, this "mechanistic" perception of the body has many limitations. This only allows us to view one perspective of the human body, when in fact there are many different levels that are important in diagnosing and fully understanding the aetiology of disease.

When observing the allopathic profession examining a patient based on this mechanistic approach, it becomes obvious why they sometimes behave in rather irrational ways. Generally, the "Medical Model of Disease" or "Biomedical Model" is based on collating the symptoms, placing them into a diagnostic category with a specific label, and then using some form of drug, surgery or radiation to eliminate the symptoms. The assumption is made that all patients are homogenous. The Biomedical model is a "wait for illness" approach.

This is a "symptom suppression" approach to dealing with disease. It rarely identifies the real causes of disease, let alone removing the causes. The fact that a diagnosis has been placed on a diseased organ does not justify the rationale that the diseased organ is the CAUSE of the diagnosis. Tonsillitis, for example, is not the cause of inflamed tonsils; Irritable Bowel Syndrome (IBS) is not the cause of an irritable bowel. The diagnostic labels themselves may be important for the medical doctors themselves, but they do little to help understand the true causes of disease.

The label given to the symptoms of an illness is *not the illness itself.* It may surprise you to hear that a cancerous tumour is not the disease, it is merely a symptom. The disease itself is all the aetiological factors that caused the body to produce the tumour in the first place.

If you put yourself in the position of a medical doctor with this perception, then it is easy to understand why they behave as they do. For example, if there is a part of the gut that is ulcerated and the symptoms cannot be eliminated using medicinal drugs, then the next "logical" step is to remove the organ itself. This may sound rather surprising to the objective onlooker, but personally I have heard from many patients who have been victims of this narrow-minded approach.

Let's Whip Out the Gut!
Late last year I was at the local general hospital seeing a young woman in her 20's who had ulcerative colitis. She was admitted to the hospital with a slight haemorrhage with diarrhoea, probably related to something that was irritating the gut. During her month's stay in the hospital, she had been taking IV cortisone with strong antibiotics (which will destroy all the protective bacteria in the gut and aggravate the inflammation), she had even had chemotherapy (what they give to cancer patients) – God knows what the logic was there – as well as a visit from the psychiatrist, who readily prescribed anti-depressants as he felt that her gut problems

were related to her depression – who would not be depressed in these circumstances?

Recently, her parents were invited to a round-table discussion by the head doctor who, with a solemn expression suggested that the gut should be removed immediately to stop the bleeding and irritation, as nothing else seems to be working!

The doctor added, in a final, desperate attempt, that they may instead decide to give Cyclosporine, a powerful immune-suppressing drug that is given to organ transplant patients to prevent rejection – this literally puts the immune system to sleep. Apart from the chances of catching a nasty bug in hospital which would be near impossible to combat without an immune system, the other side effects of this powerful drug are gum hyperplasia, convulsions, peptic ulcers, pancreatitis, fever, vomiting, diarrhoea, confusion, breathing difficulties, numbness and tingling, pruritus, high blood pressure, potassium retention and possibly hyperkalaemia, as well as kidney and liver dysfunction.[3]

I very recently saw another unfortunate tragedy, this time it was a 12-year old Swedish girl diagnosed with Crohn's Disease. She came to me about one month after the surgeons had removed a large part of her intestine and she had a colostomy bag on the side of her abdomen. If you had seen the psychological, emotional and spiritual devastation in this young teenage girl after the surgery it was a sight never to forget.

Yes, I know you are stunned, just as I was. It sounds unbelievable for a relatively simple case that is easy to bring under control simply by altering the diet (by identifying and removing food intolerances and using some healing herbs and homeopathics). Nutrition does not seem to be an issue that is of much concern to gastroenterologists, even though food is the primary material that travels through the entire gut many times per day.

The first patient in the hospital was told after querying the food she was eating, that it was a "controlled diet" that had been carefully planned by the hospital dietician – white bread, margarine, marmalade, hamburgers with spices, white macaroni and toxic chicken, as well as various dairy products and sweet foods – obviously, the hospital dietician needs to go back to school if she considers this to be a healthy diet!

I made some quick suggestions to her so that she could change her diet immediately – to eat mostly steamed vegetables, vegetable juices and fruit, while taking Omega 3 and 6 fatty acids (which help the body produce natural anti-inflammatory

---

[3] www.sideeffects.com

prostaglandins), as well as a mixture of herbs known for their anti-inflammatory effects such as curcumin (turmeric) and boswelia, as well as aloe vera juice.

Three days after implementing this simple regime she began feeling a lot better. There is also a lot more that can be done, such as identifying and removing her food intolerances, as well as optimizing her diet based on her metabolic type – which will need to wait until she is discharged from the controlled hospital environment and her dietician.

Why the Blinkers?

So, why do all these intelligent doctors who were "A" grade students at school think in this narrow-minded, blinkered and insular way? In order to understand why they are so doctrinaire in their approach to disease, let's take a step back and look at an analogy of the human being as a whole entity – I will use the analogy of an iceberg to demonstrate the point: When we look at an iceberg, we normally see about 10% of the iceberg above the waterline, the remaining 90% is below it.

Most medical doctors are trained to observe only what is above the waterline – the 10% of causative factors that involve the physical and chemical structure of disease. This is the main part of the curriculum in most medical schools. Most of the funding for research comes from the pharmaceutical companies who want the budding doctors to prescribe their drugs! They therefore have a big say in what is included in the curriculum. Nutrition, environmental medicine, energy medicine and the psychoemotional and spiritual aspects of the person make up very little of this.

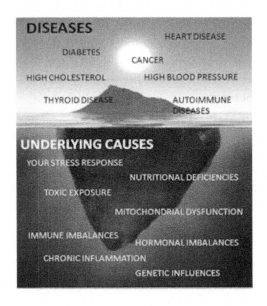

Fig 2. The iceberg analogy

100

If we return to the iceberg analogy (Fig 2), we see that just like the iceberg is composed of the 10% above the waterline, PLUS the 90% below the waterline, so is the human being composed of many different levels. Some we can see and measure and some we cannot. However, they all interact to determine whether we are healthy or not – all these levels make up the HOLISTIC MODEL OF HEALTH that this book is all about. The tip of the iceberg where doctors spend most of their time looking is based on the Biomedical Model of Disease. Doctors tend to examine the physical body for pathology or disease and are not really trained in looking at the whole health spectrum from perfect health all the way through to pathology. This is why there is very little advice that you will obtain from your average medical doctor about preventative medicine.

It is important to note that this knowledge about the physical body, and all the medical technology that has emerged over the last 30-40 years has certainly played an important role in saving many lives, particularly in emergency medicine. This needs to be respected and honoured as it is a big contribution to the health of mankind.

However, it is when the medical profession have to deal with complex, chronic diseases that have taken years to develop and are multi-causal, that they freely admit defeat – there is really not much that they can do to cure these diseases, they can treat and manage them and provide palliative care only.

Why is this? It's simply that they are only looking at one level of the body - the physical level. They can identify and label most diseases known to man, but they will not be able to eradicate those that are related to a multitude of factors on the many different levels of health.

For example, many chronic diseases are now related to the accumulating toxicity from heavy metals and xenobiotics that are ubiquitous in today's world. It is rare that you will find a medical doctor looking for these – it is not really a part of their curriculum. It is also rare that the doctor examines the diet of the person and fully understands its implications – the field of clinical nutrition or orthomolecular nutrition is again not part of their curriculum. Nor is helping patients overcome psychoemotional issues that may remain unresolved and be a major cause of the illness.

Holistic Medicine – The Whole Iceberg
This completes the analogy of the iceberg. It's clear that modern medicine practitioners who have their perception fixed on the tip of the iceberg are not going to be able to identify and eliminate ALL the causative factors of chronic diseases. Instead, they will identify ONLY the structural and biochemical

pathologies in the body and try to alleviate the symptoms using drugs, surgery or radiation.

This is one of the main reasons why modern medicine has such abysmal results in treating chronic diseases such as hypertension, diabetes, arthritis, cancer and asthma – diseases that normally have multiple causative factors. They never even look for poor nutrition which leads to gross deficiencies in nutrients, poor digestion and absorption; high levels of toxic metals and organic xenobiotics such as organochlorine pesticides, PCB's from plastics, Bisphenol-A, lead, mercury, arsenic, cadmium, as well as electromagnetic and geopathic stresses; not to mention psychological and emotional stresses from family, society and work.

If you were a patient with a chronic disease, would you not want to know what the causes of your disease were? Certainly, you would, but often we hear from medical doctors that the cause is "idiopathic" – another word for "unknown"! We also hear "psychosomatic" a lot, meaning that the causes are psychological and emotional. Genetic causes is another reason given to explain diseases that they do not know the causes of. This is not a scientific examination of the causes, but guess work which is often the "dustbin" of modern medicine where all the "unknowns" are dumped. This would include all the patients who do not get better with drugs or surgery, mainly because the true causes of their problems have not been properly diagnosed.

Modern medicine rarely asks the patient what they eat or drink, let alone look at food intolerances and allergies. I was shocked to see a 33-year old man who was referred to me by his mother – he had a heart attack two months previously, with a serious diagnosis of "deep vein thrombosis" hanging over his head; with gross oedema (swelling) of the leg. He was being treated by the medical profession with Warfarin, a blood- thinning drug, for the last month, but generally was not getting better. What I found shocking was that no medical doctor, of the numerous that he had seen, had asked him about his lifestyle habits. He was smoking 2 packs of cigarettes per day, drinking large quantities of alcohol daily (he was a barman), eating lots of junk food and drinking only 2-3 glasses of water daily!

Within 4 days of drinking more water, cutting out the junk food, stopping smoking and drinking and beginning a detoxification diet of fruit and vegetables, his swelling had greatly reduced and he was feeling so much better. This man could easily have died of his deep vein thrombosis: a very dangerous condition.

Another recent patient who was suffering from migraine attacks for 30 years, and had recently got worse, was symptom-free in one month after cutting our her food intolerances, detoxifying and drinking more water. All the drugs she had been taking all those years were simply repressing symptoms – the real causes were elsewhere.

It's important to work in a holistic fashion with these chronic patients. The therapist must begin working through the levels of the potential causative factors. This is what we do at the <u>Da Vinci Holistic Health Centre</u> in Larnaca – the IDEL Diagnostic Programme is a 5-hour testing protocol that is designed to identify and eliminate the underlying causative factors. We often identify more than 15-20 possible causative factors in a chronically-ill patient. When these are eliminated, we see all sorts of degenerative diseases cured in amazingly short periods of time.

A Modern Paradigm

In 2004, Dr. Robison wrote a paper entitled, *"Towards a New Science"*. In the paper, he argues that Holistic medicine emphasizes the relationships among the spiritual, biological, psychological, and social dimensions of the human experience, and that these are critical to a true understanding of health and healing.

He writes, *"...therefore, rather than defining health in terms of the absence of biomedical risk factors for disease or the accumulation of some ideal list of healthy behaviours, we believe that: Health can be redefined as the way we live well despite our inescapable illnesses, disabilities, and trauma."*

He continues, *"The problem is, of course, that as human beings, we all live with varying amounts of physical, psychological, and spiritual baggage."*

How many people have ever experienced or ever known anyone in optimal health? What does that mean? David B. Morris suggests in his insightful book, *"Illness and Culture in the Postmodern Age"*:

"Complete well-being is a fantasy. Health, whatever else it might be, is something that happens not so much in the absence of illness as in its presence" (Morris et al, 1998).

It is more than likely that we will all struggle with emotional, spiritual, and physical issues during our lifetimes, and it is inevitable that we will die. Understanding and living skilfully and compassionately with these struggles, rather than perpetually searching for the latest Holy Grail of optimal health, may come closer to what it truly means to be healthy.

The critical point in understanding health from a Holistic perspective is that health is connected with the manner in which we deal with what we are given in life. The concept of health therefore becomes much less black and white; more a complex and dynamic dance that is not easily quantified, controlled, or predicted. Emerging research compels us to broaden our focus to consider a wide range of psychological, social, and spiritual factors that appear to have as much, if not more, influence on our health than the more traditional biomedical risk factors for disease.

This is an interesting perspective of health and allows the person who may come into the world with genetic predispositions, or who became toxic in the womb, or who has had accidents later in life, to use the holistic model to improve their health (even genes can change their expression with the correct lifestyle changes).

In the chapter on psychological, emotional and spiritual causes of disease, we will see how important it is to forgive those that hurt us and not carry grudges in order to gain optimal health. We will also see how people that pray are much healthier compared to those that do not.

References

Hassed, C.S. (2004). Bringing holism into mainstream biomedical <u>education</u>. Journal of *Alternative & Complementary Medicine, 10*(2), 405-407.

Morris DB. Illness and Culture in The Postmodern Age. University of California Press, Berkeley, 1998.

Robison, J. (2004). Toward A New Science. WELCOA's Absolute. Advantage Magazine, 3(7), 2-5.

Strandberg EL, Ovhed I, Borgquist L, et al; The perceived meaning of a (w)holistic view among general practitioners and BMC Fam Pract. 2007 Mar 8;8:8.

Chapter 3

Toxicity: Underlying Cause of All Diseases

I first became interested in heavy metals, particularly mercury, back in 1997. After running a routine Hair Tissue Mineral Analysis (HTMA) on myself, I inadvertently discovered that I had severely high mercury levels in my system (see column 'Hg' in Fig 1 – it is off the scale)! In fact, they were about 10 times higher than the acceptable levels. That's *1,000%* higher!

This had occurred after removing about 10 amalgam fillings with the help of a holistic dentist here in Cyprus, who gave me chlorella as part of the detoxification protocol. I have since realized how misinformed the dentist was concerning toxic metal chelation protocols. I learned many years later that chlorella is simply not enough to eliminate toxic metals from the body. There are many other dentists all over the world that are inadvertently poisoning people with mercury due to their ignorance. This chapter hopefully will highlight some of the adverse effects on health mercury toxicity has.

It was no surprise that I had many health problems in those days including hand tremors, memory loss, skin irritation, ataxia (poor balance), kidney pains and neurological disturbances. I was trying so hard to keep some sort of balance to maintain my busy work schedule, not to mention bringing up a demanding family.

107

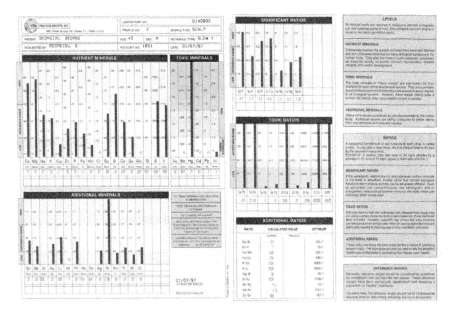

Fig 1. Dr. Georgiou's Hair Tissue Mineral Analysis results of 1997

It took me many years of study to discover how to remove this mercury from my body and regain my health. In the last few years, I have been actively involved in developing heavy metal detoxification protocols that have been scientifically proven to work. I will be discussing these, with case examples, towards the end of this chapter.

Xenobiotics

Toxic chemicals, otherwise known as 'xenobiotics' (*Greek:* 'foreign to life') which are scattered all over our planet from the North Pole to the South Pole, are constantly being researched. The conclusion is that they are *extremely* toxic to humans as well as wildlife. Even though some chemicals have been taken off the market, those that remain are even more noxious than the ones already banned.

Bioaccumulation in soils, water supplies, and the tissues of animals and humans is a real problem. It results in these chemicals lingering for many, many years even after they have been banned. DDT, for example, has been banned for more than 25 years in the Western world, yet it is still being found in the tissues of wildlife in the arctic, as well as humans in many different countries.

108

One study noted that only five organochlorine compounds, as well as mercury, were found in marine mammals in the 1960's. Today over 265 organic pollutants and 50 inorganic chemicals have been found in the same species.[4]

Other recent research has focused on how chemicals affect the thyroid and pituitary systems. Some chemicals have been identified as endocrine disrupters because they can interfere with the body's own hormones, which are secreted by the endocrine glands.

It is also emerging that endocrine disrupters can have many physiological effects not directly associated with the primary system. For example, the thyroid system is well known for regulating metabolism, but it is also a crucial component in foetal brain development in mammals. Too much or too little thyroid hormone at crucial developmental points can cause permanent damage.

The immune system is also vulnerable to hormone-mediated disruption. Chemicals can cause neurological problems, reproductive and developmental abnormalities, as well as cancers. Researchers are only just beginning to disentangle the questions about the effects of chronic low-level exposure to chemicals (as opposed to brief high doses), combinations of chemicals, and interactions between chemicals and other physiological and environmental factors.

Low Dose Exposure

Toxicologists studying chemical toxicity usually have a reference range of values which indicate the 'safe levels' of toxic chemicals. New research is showing, however, that even low-dose exposure[5] of mercury is accumulative over time and can lead to children having decreased performance in areas of motor function and memory.

Similarly, disruption of attention, fine motor function and verbal memory has also been found in adults on exposure to low mercury levels. It is an occupational hazard for dental staff, chloralkali factory workers, gold miners and those of similar professions. Mercury has been found to be a causative agent of various sorts for disorders, including neurological[6], nephrological, immunological, cardiac, motor, reproductive and even genetic. Recently, heavy metal mediated toxicity has been

---

4 O'Shea, T.J., Tanabe, S., Persistent ocean contaminants and marine mammals: a retrospective overview. In: O'Shea, T.J. et al. (Eds.), 1999. Proceedings of the Marine Mammal Commission Workshop Marine Mammals and Persistent Ocean Contaminants, pp 87-92. (cited in Tanabe, S. Contamination and toxic effects of persistent endocrine disrupters in marine mammals and birds. *Mar Pollut Bull* 2002;45:69-77.)
5 Zahir, F., Rizwi, S.J., Haqb, S.K., Khanb, R.H. Low dose mercury toxicity and human health, *Environmental Toxicology and Pharmacology*, March 2005.
http://www.detoxmetals.com/images/newsletter/Low%20dose%20Hg%20exposure.pdf
6 http://www.youtube.com/watch?v=VImCpWzXJ_w

linked to diseases like Alzheimer's, Parkinson's, Autism, Lupus, Amyotrophic lateral sclerosis, and even cancers. Besides this, it poses danger to wildlife. This low-dose toxicity and its effects on health will be the toxicologists' next goal for future research.

Let's look at some specific sources of toxins that we encounter daily:

- Cigarettes, alcohol, caffeine and drugs are all substances that the body cannot use for building and repair, so will add to the mounting waste. A lot of these toxic wastes are stored in the tissues and organs of the body.

- Heavy metals: mercury from fish and amalgam fillings; aluminium found in cheeses, baking powders, cake mixes, self-raising flour, cosmetics, toothpastes, antiperspirants and some drugs such as antacids; arsenic given to chickens as a growth promoter; cadmium found in tea and coffee, as well as cigarette smokers. Lead found in paints, fuels, rubber, plastics, inks, dyes, toys, building materials and hair restorers.

- Roxarsone - 4-hydroxy-3-nitrobenzenearsonic acid - is by far the most common arsenic-based additive used in chicken feed.[7] It is mixed in the diet of about 70% of the 9 billion broiler chickens produced annually in the U.S. In its original organic form, roxarsone is relatively benign. It is less toxic than the inorganic forms of arsenic-arsenite [As(III)] and arsenate [As(V)]. However, some of the 2.2 million lb of roxarsone mixed in the nation's chicken feed each year converts into inorganic arsenic within the bird, and the rest is transformed into inorganic forms after the bird excretes it. Arsenic has been linked to bladder, lung, skin, kidney and colon cancer. Low-level exposures can lead to partial paralysis and diabetes.

- Plastics containing Bisphenol A, the building block of polycarbonate plastics, which are everywhere; in pesticides, antioxidants, flame retardants, rubber chemicals, a coating in metals, cans and food containers, refrigerator shelving, returnable containers for juice, milk and water, nail polish, compact discs, adhesives, microwave ovenware and eating utensils.

A diet that is high in animal fats will add to the waste. There are many different drugs and chemicals that are given to animals these days; antibiotics, hormones, feed

---

[7] Hileman, B. Arsenic in Chicken Production: A common feed additive adds arsenic to human food and endangers water supplies. *Chemical and Engineering News*. Volume 85, Number 15, pp. 34-35, April 9, 2007.

concentrates, etc. All these chemicals will accumulate in the fat cells of the animals that we then eat. So, we slowly build up an accumulation of these chemicals over time.

Sluggish bowels can lead to a great deal of toxicity throughout the body. Try to imagine a 10-metre tube running from mouth to anus packed with meat, sausage, fish, fruit salad, beef burgers, sugars, milk and other goodies – all fermenting and putrefying for days on end. This fermentation produces highly toxic substances such as putrescine, neuracine, and cadaverine, which are so poisonous that a small amount injected into a laboratory animal will kill it in minutes. All these toxic substances, apart from causing disease in the body, will also act as metabolism blockers, and will therefore have consequences on weight-loss too. This process of 'self-poisoning' by these putrefying foods in the gut is called 'autointoxication.'

Refined foods such as white sugar, white flour, white rice, etc. are all deficient in nutrients, but loaded with calories. They also help to create a lot of sludge and debris in the body. If you remember from your childhood days, you probably used white flour and water to make a glue to build a kite, or to glue your coloured paper in to your exercise book at school. When you eat white flour and its products, it becomes glue in the intestine and sticks to the internal wall. When mixed with sticky sugar and fat, it becomes a rubber-like substance that blocks absorption of foods through the intestine, as well as being a constant source of toxins. If you don't believe me, read Dr. Jensen's book entitled, *Tissue cleansing through bowel management*[8]. There are also plenty of photos of what actually comes out of the intestine if you do a proper detox – disgusting!

Thousands of new, toxic chemical compounds are produced each year by the chemical industry, most of which are approved by various so-called 'Environmental Protection Agencies' (EPA's) without any serious toxicological studies. The cumulative number of toxic chemicals polluting our planet today exceeds *100,000*.

Many claim that some of these chemicals, such as the flame retardants used in children's clothing, have potentially life-saving applications. But how many of these chemicals do we ingest or are absorbed by our bodies and those of our children? And at what cost to our health? What is the capacity of the human body to eliminate them? Has anyone conducted a general contracting cost-benefit analysis as to whether the benefits offered, for example, by fire hazard protection, truly outweigh the toxicity generated within us, our children and the environment? The answer is: <u>No</u>. There are *no* comprehensive, scientific answers, other than to confirm the

---

[8] Jensen, B. Dr. Jensen's guide to better bowel care: A complete program for tissue cleansing through bowel management. USA: Avery Publishers, 1999.

obvious: toxicity levels in humans and animals across the globe are rising fast. Whether we realize it or not – we are all toxic.

In an article published in the October 2006, *National Geographic* entitled, '*The pollution within*', journalist David Ewing Duncan had himself tested for 320 synthetic chemicals and certain heavy metals at a cost of $16,000, paid for by the magazine. According to the article, Duncan was considered a healthy individual. Nevertheless, he had higher than average amounts of chemical toxins, such as flame-retardants (known as PDBE's), phthalates, Polychlorinated Biphenyls (PCBs), pesticides and dioxins, as well as heavy metals such as mercury.

Duncan's article alludes to some of the possible ways toxic chemicals may have accumulated in his body; some might have originated in childhood, while others may have been picked up in airplanes due to his extensive work-related travel. However, he and his doctors were merely speculating. Duncan also describes his pre- and post-mercury toxicity results after a fresh fish dinner and breakfast. Duncan had fresh halibut for dinner and fresh swordfish for breakfast (cooked in his toxic non-stick pan), both of which were caught in the ocean just outside the Golden Gate Bridge in the San Francisco Bay area.

He tested himself for serum mercury before and after the meals, and found that his blood mercury levels had shot up from five micrograms per litre to *over twelve*. The doctors conducting the tests advised him not to repeat that experiment ever again, yet I'm sure this dangerous diet is adhered to by thousands, unaware of the impact of toxicity on their health. After all, fish is promoted as a health food. Nevertheless, drawing conclusions on the experience of only one healthy adult is not robust, toxicological science. So, let's review the research…

It is difficult to fathom how we can live in houses that make us sick, but the term "sick building syndrome" (SBS),[9] first employed in the 1970s, describes a situation in which reported symptoms among a population of building occupants can be temporally associated with their presence in that building. Typically, though not always, the structure is an office building.

Typical complaints may include eye and/or nasopharyngeal irritation, rhinitis or nasal congestion, inability to concentrate, and general malaise-complaints suggestive of a host of common ailments, some ubiquitous and easily communicable. The key factors are commonality of symptoms and absence of symptoms among building occupants when the individuals are not in the building.

---

9 Burge, S. et al. Sick Building Syndrome: A Study of 4373 Office Workers. *Ann. Occupational Hygiene.* 31: 493-504, 1987.

There has been extensive speculation about the cause or causes of SBS. Poor design, maintenance, and/or operation of the structure's ventilation system may be at fault. The ventilation system itself can be a source of irritants. Interior redesign, such as the rearrangement of offices or installation of partitions, may also interfere with efficient functioning of such systems. Low levels of specific pollutants found in new furniture, carpeting and other furniture and fittings may also be one of the causes.

A 1984 World Health Organization report suggested that as many as 30 percent of new and remodeled buildings worldwide may generate excessive complaints related to indoor air quality.[10]

In a nationwide, random sampling of U.S. office workers, 24 percent perceived air quality problems in their work environments. 20 percent believed their work performance was hampered because of this.[11]

Toxic from Birth

In September 2005, Greenpeace International, in tandem with the World Wildlife Fund, published a document entitled, *'A Present for Life: Hazardous chemicals in umbilical cord blood.*[12] The research showed convincingly that new-borns tested for hundreds of different xenobiotics[13] showed high levels of these toxins.

Specifically, the blood tests demonstrated that these infants had an average of 287 toxins in their bodies – 180 of these, known carcinogens. Some of these chemicals included the commonly-used artificial musk HHCB, which was found in almost all blood samples at higher levels than the other artificial musk's. Musk ambrette, a chemical banned from use in cosmetics in the EU since 1995, was still found in 15 maternal and 12 cord blood samples.

Other banned alkylphenol compounds, extensively used in industrial cleaning agents, were also found. Additionally, the study quantified the antibacterial agent triclosan in human blood, which was found in almost 50% of the samples. DDT, the notorious pesticide banned from agricultural use worldwide, was found in all blood samples. Similarly, the organochlorine by-product and pesticide hexachlorobenzene – also subject to a global ban – was found in the samples. Perfluorinated compounds like

---

10 U.S. Environmental Protection Agency, Office of Air and Radiation. Indoor Air Facts No. 4: Sick Building Syndrome. revised, 1991.
11 Kreiss, K. The Sick Building Syndrome: Where Is the Epidemiologic Basis? *American Journal of Public Health* 1990; 80:1172-73.
12 Schuiling, J., van der Naald, W. A Present for Life: Hazardous chemicals in umbilical cord blood. Greenpeace International and WWF-UK, Sept. 2005.
13 A xenobiotic is an artificial or natural substance found in an organism that simply should not be present. The term covers chemicals, medical drugs, naturally occurring heavy metals and all the pollutants released into the environment from human activity.

PFOS and PFOA, used to make non-stick pans and water-repelling coatings, were present in all but one maternal sample. PFOS was detected in all cord blood samples; PFOA in half of them.

Another US-based study, *'Baby care products: possible sources of infant phthalate exposure,'* published in *Paediatrics*, February 2008,[14] concluded that phthalate toxicity is widespread in infants. Babies coming into contact with lotions, powders and shampoos had increased urinary concentrations of phthalates, in direct proportion to the number of products they had been exposed to. This association was strongest in young infants, who are more vulnerable to the developmental and reproductive toxicity of phthalates, given their immature metabolic capability and increased dosage per unit of body surface area. Thus, babies become heavily polluted with toxic and carcinogenic substances by their unsuspecting, well-meaning parents. Essentially, *we are unwittingly poisoning our own children.*

One could argue that these studies conducted in the United States – where the toxicity levels are perhaps higher than in other countries – exaggerate the problem. Perhaps in poorer parts of the world, parents use fewer of the culprit lotions and powders, or do without them. Yet, does general environmental toxicity have boundaries?

To address this question, let's examine a similar study conducted on pregnant women living well within the Arctic Circle, which most people feel is a pristine part of Earth. The research was published as an article in *The Science of the Total Environment* entitled, *'Organochlorines and heavy metals in pregnant women from the Disko Bay area in Greenland.'*[15] The study showed high concentrations of heavy metals, such as mercury, and organochlorines in the blood and fatty tissue of the Inuit population. This was attributed to their high consumption of the meat and blubber of marine mammals, which are clearly toxic.

In this study, 180 pregnant women and 178 new-born babies were sampled, amounting to 36% of the total number of births in the Disko Bay area during 1994–1996. What this study showed was that the main food supply of the native population in Greenland, that is, marine mammals, is heavily toxic. It is therefore obvious that pollution has no boundaries. While not within the scope of this book, the fact that the Inuit's were unlikely to have been the main polluters of their coastal waters raises serious additional questions of global ethics, politics and economics.

---

14 Sathyanarayana, S. Karr, CJ., Lozano, P., Brown, E., Calafat, AM., Liu, F., and Swan, SH. Baby Care Products: Possible Sources of Infant Phthalate Exposure. *Pediatrics*, Vol. 121 No. 2, pp. e260-e268, Feb 2008.
15 Bjerregaard, P., and Hansen, JC. Organochlorines and heavy metals in pregnant women from the Disko Bay area in Greenland. The Science of the Total Environment 245, 2000.

A further study published in the journal, *Environmental Research* has shown there is a correlation between the levels of methylmercury in a pregnant or lactating woman's blood and urine and that of her yet-to-be-born or new-born baby, with toxins passing from the mother to the foetus through the placenta. There has since been much research indicating the grave effects on the health of children of high mercury levels, for instance, autism and developmental delays.

The University of Cincinnati published a study in February 2008, entitled: *'Plastic bottles release potentially harmful chemicals (Bisphenol A or BPA) after contact with hot liquids.'* BPA is another synthetic chemical classified as an endocrine disruptor, widely used in plastics. The study concluded that the most important factor regarding exposure to BPA from plastic bottles is not whether the container is new or old, rather, it is the temperature of the liquid contained, that is crucial to the amount of BPA that is released. Hot liquids such as tea, coffee or milk increase the release of BPA up to *55 times*! Other similar studies have shown that if you repeatedly scrub, dish-wash, and boil polycarbonate baby bottles, these also release significant amounts of BPA.

BPA is widely used in products such as reusable water bottles, tin linings, water pipes, dental sealants and baby bottles, and has been shown to affect reproduction and brain development. Consider a baby bottle – it is supposed to be scrubbed clean and steam-sterilized before a hot liquid, such as formula milk, is poured into it and left to cool ahead of feeding a baby. The whole procedure amounts to unintentional infant poisoning! Will these infants be given the chance to naturally detoxify themselves into adulthood? The evidence indicates that this is not the case.

Mercury is a well-established, cumulative neurotoxic agent that can have serious adverse effects on the development and functioning of the human central nervous system, especially when exposure occurs prenatally.[16] Given the potential threat that methylmercury poses to the optimal development of cognitive function, clinicians and regulatory agencies are concerned about the levels of methylmercury that a pregnant women regularly ingests, as well as the levels organic mercury in diets, especially from fish containing methylmercury, which is a major source of mercury exposure to the general population. While cases in which treatment with dental amalgam resulting in elevated blood mercury concentration have been reported, other clinicians have indicated this is not the case.[17] Therefore, this issue remains controversial.

---

16 Methylmercury. Geneva: World Health Organization; Environment Health Criteria 101, 1990.
17 Behrman RE, Kliegman R, Jenson HB. Nelson Textbook of Pediatrics. 17th ed. Elsevier Science Saunders; 2004. Heavy metal intoxification; pp. 702–703.

In one study conducted by a Korean research group[18], they showed that the amount of mercury (from eating fish) in the mother's blood correlated with levels found in cord blood. Blood mercury levels in the group who ate fish more than four times per month was significantly higher than that of the group who did not consume fish ($p = 0.02$). In follow-up studies, blood mercury levels were decreased in the study group but slightly increased in the control group ($p = 0.014$). The maternal blood mercury levels in late pregnancy was positively correlated with mercury levels of cord blood ($r = 0.58$, $p = 0.047$), which was almost *twice* the level found in maternal blood. So, pregnant women who consume a large amount of fish may have high blood mercury levels.

North Americans are also Toxic
In July 2005, the US Department of Health and Human Services, Centers for Disease Control and Prevention, published a 475-page document entitled, *Third national report on human exposure to environmental chemicals*[19], which clearly indicates the growing number of chemical toxins present in all age groups in North America.

A Canada-based study has also compared heavy metal intake in different age groups and their corresponding intake guidelines. The report: *Metallic lunch: an analysis of heavy metals in the Canadian diet*[20], showed that Canadians young and old are ingesting unhealthy levels of toxic substances, such as cadmium and lead. In addition, Canadian children are also being exposed to potentially unsafe levels of copper, manganese, molybdenum and nickel.

Europeans of All Age Groups are Toxic
A study conducted by the World Wildlife Fund set out to explore whether there was any link between the types and levels of contamination found in three generations of families. They wanted to examine possible links between contamination and a family's lifestyle, consumption patterns and use of everyday products.

The study entitled, *Contamination: the next generation - Results of the family chemical contamination survey*[21], summarizes the findings of an analysis of 104 different chemicals in the blood of 33 volunteers from 7 families living in England, Scotland, and Wales. The volunteers in each family spanned 3 generations, comprising a grandmother, mother, and 2 children. In all, 14 children, 13 adults, and 6 grandmothers took part in the study. The ages of the volunteers ranged from 9 to 88.

---

18 Kim, EH., Kim, IK., Kwon, JY., Kim, SW., and Park, YW. The Effect of Fish Consumption on Blood Mercury Levels of Pregnant Women. *Yonsei Med J.* 31; 47(5): 626–633, Oct 2006.
19 A full colour report can be downloaded from http://www.cdc.gov/exposurereport/pdf/thirdreport.pdf
20 Download the full report at
http://www.environmentaldefence.ca/reports/Metallic%20Lunch%20Report_final.pdf
21 WWF-UK. Contamination: the next generation. Results of the family chemical contamination survey.
October 2004.

On analysing the results, all 3 generations were shown to be contaminated by a cocktail of hazardous artificial chemicals, some of them every day domestic products. Every child carried in his or her body the same range of toxic substances: organochlorine pesticides, PCB's, brominated flame-retardants, phthalates and perfluorinated ('non-stick') chemicals. Five such substances found in each parent and grandparent, were also found in every child.

While it might be expected that the chemical load increases with age, the study demonstrated that this is not always true. Children can be more contaminated by higher levels of certain newer chemicals than their parents or even their grandparents, despite being exposed to these chemicals for only a fraction of the time.

Another interesting report compiled by the World Wildlife Fund UK (2005), *'Still dirty: a review of action against toxic products in Europe,'* highlights the occurrence of hazardous chemicals in everyday products and notes which EU member states have taken measures to help protect their citizens and wildlife. One of the report's observations is that phthalates used in plastics and cosmetics have been linked to reduced sperm counts. The report also documents that lead is still in use in the EU, despite its proven toxicity to children and wildlife.

Other chemicals found, such as alkyl phenols and alkyl phenol ethoxylates – industrial chemicals used in plastics, pesticides, and detergents – are toxic and mimic the female hormone oestrogen, causing feminization of male fish. Brominated flame-retardants - chemicals widely used in electronic equipment, fabrics and plastics - are now found in human breast milk and wildlife, even in remote areas.

Cosmetics Beautify but They Also Poison

Are hair dyes worth perishing for? Is your lipstick making you sick? What about beauty creams and other cosmetics? Over 50% of women of all ages colour their hair. Men increasingly dye their hair, too. Research shows a connection between the use of commercial hair dyes and various diseases, including cancer.[22] Newer studies state that because of the prevalence of hair dye use, further studies are necessary to address the effects of specific colours and types of hair dyes with the possible role of individual susceptibility. So, are *you* susceptible?

I have seen and tested several patients who were suffering from many serious, inexplicable symptoms whose doctors were mystified as to the reasons for their deteriorating health. One 34-year-old lady came up really high on tin toxicity, with all

---

22 Ames, BN, Kammen, HO and Yamasaki, E. Hair dyes are mutagenic: identification of a variety of mutagenic ingredients, 1975. See also Watanabe T, Hirayama T, Fukui S, Mutagenicity of commercial hair dyes and detection of 2,7-diaminophenazine, Kyoto Pharmaceutical University, Japan, 1990.

the accompanying symptoms – skin rash, stomach complaints, nausea, vomiting, diarrhoea, abdominal pain, headaches and palpitations. As she was not eating anything from tin cans, but she investigated and found it in her lipstick. Stannous fluoride or tin fluoride is also found in some toothpastes.

Independent laboratory testing initiated by the 'Campaign for Safe Cosmetics' in 2007, found that lipsticks from top brands contain lead also. *Two-thirds* of the 33 cosmetics samples tested contained detectable levels of lead.[23] It was lucky that this lady's lipstick only contained tin, which was eliminated using the heavy metal detox agent HMD[®3].

Almost all cosmetics can cause allergic reactions in certain individuals. Nearly one quarter of the people questioned in the FDA's 1994 cosmetics survey responded 'Yes' to having suffered an allergic reaction to personal care products including moisturizers, foundations, and eye shadows. In the book, *'Drop dead gorgeous: protecting yourself from the hidden dangers of cosmetics*[24], Kim Erickson, with a forward by Dr Samuel Epstein, reveals how manufacturers exploit loopholes in legislation designed to protect the public. So, cosmetic users: beware.[25]

Given that just about everything you put on your skin gets absorbed into your bloodstream, it is interesting that there is such a lack of regulation of carcinogenic ingredients in skin care products. There are over 150 toxic, cancer-causing ingredients currently used in cosmetic products alone. Sunscreens are particularly suspect given that they are recommended, without serious research, as cancer prevention products, whereas in fact they contain many chemicals that *promote* cancer. Another book worth reading that describes the consequences of many of these chemicals on cosmetics is Judi Vance's book entitled, *'Beauty to Die For: The Cosmetic Consequence.'*[26]

Mercury is Everywhere
One of the causative factors that led to my health saga (which I discussed in chapter one), was the extraction of over 10 mercury amalgam fillings several years back. My holistic dentist and I at the time were not so knowledgeable, and we proceeded to remove all the amalgams as quickly as possible. THIS IS A CRITICAL MISTAKE! Notice that this is CAPITALIZED! Removing mercury amalgams quickly, particularly when not using a chelation protocol to remove the mercury released, is

---

23 For more details see: http://www.safecosmetics.org
3 See http://www.worldwidehealthcenter.net/product-category/detox/
24 Erickson, K. Drop-Dead Gorgeous: Protecting Yourself from the Hidden Dangers of Cosmetics, McGraw Hill, 2002.
25 In response to the toxic onslaught from cosmetics, the Environmental Working Group began an initiative to register the fairly safe cosmetics, which can be accessed at: http://www.cosmeticdatabase.com.
26 Vance, J. Beauty to Die For: The Cosmetic Consequence. USA: iuniverse.com, 1999.

the best way of making you so toxic with mercury that the chances of developing a chronic disorder such as cancer or multiple sclerosis increases exponentially. After poisoning my own self out of ignorance, I have consequently spent many years studying and developing natural products for detoxification that also work for mercury – one of the products is the above mentioned, **HMD®**, that we will discuss a little later.

Mercury in Amalgam Fillings

Mercury used in amalgam tooth fillings remains a big issue of dispute. Amalgam was found to be a cheap and long-lasting substance to fill teeth with, but the danger of mercury poisoning was overlooked and ignored. The use of amalgams is now prohibited in many countries. Norway recently announced a ban on the use of mercury, including dental amalgam, that took effect on January 1, 2008. Sweden announced a similar ban and dentists in Denmark will no longer be allowed to use mercury in fillings after April 1, 2008.[27]

The biomedical literature contains numerous articles on the adverse health impact before and after amalgam removal. The International Academy of Oral Medicine and Toxicology[28] has even produced video evidence showing mercury vapour released from amalgam fillings, even though they may be over 30 years old.

Chewing gum, drinking hot beverages, brushing teeth and dental polishing increase the methylmercury released from amalgam fillings.[29] If you doubt how lethal mercury can be, particularly for the nervous system and the brain, a video produced by the University of Calgary Faculty of Medicine, entitled *'How mercury causes brain neuron degeneration*[30] may persuade you. It clearly shows how mercury degrades neural fibres in a petri dish in zero time. Despite all this damning evidence, in the USA alone around 180 million mercury amalgams are placed in peoples' mouths every year.

Before we leave the topic of mercury amalgams, I would like to broadcast a loud warning AGAIN to all those reading this – PLEASE DO NOT REMOVE YOUR AMALGAMS UNLESS YOU ARE FOLLOWING AN ADEQUATE CHELATING PROTOCOL!! There is research which clearly shows that once the dentist's drill is on the amalgams, there are huge mercury deposits released into the blood – up to *100 times* the initial level before the dentist starts working on your amalgams.[31]

---

27 www.mercurypolicy.org
[28] www.iaomt.org
29 Gebel T, Dunkelberg H. Influence of chewing gum consumption and dental contact of amalgam fillings to different metal restorations on urine mercury content. Zentralbl Hyg Umweltmed. 199(1):69-75, Nov 1996.
30 http://commons.ucalgary.ca/mercury
31 Bjorkman, L, Sandborgh-Englund, G, Ekstrand, J: Mercury in saliva and faeces after removal of amalgam fillings. Toxicol Appl Pharmacol 144(1): 156-162, 1997.

Mercury in Vaccines

Many vaccines and inoculations use Thimerosal as a preservative. Following a 1999 recommendation in the US, this is generally being phased out, though it remains in use in several countries. Thimerosol contains around 50% toxic mercury; often linked to Autism. There is an interesting article published in *Medical Hypotheses*: *'Autism: a novel form of mercury poisoning*[32], showing how exposure to mercury can cause immune, sensory, neurological, motor and behavioural dysfunctions, like traits defining or associated with Autism.

The authors of this paper conclude: *"A review of medical literature and U.S. government data suggests that: (i) many cases of idiopathic autism are induced by early mercury exposure from thimerosal; (ii) this type of autism represents an unrecognized mercurial syndrome; and (iii) genetic and non-genetic factors establish a predisposition whereby thimerosal's adverse effects occur only in some children."*

The similarities extend to neuroanatomy, neurotransmitters and biochemistry. By the age of 10, a child may be many hundreds of times over what is considered a 'safe' dose of mercury poisoning from injections. There is no safe dose of mercury.

There are a variety of chemicals that have been found in vaccinations such as:

- ❖ Mercury - the heavy metal used in the disinfectant and preservative, Thimerosal, known to cause brain injury, Autism, attention deficit hyperactivity disorder (ADHD) and autoimmune diseases.
- ❖ Aluminium - a toxic metal additive used to promote antibody response, associated with Alzheimer's disease, brain damage, seizures and cancer.
- ❖ Formaldehyde - a preservative, as well as a nerve-damaging and cancer-causing agent.
- ❖ Ethylene glycol - (antifreeze).
- ❖ Monosodium glutamate (MSG) - a breakdown product of protein, and common flavour enhancer well known for poisoning brain cells.
- ❖ Sulphites - cause genetic damage.
- ❖ Neomycin - an antibiotic, also previously registered for use in US pesticides, known to cause reproductive and developmental harm such as birth defects, infertility, sterility and impairment of normal growth and development.

Servicemen and women who are subjected to many different injections during their tours of duty are at risk of toxic poisoning. Most fish are contaminated with mercury

---

32 Bernard, S., Enayati, A., Redwood, L., Roger, H., Binstock, T. Autism: a novel form of mercury poisoning. *Medical Hypotheses* 56(4), 462–471, 2001.

and other toxic substances, as the *National Geographic* reporter (mentioned above) easily discovered. Even polar bears living in the Arctic, thousands of miles away from any industry, have been found in poor health and even dying because of toxic poisoning.[33,34] No animal or human living on planet Earth is free from the risk of contamination.

Toxins accumulate in the body over time. Some people experience toxicity symptoms from birth, while others experience symptoms gradually. Children with Autism, Attention Deficit Disorder and similar neurological problems are usually found to have high levels of mercury, which is thought to be a major contributory factor in these conditions. Disruptions of the endocrine system and other metabolic functions develop over time, leading to chronic diseases, including multiple sclerosis and cancer.

Toxicity and the Fertility Threat

In 1992, a study in the *British Medical Journal* entitled, *'Evidence for decreasing quality of semen during the past 50 years*[35], reported that semen quality is seriously declining. In 1997, Dianne Dumanoski and others published a book entitled, *'Our stolen future: are we threatening our fertility, intelligence and survival?*[36] This ground-breaking book revealed that chemicals in the environment have affected human reproductive patterns in ways that may threaten the survival of the species. Yueliang Guo and others in 2000 published a study in the *Lancet*: *'Semen quality after prenatal exposure to polychlorinated biphenyls and dibenzofurans.*[37] The study reported that boys prenatally exposed to such chemicals have sperm with abnormal morphology, reduced motility and reduced strength. These results are consistent with studies on animals exposed in the womb to such toxic chemicals.

Another study entitled, *'Chlorinated pesticides and heavy metals in human semen*[38], published in 2000, measured concentrations of chlorinated pesticides and heavy metals (lead and cadmium) respectively, in semen samples collected from men amongst the normal population in India. The study concluded that the presence of these xenobiotics in human semen related to the use of pesticides, emissions of exhausts from motor vehicles and industrial operations.

33 Brown, V. Toxic Chemicals: A Threat to Wildlife and Humans. WWF. December 2003.
34 WWF International Arctic Programme. The Tip of the Iceberg: Chemical Contamination in the Arctic. 2006.
35 Carlsen E, Giwercman A, Keiding N, Skakkebaek NE. Evidence for decreasing quality of semen during past 50 years. *BMJ.* 12;305(6854):609-13, Sept 1992.
36 Theo, C., Dumanoski, D., Myers, JP. Our stolen future: are we threatening our fertility, intelligence and survival? Penguin, USA: 1999.
37 Guo YL, Hsu PC, Hsu CC, Lambert GH. Semen quality after prenatal exposure to polychlorinated biphenyls and dibenzofurans. *Lancet.* 7;356(9237):1240-1, Oct 2000.
38 Kumar R; Pant N; Srivastava S P. Chlorinated pesticides and heavy metals in human semen. *International journal of andrology* 23(3):145-9, 2000.

A 2006 study entitled, *Persistent pesticides in human breast milk and cryptorchidism*[39] investigated a possible association between maternal exposure to 27 organochlorine compounds used as pesticides and cryptorchidism among male children. The study concluded that the link between congenital cryptorchidism and certain persistent pesticides in breast milk, as a proxy for maternal exposure, suggests that testicular descent in the male foetus may be adversely affected.

There are, of course, other concurrent reasons for human reproductive decline, but the toxicity explanation is the most compelling. And yet, most of these women and men could reclaim their lost fertility simply by removing toxins. It is a cheaper and less risky solution, and offers other health benefits as well – just think about it.

The Toxic Onslaught in a Nutshell

There are countless toxicological studies on pregnant and lactating women, infants, as well as young and old members of both genders confirming that we are all toxic. How much more scientific evidence do we need to be convinced of the obvious? The problem has been well identified. In a nutshell, it can be stated as follows:

We have converted our world into a toxic waste dump.

Even before we are born, we accumulate several toxins, which are passed on to us in the womb. After our birth, our bodies keep on accumulating and storing up all types of toxins. From the food we eat, the water we drink, the air we breathe and nearly everything we put in and on our bodies.

This includes cigarettes, caffeine, medical drugs including over-the-counter drugs, alcohol, deodorants, shampoos, tap water, plastic-bottled water, plastic food containers, insecticides, pesticides, herbicides, ordinary food, junk food, fast food, processed food, gourmet food, 'Health' food, beauty creams, shaving creams, tin and lead-contaminated lipsticks; nickel ear/nose/nipple rings, artificial cleaning materials, swimming pools loaded with chemicals, dental mercury amalgams, other toxic dental restoration materials, root canals, dental implants and dentures, childhood vaccinations, adult vaccinations, food additives, flavour-enhancers, food preservatives, hormones, antibiotics and God-only-knows what else.

Unfortunately, there is a lot of medical ignorance that could be exacerbating the situation. Despite the growing number of press reports linking chemicals with disease, and the increasing number of urgent warnings from scientists specializing in

---

39 Damgaard, IN., Skakkebæk, NE., Toppari, J., Virtanen, HE., Shen, H. Schramm, K., Petersen, JH., Jensen, TK., Main, KM. Persistent Pesticides in Human Breast Milk and Cryptorchidism. *Environmental Health Perspectives* Volume 114, Number 7, July 2006.

environmental medicine, the medical world appears to be oblivious to these warnings.

The problem begins in medical schools. Few doctors are taught about modern-day chemicals and their sources, let alone their health effects. Therefore, during the taking of a medical history, the aspect of toxicity that often manifests itself in the patient's symptoms, and the reporting of it, are completely ignored. Maybe one of the reasons why none of this is taught in medical school is that there is no drug they can give to remove these toxins; not to mention this is not good for the profits of the pharmaceutical companies who have a strong influence within the medical faculties. In addition, many of these chemicals are present in foods, cosmetics, vaccinations, herbicides and the like – which involve large international corporations. The topic is controversial if one does not want to stir the waters.

Toxins Versus Nutrients: The Uneven Battle

The body puts up a good fight for survival against the toxic onslaught. But the capacity of the body to deal with and eliminate these toxins is limited. It has several primary and secondary defence lines; namely its excretory and immune systems. These systems need 'ammunition' to keep up the fight, that is, a continuous intake of high-quality nutrients. Sadly, while the amount and varieties of toxins are increasing, the nutrient intake in humans is declining. The nutrient content of the average modern meal has been on the decline for some decades now.

Only a small part of the globe's population has access to – and the inclination for – wholesome, nutrient dense, organic products. The rest of us struggle to survive on the conventional produce available in the typical grocery store. Even worse, a large percentage of the population feeds on junk, toxic, denatured and heavily-processed food – a recipe for a health catastrophe. And the toxins are rising fast, while the nutrients (or antitoxins) are declining equally swiftly. Chronic degenerative diseases are largely the direct outcome of this uneven battle between nutrients and toxins.

The least you can do to help the imbalance is to try to eat a much organic food as possible, while supplementing with a good quality, high-potency multivitamin and mineral formula.

New 21st Century Theory of Disease

Dr. Miller, of the Department of Family Practice, University of Texas Health Science Center at San Antonio, USA, believes that we are on the threshold of the new theory of disease that is based on the toxicity of chemicals. She states in one of her papers,[40] *"In the late 1800's, physicians observed that certain illnesses spread from sick, feverish*

---

[40] Miller C. Are We on the Threshold of a New Theory of Disease? Toxicant-induced Loss of Tolerance and its Relationship to Addiction and Abdiction. *Tox. Ind. Health.* 15:284-294, 1999.

individuals to those contacting them, paving the way for the germ theory of disease. The germ theory served as a crude but elegant formulation that explained dozens of seemingly unrelated illnesses affecting literally every organ system."

She continues: *"Today we are witnessing another medical anomaly – the unique pattern of illness involving chemically exposed people who subsequently report multisystem symptoms and new-onset chemical and food intolerances. These intolerances may be the hallmark for a new disease process, just as fever is a hallmark for infection."*

I strongly agree with Dr Miller and believe that many of the new diseases that we are seeing today such as Gulf War Syndrome,[41] Chronic Fatigue Syndrome, Myalgic Encephalomyelitis (ME), fibromyalgia, childhood diabetes, attention deficit hyperactivity disorder and others are all chemically related disorders.[42]

How exposed are you to these chemicals?
Check out below how prone you are to developing a chemically-triggered, 21st century disease, by checking off the various categories – the more of these that apply to you, the higher your risk if you:

- ❖ work with chemicals
- ❖ use pesticides around the house and garden such as fly spray, weed killer or flea powder
- ❖ use non-environmentally friendly cosmetics, toiletries and household cleaners
- ❖ you are responsible for disposal of chemicals used in medicines such as mercury preservatives in vaccines and flea shampoo
- ❖ eat nonorganic fruit, vegetables and meat products
- ❖ eat contaminated seafood, usually containing mercury
- ❖ eat too many processed foods, full of preservatives, colourings, flavourings and other additives
- ❖ drink unfiltered tap water containing aluminium and fluoride
- ❖ consume soft drinks from aluminium cans
- ❖ have mercury amalgam fillings in your mouth
- ❖ live in a major city with air pollution

---

[41] Miller, C. and Prihoda, TA Controlled Comparison of Symptoms and Chemical Intolerances Reported by Gulf War Veterans, Implant Recipients and Persons with Multiple Chemical Sensitivity. *Tox. Ind. Health* 15:386-397, 1999.
[42] Miller, C. Prihoda, T. The Environmental Exposure and Sensitivity Inventory (EESI): A Standardized approach for measuring Chemical Intolerances for Research and Clinical Applications. *Tox. Ind. Health* 15:370-385, 1999.

These chemicals are accumulative, so do not think that a little exposure will do you no harm – it simply takes longer to reach critical levels in the body before symptoms appear.

Mercury: 'The Big One'

Let us take a closer look at mercury – which I refer to as the 'Big One' as it is omnipotent and ubiquitous. There is probably not a living person on this planet, or living animal – whether domesticated or wild – that does not have their share of mercury toxicity. Mercury is a very toxic substance; more toxic than lead, cadmium, or arsenic.[43]

Mercury is listed as one of the top six most poisonous metals on Earth, with known human toxicity occurring at minimal doses, producing urine levels of 5 mcg/l – which is another way of saying 5 millionths of one gram.

Many Forms of Mercury

Mercury's elemental symbol is *Hg*, which is derived from the Greek word *hydrargyrias*, meaning 'water silver.' As stated above, mercury is found in organic and inorganic forms. The inorganic form can be further divided into elemental mercury and mercuric salts. <u>Mercury in any form is toxic</u>. The difference lies in how it is absorbed, the clinical signs and symptoms and the response to treatment modalities. Mercury poisoning can result from vapour inhalation, ingestion, injection or absorption through the skin.

Elemental mercury is found in liquid form, which easily vaporizes at room temperature (the only metal to do so) and is well absorbed through inhalation. Its lipid (fat)-soluble property allows for easy passage through the alveoli into the bloodstream and red blood cells. This inorganic form has similar properties to organic mercury. Small amounts of non-oxidized elemental mercury continue to persist and account for CNS toxicity.

Mercury in Surprising Places

The use of mercury in Medicine predates its use in dentistry by centuries. Mercury has been found in Egyptian tombs, indicating that it was used as early as 1500 BC. As far back as 500 BC there is evidence that India was using mercury as a drug.

However, Arabic physicians first studied mercury as a drug and introduced the use of a mercurial ointment in the 10th century AD. It was towards the end of the 18th century that mercury found its way into medical practice in the US as a prescription item. In the late 18th century, antisyphlitic agents contained mercury. For centuries,

---

43 Sharma, RP; Obersteiner, EJ., Metals and Neurotoxic Effects: Cytotoxicity of Selected Metallic Compounds on Chick Ganglia Cultures, *J Comp Pathol,* 91(2):235-44 (1981).

mercury was an essential part of many different medicines such as diuretics, antibacterial agents, antiseptics and laxatives.

The number one source of human contamination of *inorganic* mercury today is coal-burning plants. However, the primary source of *organic* mercury contamination is right in your mouth – dental fillings composed of an amalgam, which about 50% of is the metallic form of mercury. A small, tenth-of-a-gram mercury filling would release enough organic mercury to last *27 years*, which is pretty much a consistent chronic toxic exposure for the life of most fillings.

At least seventeen separate studies have confirmed that dental patients absorb a daily dose of mercury derived from their mercury fillings.[44] Mercury poisoning is usually misdiagnosed because of its insidious onset, nonspecific symptoms and lack of knowledge within the medical profession. In medicine today, mercury is still used in various antiseptic agents as well as amalgams.

Mercury is found in many industries such as the manufacture of batteries, thermometers and barometers. It can also be found in fungicides used in the agricultural industry. Before 1990, paints contained mercury as an antimildew agent. On July 7, 1999, a joint statement by the American Academy of Paediatrics and the US Public Health Service was issued, alerting clinicians and the public to the dangers of *thimerosal*, a methylmercury[45]-containing preservative used in vaccines.

Although several sources contributing to the domestic mercury concentrations have been identified, human waste (faeces and urine) from individuals with dental amalgam fillings is believed to be the most significant source – greater than 80 percent.

Mercury is also in many of the foods we eat and it is contained many over-the-counter drugs and cosmetics; e.g. mascara, contact lens solution, haemorrhoid preparations, etc. The mercury ingredients used are *thimerosal, phenylmercuric acetate, phenylmercuric nitrate, mercuric acetate, mercuric nitrate, MB for merbromin* and *mercuric oxide yellow*.

Mercury Toxicity in Fish
About 95% of methylmercury ingested in fish is absorbed into the gastro-intestinal tract, although the exact site of absorption is not known. It is distributed to all tissues in a process completed in about 30 hours. About 5% is found in the blood

---

44 Richardson, G.M., Inhalation of Mercury-Contaminated Particulate Matter by Dentists: An Overlooked Occupational Risk, *Human and Ecological Risk Assessment*, 9:1519-1531 (2003).
45 Ethylmercury – an organic form of mercury widely used as an antifungal agent

components and about 10% in the brain. The concentration in red blood cells is about 20 times the concentration in the plasma.

Guidelines for Minimizing Mercury Exposure from Fish and Shellfish

Fish and shellfish are an important part of a healthy diet. Fish and shellfish contain high-quality protein and other essential nutrients, are low in saturated fat, and contain omega-3 fatty acids. A well-balanced diet that includes a variety of fish and shellfish can contribute to heart health and children's proper growth and development. So, women and young children should include fish or shellfish in their diets due to the many nutritional benefits.

By following these 3 recommendations for selecting and eating fish or shellfish, women and young children will receive the benefits and be confident that they have reduced their exposure to the harmful effects of mercury:

❖ Do not eat shark, swordfish, king mackerel, or tilefish because they contain high levels of mercury.

❖ Eat up to 12 ounces (2 average meals) a week of a variety of fish and shellfish that are lower in mercury.

❖ Five of the most commonly eaten fish that are low in mercury are shrimp, canned light tuna, salmon, pollock and catfish.

❖ Another commonly eaten fish – albacore ('white') tuna - has more mercury than canned light tuna. So, when choosing your two meals of fish and shellfish, you may eat up to 6 ounces (one average meal) of albacore tuna per week.

❖ Check local advisories about the safety of fish caught by family and friends in your local lakes, rivers, and coastal areas. If no advice is available, eat up to 6 ounces (one average meal) per week of fish you catch from local waters, but don't consume any other fish during that week.

Follow these same recommendations when feeding fish and shellfish to your young child, but serve smaller portions.

On January 12, 2001, government health officials issued new advisories warning women to limit fish consumption during pregnancy to avoid exposing their unborn children to unsafe levels of methylmercury.

In February 2009, the Zero-Mercury Working Group[46] published a report entitled *"Mercury in Fish is a Global Health concern.[47]"*

---

46 The Zero Mercury Working Group is an international coalition of more than 75 public-interest non-governmental organizations from around the world, formed in 2005 by the European Environmental Bureau and the Mercury Policy Project/Ban Mercury Working Group. The aim of the group is to continually reduce

"Mercury contamination of fish and mammals is a global public health concern," said Michael Bender, co-author and member of the Zero Mercury Working Group. *"Our study of fish tested in different locations around the world shows that internationally accepted exposure levels for methylmercury are exceeded, often by wide margins, in each country and area covered."*

The Food and Drug Administration (FDA), which regulates commercially sold fish, recommends that pregnant and nursing women and young children don't eat any shark, swordfish, tilefish, or king mackerel; but does recommend 12 ounces per week of any other fish.

The Environmental Protection Agency (EPA), which makes recommendations to states about safe mercury levels in sport fish, allows up to 8 ounces of any fish per week for pregnant women with no prohibitions on consumption of any individual fish caught recreationally.

These restrictions are steps in the right direction, but they need to be tightened significantly to adequately protect women and their unborn children from the toxic effects of methylmercury.

The nutritional benefits of fish complicate the task faced by health officials when protecting the public from methylmercury. Protein, omega-3 fatty acids, Vitamin D, and other nutrients make fish an otherwise exceptionally good food for pregnant mothers and their developing babies.

Some research suggests that the risk of cardiovascular disease increases with methylmercury exposure.[48] In extreme cases, methylmercury poisoning can lead to paralysis, coma and even death.

A new Mercury Policy Project (MPP) report recently published entitled, Mercury in Fish: An Urgent Global Health Concern,[49] explains that the mercury risk is greatest for populations whose per capita fish consumption is high, as well as in areas where pollution has elevated the average mercury content of fish. But methylmercury hazards also exist where per capita fish consumption and average mercury levels in fish are comparatively low. In cultures where fish-eating marine mammals are part of the traditional diet, mercury in these animals can add substantially to total dietary exposure.

---

emissions, demand and supply of mercury from all sources we can control, with the goal of eliminating mercury in the environment at EU level and globally. See www.zeromercury.org

47 http://www.zeromercury.org/press/090210-MercuryFishRelease.pdf

48 Konig, A., et al. (2005), A Quantitative Analysis of Fish Consumption and Coronary Heart Disease Mortality. *Am J Prev Med* 29 (4): 355-346.

49 Mercury in Fish: A Global Health Hazard, Zero Mercury Working Group, *Mercury Policy Project*, Feb. 2009.

Toxicity caused by excessive mercury exposure is now becoming recognized as a widespread environmental problem and is continuing to attract a great deal of public attention. A National Academy of Sciences study [50] published in July 2001 estimates that up to 60, 000 children born in the US each year may be affected by mercury toxicity. In March of 2002, an environmental group charged the FDA with failing to warn the public of the dangers of mercury contamination from eating tuna, which contains high levels of mercury.

The World Health Organization reports that the amount of mercury absorbed daily by the average human body is 0.3 micrograms (mcg) from water and air; 2.61 mcg from fish; and 17 mcg from dental amalgams (silver fillings). Uptake of up to 100 μg daily has been observed in extreme cases. Research points out that mercury vapour is 80% absorbed into the blood, and that in animal studies, mercury vapour goes directly from the nose to the brain, following nasal nerve pathways. Amalgam fillings release mercury for as long as *70 years*. Someone with 8 amalgams could release 120 mcg into the saliva per day.

The maximum mercury exposure allowable by the US Environmental Protection Agency (EPA) is less than 0.1mcg per kilogram of body weight per day to be absorbed.

Dental Amalgams: A Closer Look

> *"The mercury uptake from amalgam is the dominating source for inorganic mercury in the central nervous system and is the major source of total mercury uptake in the population."*
>
> – Maths Berlin, a leading Swedish toxicologist

So, what is an amalgam? It was dentists who, over 150 years ago, discovered a new, less expensive way to fill cavities in teeth, rather than using gold and silver alone. This was a mixture of an assortment of metals such as mercury (45% - 52%),[51] silver (30%) and small amounts of copper, zinc and tin.

---

50 NAS (2000). National Academy of Sciences Report: Toxicological Effects of Methylmercury. C. R.A. Goyer, National Academy Press: pp. 344.
51 Sandra Denton MD : Proceedings of the First International Conference on Biocompatibility 1988.

Mercury causes adverse health effects in dentists and dental personnel[52,53,54,55]. Dentists have 4 times as much of a body burden of mercury as an average non-dentist. Dental workers show 50-300% more mercury in hair and fingernails than the average population.

Denying the Truth About the Dangers of Amalgam Toxicity
Initially, back in the early days, the American Society of Dental Surgeons opposed its use because they knew that mercury was so toxic. However, so many dentists were using it that the original society collapsed and the rogue dentists replaced it with a new one: the American Dental Association (ADA), which is still in existence. This has now grown to be a powerful lobby in Washington and other states. After 150 years, the ADA is still allowing over 180 million mercury-containing amalgam fillings to be placed in people's mouths, including young children!

The ADA has been covering up the danger by saying that the mercury is 'locked in' to the tooth and is not released from the filling itself. The scientific evidence is now so overwhelmingly against this lie, that the ADA had to eventually admit that mercury is released from amalgam fillings (as a vapour) and that over 80% of this is absorbed into the body.

Amalgams release mercury even quicker when a person chews or drinks hot liquids. This is a shocking realisation given that everyone alive today will chew and drink hot liquids on occasions![56]

Consumers aren't being told the truth: <u>Amalgam fillings contain 50% mercury – a known neurotoxin.</u> Worse, they are deceived. The ADA still uses the deceptive word 'silver' to describe a product that is mainly mercury, thus hiding the product's main ingredient.

In previous years, the ADA had managed to de-license various dentists who proclaimed amalgams to be dangerous, and strictly enforced a Gag Rule[57]. In response, these dentists have taken the issue to court, protecting their right, among

52 Ngim, CH; et al., Chronic Neurobehavioral Effects of Elemental Mercury in Dentists, *Brit J Indust Med*, 49:782-90, 1992.
53 Echeverria, D; et al., Behavioral Effects of Low-Level Exposure to HgE Among Dentists. *Neurotoxicol Teratol*, 17(2):161-8 (1995).
54 Shapiro, I.M., et al., Neurophysiological and neuropsychological function in mercury-exposed dentists. *The Lancet* 1, 1147-1150 (1982).
55 Uzzell, B.P., et al., Chronic low-level mercury exposure and neuropsychological functioning. *J of Clin and Exper Neuropsych.* 8, 581-593.
56 http://www.iaomt.org/videos/
57 The Gag Rule is a pillar of the ADA's agenda to block consumers from learning that the major component of amalgam is Mercury. The Gag Rule instructs dentists to abandon their allegiance to patient health care - to remain silent or face disciplinary action.

others, to Free Speech. And yet today, member dentists of the ADA who talk against mercury, or even mention that mercury 'might' be toxic, run a high risk of being expelled as well as having their licenses revoked. The ADA even calls it 'unethical and unprofessional conduct' to inform patients of the potential dangers of the most hazardous metal known to mankind. Yet European countries like Sweden[58] have legislated a total ban on all amalgams and other products containing mercury, after spending years reviewing the scientific research.

Yielding to scientific pressures, the ADA now admits that mercury is indeed released from amalgam fillings, even after placement, but state that it is perfectly safe and still support the use of amalgam fillings. They claim their use is safe, based on over 150 years of use, and that no scientific evidence shows mercury exposure from dental fillings causes any known diseases. Yet the ADA does admit there is a potential hazard for dental office personnel with the handling of dental amalgam and recommend that dentists use a 'no-touch' technique, because dentists and their staff might become contaminated. They admit that the 'scrap' amalgam – the excess amalgam left over after filling a tooth – also constitutes a hazardous threat because of continuous vapour release.

There is no scientific evidence showing amalgam's safety, and mixed dental amalgam has never had US Food and Drug Administration (FDA) research or approval. If it were to be classified as a *class II* medical device and made to undergo the rigorous testing needed to prove safety, it would *never* pass.

After filing petitions, testifying at Congressional hearings, providing state fact sheet laws, testifying at Scientific Advisory Committee hearings, and writing hundreds of letters, the Consumers for Dental Choice (CDC)[59] eventually won their ten-year battle to get the FDA to comply with the law and recently (2008) reclassify mercury amalgam. The FDA website[60] now states:

> *"Dental amalgams contain mercury, which may have neurotoxic effects on the nervous systems of developing children and fetuses.[61] ... Pregnant women and people who may have a health condition that makes them more sensitive to mercury exposure, including individuals with existing high levels of mercury bio burden, should not avoid seeking dental care, but should discuss options with their health practitioner."*

---

58 http://www.sweden.gov.se/sb/d/11459/a/118550
59 www.toxicteeth.org
60 www.fda.gov
61 Mercury has been removed from thermometers and vaccines, controls have been tightened on mercury emissions from coal power plants, and pregnant women have been warned about consuming fish tainted by mercury.

Each amalgam filling has as much mercury as a thermometer, and its poisonous vapours are constantly emitted from the teeth to the brain. A particular risk, according to the US government, to the developing brain of the child. As mentioned earlier, the foetus is at the greatest risk of all if the pregnant woman has dental fillings drilled out or implanted, because of the proven transport of mercury through the placenta. So too is the nursing infant of a woman with amalgam dental fillings, because of the transport of mercury into the breast milk.

Confirmation of the escape of mercury vapour and ions from amalgam dental fillings is provided by The World Health Organization (WHO) Environmental Health Criteria 118 document (EHC 118) on inorganic mercury. It clearly states that the largest estimated average daily intake and retention of mercury and mercury compounds in the general population is from dental amalgams, not from food or air.

The Nuts and Bolts of Mercury Vapour Inhalation from Amalgams

> *"Worldwide there are over 4,000 research papers indicating that mercury is a highly toxic substance. How can dentists be so thoughtless as to place one of the deadliest toxins in existence two inches from our brains?"*
>
> *– Tom Warren*

Mercury vapour inhaled into the lungs is absorbed almost 100 percent and immediately passes into the bloodstream. It takes approximately four minutes before mercury is converted or oxidized into an ionic state from its elemental vapour state. While in its elemental form, mercury vapour is lipid (fat) soluble and readily passes through the blood-brain barrier or the placental membrane.

It can also accumulate in other organs and tissues of the body. The estimated average daily intake of mercury from dental amalgams is 3.8 - 21 micrograms per day. Two-thirds of the body burden of mercury is derived from the mercury vapour released from amalgams. The static release of mercury vapour from amalgam fillings that is not being stimulated, which goes on 24 hours a day, 365 days a year, is a major contributor to the total mercury body burden. A large amount of mercury vapour is released during chewing. After only ten minutes of gum chewing, there is an average increase in mercury release of 15.6 times more than during the resting state in test subjects. That converts to a *1,560% increase* in mercury release.

Increased amounts of mercury are excreted in the faeces of individuals with amalgam fillings. Engqvist et al.[62] found that only 25% of the total mercury in fecal samples was in the form of amalgam particles, in samples taken from six adults with a moderate load of amalgam fillings. About 80% of an oral dose of amalgam particles or mercuric mercury attached to sulfhydryl groups was excreted in the faeces. Interestingly, 60% of an oral dose of vapor dissolved in water was retained. Previously it had been assumed that intake of vapor was due solely to inhalation.

Mercury readily mixes with food and is swallowed with it. The body uptake from inorganic mercury, swallowed with saliva, can be as much as hundreds of micrograms per day for individuals with many amalgam fillings. Urinary excretion is a common indicator of mercury toxicity, even though faecal excretion of mercury is twenty times greater than the corresponding urinary excretion.

There is a statistical correlation between the mercury concentration in saliva and the number of amalgam fillings. The United States government has determined and ruled that the continual exposure to mercury from amalgam fillings is not without risk to patients.

> *"You wouldn't take a leaky thermometer, put it in your mouth, and leave it there 24 hours a day, 365 days a year. Yet that's exactly what happens when an amalgam filling is installed in your mouth."*
>
> – Dr. Michael Ziff

If other dental work is also present in the mouth, such as gold crowns, nickel crowns and removable bridges or braces, the mercury emission further increases from the amalgam. This is due to the electrical current generated by the presence of dissimilar metals in an electrolyte medium such as saliva.

Chronic inhalation of mercury vapour from amalgam fillings for twenty years or more can result in the accumulation of pathologic quantities of mercury in the brain and other critical organs and tissues. Human autopsy studies of accident victims have shown a positive correlation between the numbers of mercury amalgam dental fillings and the concentration of mercury in the brain. The onset of clinically observable signs or symptoms of mercury toxicity may take as long as 20-30 years to appear, depending on a person's biochemical individuality.

---

62 Engqvist A, Colmsjo A, Skare I. Speciation of mercury in faeces from individuals with amalgam fillings. Arch Environ Health 53:205–213 (1998).

Several recent reviews have discussed in detail the uptake, distribution, excretion, metabolism, and kinetics of inhaled mercury vapour.[63,64,65] About 80% of inhaled mercury vapour is retained in the body. However, approximately 7-14% is exhaled within a week after exposure.

Diagnosis of Heavy Metal Toxicity

The diagnosis of heavy metal toxicity must consider the exposure history, clinical signs and symptoms and laboratory tests. While the US Centers for Disease Control has steadily dropped the 'allowable level' of lead in the blood over the last fifteen years, there remains a problem with using blood levels to evaluate toxicity in the first place. Blood levels may not accurately reflect the *total* body burden of toxic metals. High blood levels are usually only found in acute toxic metal exposure, or in people exposed to high levels of toxins over a long period. In chronic low level exposure, however, the blood levels may actually be low, due to redistribution of the toxins throughout the body, while bone and other tissue levels remain high.

Hair Tissue Mineral Analysis (HTMA)

Hair analysis is a method of determining toxin exposure which is popular with many clinicians. The amount of mercury in the hair is determined by first digesting the hair in acids and then using a spectrometer such as ICP-MS to measure accurately, to parts per billion, the levels of mercury.

What are we measuring from hair, and why? When the body has toxic metals circulating in the blood, the first thing that it tries to do is remove them from circulation. This is because the toxic metals are prone to do a lot of damage to different cells of the body through their vicious free radical activity. The first place that the body stores these metals is in inert tissues, such as the hair and nails, which are situated outside the body and therefore would do the least harm. When these storage sites are full, the body will start distributing and storing the metals in other less inert tissues and organs, such as fat, liver, kidneys, thyroid, brain and other organs.

The hair sample taken represents about a two month 'history' of what has been circulating in the blood – the typical sample of hair is about 1 inch long, which takes

---

63 U.S. EPA. Mercury Report to Congress Office of Air Quality and Standards. Washington, DC:U.S. Environmental Protection Agency, 1997.

64 ATSDR. Toxicological Profile for Mercury. Atlanta, GA:Agency for Toxic Substances and Disease Registry, 1999.

65 WHO. Environmental Health Criteria 118. Inorganic Mecury. International Program on Chemical Safety. Geneva: World Health Organization, 1991.

about two months to grow. Therefore, the levels of metals in the hair correlate quite well with the levels in the circulating blood. If there are no metals circulating in the blood during the last two months, then there is a good probability that none will appear in the hair either.

This is a far more clinically significant test that facilitates the practitioner's clinical decision-making, which shows a timeline or history of progress, not simply a snapshot. There are also many advantages to using this over the urine pre-post provocation test using chemical provocation agents:

- ❖ It is a 'gentle' way to proceed as there is no aggressive mobilization and release of large quantities of metals – as with the chemical chelators[66] – which can greatly exacerbate symptoms of neurological problems such as MS, cancer, autism, cardiovascular diseases and others.
- ❖ The history of progress can be mapped over time. The decline in toxic metals shown on the HTMA is an indication that the storage sites in the body are also diminishing. If the levels are still high on the HTMA, then this is an indication that the storage sites are still loaded and that HMD® chelation should be continued for longer. HMD® is a natural, heavy metal chelator that we will talk about more below.
- ❖ It is not a 'snap-shot' picture provided by urine tests, which are difficult to interpret over time.
- ❖ The HTMA is far more cost effective than the urine tests – costing the patient about $120 every two months.[67]
- ❖ The HTMA is very quick, and easily implemented by an assistant in any clinical setting. It also negates the compliance problems often faced by practitioners when they ask the patient to collect urine over a 24-hour period.

Urine and Faeces Testing

Urine and faeces testing can also be used, but as we have already mentioned, these are only 'snapshots' of metabolic activity in the body at the time of collection, which usually runs over a 24-hour period. The differences between the baseline sample and the post-provocation sample when a provocation agent such as EDTA or DMSA is used are not comparable; they are arbitrary figures. These tests are fine for research purposes but don't really help the practitioner make clinical judgements for the best interest of the patient.

---

66 The word 'chelation' comes from the Greek word 'chelos' which stands for 'claw' – these are chemical or natural substances that attach to toxic metals and help in their removal from the body.
67 http://www.worldwidehealthcenter.net/product-category/hair-mineral-analysis/

What Can We Do to Protect Ourselves?

The answer to this question is two-fold. Firstly, we can push for legislation to ban a lot of the harmful chemicals which are known to be detrimental to animals and humans. Secondly, we need to be able to detoxify our bodies to eliminate many of these chemicals. Given that we are exposed to these literally *daily*, this process must be an ongoing one.

Treating Heavy Metal Toxicity Using Conventional Chelators

Many health practitioners use synthetic chelating agents such as DMPS, DMSA, EDTA and others to mobilise and eliminate heavy metals from the body. One advantage of these is the power of their mobilising activity. They are quick to mobilise and eliminate certain metals in the body. However, this may place a huge burden on the body's detoxification systems. Furthermore, symptoms have been reported by natural medical physicians throughout the US, such as intractable seizures in paediatric patients and multiple sclerosis in adult patients, due to taking high doses of DMSA, (also known as Succimer), over extended periods of time.[68,69,70]

The above are valid reasons to at least be cautious of using DMSA for the treatment of mercury-toxic paediatric patients. The fragile brains and nervous systems of children, and particularly those with autism, PDD and seizure disorders, should be handled with considerable care so as not to increase the damage. As of March 2009, as I write, the Federal Drug Administration (FDA) in the USA is considering removing DMSA from the market, but the motives for this move remain unclear.

DMSA and DMPS can certainly be life-saving drugs in cases of ACUTE metal poisoning. Toxicologists have noted that synthetic chelators should only be used in cases of ACUTE metal poisoning, or as a last resort for intractable chronic poisoning. Natural methods are preferable and should be exhausted first.

Natural Heavy Metal Chelators: Do They Work?

It is not safe to use chemical chelators on an ongoing basis. Natural ones can be used instead, much like a supplement, daily. There are several purported natural heavy metal chelators on the market, but literally none of these have been investigated in depth using double blind, placebo controlled trials; except one.

---

68 Smith, DR., et al, Succimer and the urinary excretion of essential elements in a primate model of childhood lead exposure, *Toxicological Sciences*, 2000, Apr, 54 [2] 473-80.
69 Mann, KV. and Travers, JD., Succimer, an oral lead chelator, Clinical Pharmacology, 1991, 10 [12] 914-22.
70 Jorgensen, FM., Succimer: the first approved oral lead chelator, *American Family Physician*, 1993, 48 [8] 1495-1502.

The natural product called HMD®,[71,72,73] has undergone a 'gold standard' double blind, placebo-controlled study using 350 people, at a cost of over one million US Dollars.

It can be used safely over long periods of time with no side effects and is presently being tested to see its efficacy in eliminating some of the xenobiotics mentioned in this chapter.

HMD® is a Patent-Pending, proprietary synergistic blend of three natural ingredients:

- ❖ Chlorella Growth Factor (CGF)
- ❖ Organic Coriandrum sativum leaf tincture
- ❖ Homaccord of cell-decimated, energized Chlorella

Research on HMD®

The research initially began as a health impact study to determine the levels of heavy metals in 374 metal foundry workers in Russia. These were randomly chosen from a workforce of 2,000 people and screened using Hair Tissue Mineral Analysis (HTMA) in a reputable US laboratory specializing in this type of analysis, using Inductively Coupled Plasma–Mass Spectrometer (ICP-MS) technology. There were four major heavy metals identified in this sample that were present at very high levels and were common to the entire workforce (they were by-products of the production process): lead, antimony, cadmium and arsenic.

The research design was a double blind, placebo-controlled study. Neither the participants, researchers, nor the analytical chemists doing the spectrometry analysis knew which treatment protocol each participant belonged to. The coding was stored in the co-ordinator's safe until it was time to interpret the statistical data. All participants signed an Informed Consent Form after discussion of the research protocols. There was a medical team on 24-hour standby to deal with any potential side-effects.

Each participant had to acquire a baseline sample of urine (24-hour collection) and faeces before taking HMD®. Both urine and faeces samples were taken to determine the excretory route used by the various substances tested. These samples were

---

71 Georgiou, G.J. The Discovery of a Unique Natural Heavy Metal Chelator. Explore! Volume 14, Number 4, 2005.
72 Georgiou, G.J. Natural Heavy Metal Chelators. Explore! Volume 16, Number 6, 2007.
73 Georgiou, G.J. A Natural Heavy Metal Chelator Is Born: It's Use With Paediatric Cases. Volume 24, Number 1, 2007.

returned to the research team and circumspectly recorded in preparation for spectrometry, using the foundry's in-house instrument. Further ICP-MS analyses were conducted using two independent laboratories in Russia and the USA.

Table 1 below shows the summarized results of several different trials over a 3-year period. To make sense of the data, there was a group of people who were in the placebo group; these people took an initial urine and faeces sample, then they began taking a weak solution of chlorella (the same dosage used for the experimental group mentioned below). The chlorella solution had been shown in previous trials to not mobilize metals in any way.

After a 24-hour period, another urine sample was taken, and after 48-hours another faeces sample was taken. The difference between the baseline sample and the final sample is expressed in Table 1 below as the mean percentage increase of toxic metals after provocation – this is given for both the placebo group that took the inert chlorella as well as the experimental group that took the HMD®. 'U' denotes the Urine samples and 'F' the Faeces samples. The Mercury results are from a recent independent trial which is discussed in more detail below.

The experimental group followed the same protocol as the chlorella group, as mentioned above, but they took the HMD® - 40 drops in the morning, 50 drops at lunch and 60 drops in the evening; all taken in a little water before food for both groups. Further research showed that similar results were achieved when taking 50 drops x 3 daily which is the present dosage recommended.

The mean percentage increase of heavy metals after provocation with HMD® is compared with the elimination while using a placebo (a mild chlorella tincture).

METALS	Mean % increase after provocation (Experimental group)	Mean % increase after provocation (Placebo group)	Number in sample	t-test results	Degrees of Freedom	Sig. (p =)
ARSENIC-U	7,409.00	11.16	84	-	-	p<0.0005
ARSENIC-F	59.83	61.13	84	-	-	p<0.05
LEAD-U	466.47	-16.95	84	-	-	p<0.005
LEAD-F	142.16	-6.012	84	-	-	p<0.05
CADMIUM-U	67	-27.91	84	-	-	p<0.05
CADMIUM-F	43.13	22.62	84	-	-	p<0.05
ANTIMONY-U	59.16	14.91	84	-	-	p<0.05
ANTIMONY-F	50	6.61	84	-	-	p<0.05
NICKEL-U	80	5.52	77	t = 1.425	76	p<0.158
BISMUTH-U	564	7.95	19	t = 2.109	18	p<0.04
URANIUM-U	707	18.23	76	t = 1.015	75	p<0.03
MERCURY-U *	448	0.799	56	t = 5.395	55	p<0.0005

Table 1: HMD® data over several trials conducted over a 3-year period
* Mercury trial was conducted separately and the results of this are discussed below.

There were no serious side effects during the trials. Two people complained of a minor, transitory headache. Kidney, heart, liver and electrolyte blood tests showed that there were no pathological parameters in the post urine and faeces samples in all people tested, suggesting that HMD® is a 'gentle' chelator that does not place undue stress on the kidneys and liver.

Moreover, Heart Rate Variability Testing (HRV), a measure of the functioning of all the physiological systems of the body, showed a significant increase in 40% of the people tested, only 48 hours after provocation with the HMD®. It is predicted that HRV scores would be greatly improved if the HMD® were taken for much longer periods of time.

Independent Mercury Trial Using HMD®

Over the last year, a voluntary group of clinical patients from the Da Vinci Holistic Health Centre in Cyprus were used to test the efficacy of HMD® on mercury. All urine analyses were conducted on a mercury-dedicated PSA Atomic Fluorescence Spectrometer, measuring levels of parts per billion. This involved a total of 56 patients who participated in a 24-hour provocation trial using HMD® at dosages of 40, 50 and 60 drops throughout the day. Initial 6-hour baseline pre-urine samples were collected, along with a 24-hour collection for the post-urine sample.

There was a 448% increase in eliminated mercury in the post-test after 24-hour provocation with HMD® in the 56 people tested, as compared with the pre-test baseline sample. Moreover, there was a negligible increase in mercury in the control group that were given only powdered chlorella in a little alcohol as a placebo. There was a statistically significant difference between the percentage increase of mercury in the post-sample as compared with the controls (t = 5.395, df = 55, p<.0005).

Percentage Increase of Mercury in Pre-Post Test and Controls

Mean % Increase of Hg

Liver and kidney serum test results during the HMD® pre-post provocation trials:

During the HMD® research trials, blood samples were taken from a small group of people (N=16) to determine the effects of the HMD® provocation on liver and kidney function. The average percentage increase was calculated from the pre-and post-sample figures of these biochemical tests.

Table 2 below shows the percentage increase of these biochemical parameters in the post-serum samples when taking of HMD®, as compared with the baseline serum sample before HMD® was taken. Overall, there are small average increases in creatinine, bilirubin, urea, ALT and AST, but nothing that surpassed pathological parameters. The minimum and maximum levels are also shown, but generally the higher levels were present in one individual only.

LEVELS OF LIVER & KIDNEY FUNCTION TESTS DURING HMD® PROVOCATION					
	CREATININE	BILIRUBIN	UREA	ALT	AST
% INCREASE	11.95	3.15	25.35	16.74	5.25
MINIMUM	0	0	0	0	0
MAXIMUM	42.80	20.19	53.73	75.00	38.46
N=	16	16	16	16	16

Table 2: Details of the liver and kidney function tests

It can be concluded from these tests that HMD® is a gentle chelator that does not adversely affect liver and kidney function tests and is tolerated by most people of all ages.

However, based on clinical use of HMD® over the last 5 years, it would be advisable for the practitioner to use a universal drainage remedy that can work concomitantly on all detoxification systems including the liver, kidney, skin, lymph and blood. I have formulated such a natural herbal drainage remedy called Organic Lavage.[74]

Natural Heavy Metal Chelation Protocol
I have been working on a natural, heavy metal chelating protocol based on scientific and clinical evidence for over five years now. This is what I suggest can be used for most cases of heavy metal toxicity – I have called it the HMD ULTIMATE DETOX PROTOCOL and it consists of the following:

---

74 See http://www.worldwidehealthcenter.net/product/hmd-lavage-drainage-remedy-2oz-60ml/ for more details

❖ **HMD®** – 50 drops x 3 daily for adults[75] – sensitive adults who have chronic diseases or compensated detoxification organs, as well as people with neurological diseases such as multiple sclerosis and the like, as well as autistic people, should begin with half this dose or less, and increase by one drop x 3 daily, every day until they reach a comfortable level.

❖ **ORGANIC LAVAGE** – this is a herbal formula of wild-crafted and organic herbs such as Silybum marianum (Milk Thistle Seed), Taraxacum officinale (Dandelion Root), Arctium lappa (Burdock Root), Trifolium pratense (Red Clover Tops), Curcuma longa (Turmeric Root), Hydrangea arborescens (Hydrangea Root) and Arctostaphylos uva ursi (Bearberry Leaf). This herbal formula is designed to facilitate detoxification of the liver, kidneys, lymphatics and skin, as well as cleanse the blood and act as a natural anti-inflammatory. Adult dosage: 25 drops x 3 daily for adults, or more as directed by a practitioner.

❖ **ORGANIC CHLORELLA** – there are many concerns about finding good quality, clean Chlorella that is void of heavy metals and xenobiotics. We have searched and travelled far and wide, and found an excellent source that is provided with a Certificates of Analysis with each pot. This chlorella comes from the western coast of Hai-Nan Island, China's southernmost island. Hai-Nan Island is a tropical island with an excellent climate and lies on the same latitude as Hawaii. The non-industrialized, pollution-free, tropical island offers favorable growth conditions for chlorella, including intense sunlight, pure water, and clean air. Available in 500mg tabs, adult dosage should be 2 tabs x 3 daily.

❖ **LIPOIC ACID** – I believe that when metals and other xenobiotics are mobilized in the body, there should be some protection against free radical damage. Lipoic acid is that extraordinary antioxidant which is both water and fat soluble, able to penetrate the brain and other nervous tissues, and is therefore able to protect all parts of the body against free radical damage.

❖ **MINERALS** – flushing the body with high levels of most of the minerals and trace elements will prevent the metals from re-entering the cell, as well as providing the raw materials for enzyme systems to reactivate, including detoxification systems. The easiest way is to take a colloidal multi-mineral formula in solution. Otherwise, a good-quality, high-potency, multi-mineral capsule will suffice.

---

75 See *http://www.worldwidehealthcenter.net/hmd-dosage-guidelines/ for full details*

I will often fine-tune this protocol depending on the needs of the patient, but generally this works well for most cases as a basic protocol.

Further Research

During the 5 years of experience with HMD® we have had many reports from women of all ages who have suffered from chronic endocrine problems coming back into balance while using HMD® for 2-3 months. Many of these women suffered from irregular periods, heavy bleeding, PMS and other hormonal imbalances.

Based on this anecdotal evidence, we believe that HMD® is eliminating other chemicals (xenobiotics) such as Bisphenyl A and Phthalates which are known endocrine-disrupting chemicals, as described above.

Preliminary trials have already been done which have shown that indeed this is the case – HMD® is eliminating the xenobiotics through the urine. However, the sample of people tested is small, so further trials need to be conducted in this area before any scientific papers can be written.

Conclusion

There is an overwhelming amount of scientific evidence to support the relationship between heavy metal toxicity and chronic diseases in general.

This is why these toxic metal detoxification protocols detailed in this chapter are relevant to ALL diseases, without exception. So, these protocols need to be assimilated and practiced regularly. We are continuously accumulating toxins; it doesn't matter where we live these days, toxins are *everywhere!*

If you wish to see the progress of your own toxicity, then a good starting point is to run a Hair Mineral Analysis on yourself to determine the amount of toxic metals in circulation, and begin taking the HMD ULTIMATE DETOX PACK for 2 months, before running the hair test again.

If there is a percentage increase of toxic metals in the second test, then you will know that you have accumulated a number of toxic metals and will need to continue detoxing.

All these supplements can be obtained from www.worldwidehealthcenter.net.

Chapter 4

Food Intolerances, Inflammation and Disease

"One man's food is another man's poison" is a centuries-old saying that implies that different people can have different reactions to exactly the same food. This has been known for eons, but modern medicine is still in the dark regarding this very important cause of many health issues and symptoms. One of the greatest enigmas in modern medicine is food intolerances.

The reason that food is extremely important to health is that the body can react to certain foods in a negative way, causing the body to have an inflammatory reaction.

There are basically two levels of reactions. One is the life-threatening FOOD ALLERGIES, which can cause anaphylactic shock and difficulty breathing which requires immediate medical attention.

The other is FOOD INTOLERANCES, that still cause a reaction, but it is much slower and more prolonged. The symptoms are not so life-threatening, even though they can cause chronic diseases over time.

We will not spend much time discussing food allergies per se, as these only involve about 1% of the population. This chapter is more devoted to food *intolerances*, that involve far more people. According to research by the charity Allergy UK, up to 45% of the population suffer from food intolerances, otherwise known as *Food Hypersensitivity*.

Before we leave the topic of food allergies and concentrate on food intolerances, let's look at the difference between FOOD ALLERGIES and FOOD INTOLERANCES/HYPERSENSITIVITIES.

Food Allergies

Over 140 different foods have been identified as causes of allergic reactions. According to a recent report by the U.S. Centers for Disease Control, 90% of food allergies are associated with only 8 food types:

- ❖ Cow's milk
- ❖ Hen's eggs
- ❖ Peanuts
- ❖ Soy foods
- ❖ Wheat
- ❖ Fish
- ❖ Crustacean shellfish (such as shrimp, prawns, lobster, and crab)
- ❖ Tree nuts (such as almonds, cashews, walnuts, pecans, pistachios, Brazil nuts, hazelnuts, and chestnuts)

When people with these food allergies consumed the food, can go into anaphylaxis and can die within minutes if they ingest even one molecule of their allergic food. This is a serious issue requiring immediate medical attention.

Should such a reaction occur, taking **Sodium Cromoglycate,** a non-steroidal anti-inflammatory commonly used with asthmatic patients, or the natural bioflavonoid **Quercetin,** are both effective agents in blocking mast cell degranulation and slowing down the adverse reaction until medical help arrives. Under no circumstances, however, should you try treating such food allergic reactions at home, even if you are a practitioner. Immediate medical intervention will most likely be required.

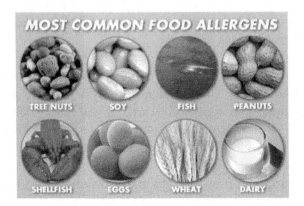

So, what actually happens in the body when we ingest a food that we are allergic to? During an allergic response, the body reacts to the allergen by producing a number of antibodies. In the case of food allergies, it is called Immunoglobulin E (IgE). This is a Type 1 allergic reaction.

Diagram 1 demonstrates how the allergen or food is detected by a white blood cell called a **B-lymphocyte cell (Plasma cell).** This plasma cell will produce an IgE antibody.

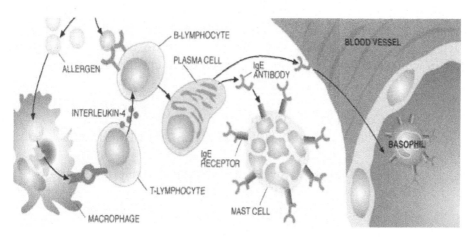

Diagram 1. Classic allergy response

This IgE antibody will then attach itself onto a **mast cell** (another type of white blood cell), which releases potent inflammatory chemicals. This action signals the mast cells and the Basophil cells to begin disintegrating, thereby releasing **histamine** and other chemicals such as proteoglycans (e.g. heparin and chondroitin), and proteolytic enzymes (e.g. elastase and lysophospholipase).

They also secrete lipid mediators like leukotrienes, and several cytokines that contribute to inflammation.

Immediate reaction to foods may involve the **skin, respiratory tract, GI mucosal and cardiovascular system.** Usually the throat or pharynx that begins to constrict and the person has difficulty breathing.

Table 2 shows a comparison between food intolerances and food allergies:

Food Intolerances
Food intolerances do not involve an immediate response. There is a delay in symptoms that can take from 45 minutes to several days for them to become apparent.

The delayed onset of symptoms and complex physiological mechanisms involved in food intolerances make them an especially difficult puzzle to try to solve either

147

on your own or with most laboratory tests. In fact, food sensitivities often go undiagnosed or misdiagnosed.

The medical name for FOOD INTOLERANCES is "Non-IgE mediated food hypersensitivity", which is sometimes loosely referred to as "food hypersensitivity". This is also known as a "Type III Allergy" and is IgG-mediated, characterised by the production of IgG antibodies and the gradual formation of antigen/antibody complexes which are deposited in tissues, which cause chronic inflammation.

Item Compared	FOOD INTOLERANCES	FOOD ALLERGIES
Body Organs Involved	Any organ system in the body can be affected	Usually limited to airways, skin, gastrointestinal tract
Rate of Response	From 45 min up to 3 days after ingestion	From seconds to 1 hour after ingestion
Severity	Not life-threatening	Can be fatal
Are symptoms acute or chronic?	Usually chronic, sometimes acute	Usually acute, rarely chronic
Percentage of Population Affected	30 - 45%	1-2%
Permanence	Can last a lifetime	Can be reversed or reduced after eliminating problem foods
Immunologic Mechanisms	White blood cells – rapid release of histamine IgG antibodies	Gradual formation of Antigen/Antibody complexes IgE antibodies

148

Non-Immunologic Mechanisms	Toxic, pharmacologic	None
How much food is needed to trigger the allergy?	From small amount to large amount; often dosage dependent	1 molecule of allergic food needed to trigger reaction
Half-life of Immunoglobulins	IgG – 21 days – 3 months	IgE – 1 – 14 days

Table 2. Food intolerances vs food allergies

The best example of food intolerance is lactose intolerance. This condition is characterized by bloating, loose stools, diarrhoea and gas. Lactose intolerance is caused by an inability of the body to produce enough of the enzyme *lactase*, which breaks down lactose, the primary sugar found in milk. Avoiding milk products or supplementing the diet with lactase enzyme is the best way for a person with lactose intolerance to overcome the problem.

Signs and Symptoms

Food intolerance is more chronic, less obvious in its presentation, and often more difficult to diagnose than a food allergy. Symptoms of food intolerance vary greatly, and can be mistaken for the symptoms of a food allergy. While true food allergies are associated with fast-acting immunoglobulin IgE responses, it can be difficult to determine the offending food causing a food intolerance because the response generally takes place over a prolonged period of time.

Food intolerance symptoms usually begin about half an hour after eating or drinking the food in question, but sometimes symptoms may be delayed by up to 48 hours. Diagram 2 shows some of the symptoms that are commonly encountered in cases of food intolerances.

The most common symptoms include: irritable bowel (Jones, VA, 1982; Nanda, R et al, 1983), headaches, migraines, fatigue, behavioural problems (Pelsser, LMJ et al, 2008; McCann D et al, 2007; Bateman, B et al 2004; Breakey, J. 1997; Swain, A et al, 1985) or urticaria (Di Lorenzo, G et al, 2005). Asthma symptoms can also be triggered in some patients and, occasionally, anaphylactoid reactions occur.

149

Withdrawal, super-sensitivity, tachyphylaxis and tolerance are often observed (Loblay, RJ, 1982). Food chemicals implicated include artificial food colours, preservatives, flavour enhancers, glutamates, vasoactive amines and salicylates (Loblay, RH, 1986; David, TJ, 2000; Perry, CA et al, 1996). It is common for patients with food intolerance to react to several chemicals – all of which can be found in a wide range of foods. A family history of symptoms and specific chemical intolerances is common (Loblay, RH et al, 1986).

Food intolerances can present with symptoms affecting the skin, respiratory tract, and gastrointestinal tract (GIT), either individually or in combination. Skin problems may include rashes, urticaria, angioedema, dermatitis and eczema.

Respiratory tract symptoms can include nasal congestion, sinusitis, pharyngeal irritations, asthma and an unproductive cough. GIT symptoms include mouth ulcers, abdominal cramp, nausea, gas, intermittent diarrhoea, constipation, irritable bowel syndrome and anaphylaxis.

Food intolerance has been found to be associated with Irritable Bowel Syndrome and inflammatory bowel diseases such as Crohn's disease.

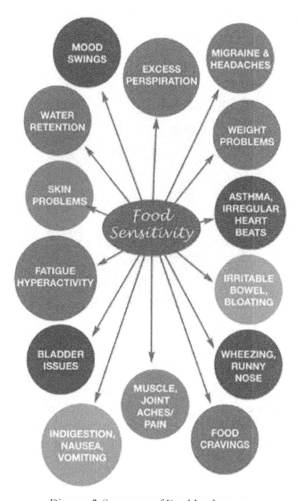

Diagram 2. Symptoms of Food Intolerances

Other general symptoms include chronic constipation, chronic hepatitis C infection, eczema, NSAID intolerance, respiratory complaints, asthma, rhinitis, headaches, functional dyspepsia, eosinophilic esophagitis and ENT illnesses, as well as a myriad of other symptoms. This is why it is very difficult to find a correlation between these symptoms and foods that we eat.

Apart from these symptoms, food intolerances may also cause commonly encountered symptoms that most people feel are "normal," given that so many people have them. These include symptoms such as fatigue, gas, bloating, mood swings, nervousness, migraines and eating disorders.

151

Clinical research is accumulating evidence that food intolerances can also increase the severity of the symptoms of rheumatoid arthritis, asthma and other diseases normally not considered food related.

Mechanisms of Food Intolerances

The mechanism of food intolerance involves the production of antigen/antibody complexes which are deposited in the tissues, triggering the release of inflammatory chemicals causing damage and inflammation in that particular tissue. This could be in any part of the body, for example, the gut, causing IBS symptoms or Crohn's; in the joints, producing symptoms of arthritis; in the head producing migraines and so forth.

The sequence of events is as follows (diagram 2 shows this diagrammatically):

- ❖ Partially digested foods pass between gut cells into the blood.
- ❖ These proteins are recognised as 'foreign' and food specific IgG are produced in response.
- ❖ Antigen/antibody complexes form between the partially digested foods and the IgG antibodies. The symptoms of food intolerance tend to be delayed because this formation of complexes is a gradual process – it does not happen immediately.
- ❖ The complexes are deposited in tissues (could be anywhere in body such as gut, head, skin etc.).
- ❖ Complement is activated which causes respiratory burst in neutrophils, release of proteolytic enzymes, mast cell mediators and vasoactive peptides, and aggregation of platelets.

❖ Complement and macrophages stimulate inflammation, although complement helps to prevent smaller complexes going on to form larger complexes.

❖ C2 and C5 (part of the enzyme cascade) can release histamine too.

❖ Macrophages release inflammatory mediators such as interleukin-1, tumour necrosis factor, reactive oxygen species and nitric oxide (N.B. The complement system is an enzyme cascade that helps defend against infection).

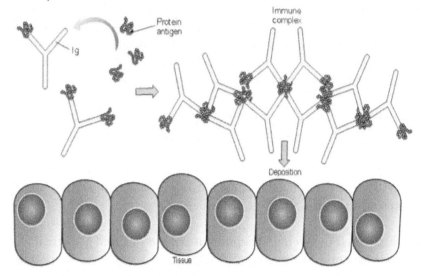

Diagram 2. showing IgG Response

Tests for Determining Food Intolerances

In clinical practice, I use Bioresonance testing to determine what foods the patient may be intolerant to. I have been doing this for over 20 years now; it is possible to test for over 100 foods in less than 15 minutes, and the accuracy is around 85% which is akin to the IgG tests already discussed. It is a quick, easy, efficient and cost effective way of testing for this critical health parameter that is important to identify and eradicate.

I have always said to my friends that if I were ever stranded on a remote island somewhere in the Pacific and had to work as a therapist, the only piece of equipment I would take with me would be my Bioresonance device and some testing ampoules. I personally use the German VEGA Bioresonance device, as well as the Russian Deta Elis PROFESSIONAL. This has its roots in the work of Dr. Reinhold Voll, MD, who ingeniously merged and transformed traditional Chinese acupuncture into a modern form of electromedicine called EAV (Volls' so-called Electro Acupuncture).

153

In the early 1950s, Reinhold Voll (76), a German medical doctor, developed an electronic testing device for finding acupuncture points electrically. He was successful in demonstrating that specific acupuncture points, known to Chinese acupuncturists for millennia, had a different resistance to a tiny electrical current passing through the body, compared to the adjacent tissues (77). Many other researchers have also verified that electrical conductance at the acupuncture points is significantly greater than the surrounding tissue.

Voll then began a lifelong search to identify correlations between disease states and changes in the electrical resistance of the various acupuncture points. He thought that if he could identify electrical changes in certain acupuncture points associated with certain diseases, then he might be able to identify those diseases more easily, or earlier, when treatment intervention was likely to be more effective.

Voll was successful in identifying many acupuncture points related to specific conditions and published a great deal of information about using acupuncture points diagnostically (78). He found, for example, that patients with lung cancer had abnormal readings on the acupuncture points referred to as 'lung points'. Changes also occurred in the electrical conductance of the acupuncture points supplying musculoskeletal structures that were inflamed.

Voll also discovered that certain acupuncture points showed abnormal readings when subjects were reacting allergically (79). He made several serendipitous discoveries related to "allergy" testing. He noted some unusual readings on certain acupuncture points when a patient had a bottle of medicine in his pocket. He could remove the bottle and consistently get different readings when the bottle was in his pocket compared to when it was not.

At first, he was baffled as to how a closed bottle of medicine outside the body could affect the acupuncture readings. It was even more baffling when he discovered that the glass bottle of medicine could change the readings when it was in contact anywhere along the closed electric circuit involved with the testing procedure (80).

---

76 Voll, R. 1980. The phenomenon of medicine testing in electro-acupuncture according to Voll. American Journal of Acupuncture 8:97-104.

77 Voll R.: Topographic Positions of the Measurement Points in Electroacupuncture. (Illustrated Vol. I). Med. Liter. Verlagsgesellschaft, Uelzen, 1977.

78 Voll, R: Twenty Years of Electroacupuncture Therapy Using Low Frequency Current Pulses. *Amer. J. Acupuncture*, 3(4): 291-314, 1975.

79 http://www.youtube.com/watch?v=Jltzy072hxY

80 Kenyon JN. 21st century medicine: a layman's guide to the medicine of the future. Wellingborough, Northants: Thorsons, 1986.

Personally, I have spent more than 20 years working with the VEGA (81) machine and I can say that I truly resonate with it. The analogy that I give to illustrate this is that the VEGA is akin to a musical instrument. We often see a maestro playing a guitar so beautifully that we are in awe - how beautiful those notes seem to flow and with such ease the maestro plays. Of course, if we take the same instrument that the maestro is playing in to our own hands, without devoting a lot of time and arduous effort in really learning to play it, then our attempts to perform like the maestro will be in vain.

This is really what happens with the VEGA machine, or any other Bioresonance testing device using VRT testing. In the wrong hands it can make more wrong predictions than pure guesswork – in the maestro's hands it can be as accurate as any medical scanning device at determining anything that you ask of it. It will accurately determine what food intolerances a person has; as well as whether they have viruses or residual particles of viruses in their tissues that may have been left from an old infection or vaccination.

It can identify bacteria, parasites, fungi and moulds and tell what drugs or remedies a person is adversely reacting to. It can also identify organ weaknesses and prioritise them; it can identify whether the person has electromagnetic stress, X-ray stress, mobile phone stress, geopathic stress and the like; as well as being able to identify the specific potency of any remedy that a person needs to take.

All these tests can be done quickly and in less than an hour. It is not difficult to scan all the organs of the body; test for food intolerances (82); identify the weak organs; identify the specific potency required to make a homeopathic sarcode in order to strengthen a weak organ; as well as scan for vaccination stress, viruses, bacteria, fungi, Candida and parasites.

The Bioresonance device helps the practitioner to take the guesswork out of working out the pathogenesis of disease, as well as guessing which dosage or homeopathic potency the patient is resonating with. It is my belief that when there is a paradigm shift in thinking from mechanistic to *holistic*, then most health practitioners of all disciplines will be proud owners of a Bioresonance testing device.

In the early days when I began using the VEGA, I was astounded by its accuracy as I was testing the organ systems of an athlete who wanted to optimize his health and sports performance. I really did not find much as this athlete was fairly healthy and was on an optimal diet and supplement programme. But one thing that came up on

81 Fehrenbach J, Noll H, Nolte HG, et al. Short manual of the Vegatest-method. Schiltach: BER, 1986.
82 Krop J, Swiertzek J, Wood A. Comparison of ecological testing with the Vega test method in identifying sensitivities to chemicals, foods and inhalants. *Am J Acupuncture* 13 253-259, 1985.

the VEGA was the reproductive system – it was showing weaknesses in the testes, epididymis and prostate.

It turned out that he was indeed sterile but did not mention this in his history as he was ashamed and embarrassed; this was a real blow to his vision of having a family with his wife. Further testing showed that he was afflicted with systemic Candidiasis and certain protozoa, along with vaccination stress. When these issues had been addressed with a 90-day protocol, his wife became pregnant a couple of months later. This was a professional athlete who had consulted at least 5 doctors about his sterility problem, but no amount of medical testing could determine what the VEGA had helped me to diagnose in less than 30 minutes.

I also use other Bioresonance testing devices which I have found to be just as good, but more cost effective as they have over 20,000 digitized ampoules already programmed into the device. One such device is called the DETA PROFESSIONAL from the Russian company Deta Elis. This has the capabilities of treating using Bioresonance and other treatment modalities – see www.deta-elis-uk.com.

The Link with Chronic Disease

Food intolerance (as defined by elevated levels of IgG food antibodies), is being increasingly associated with the low-grade inflammation which characterises most chronic conditions such as Crohn's, Irritable Bowel Syndrome, atopic allergies, obesity and arthritis.

Research supports this with studies showing how testing for IgG antibodies has helped in improving conditions like obesity, migraines, arthritis and IBS.

The mechanisms behind this link are thought to include the following:

1. Formation of antigen/antibody immune complexes. The immune system may occasionally react to substances, including foods that adversely affect it. Under normal conditions, the formation of antigen/antibody complexes are dealt with and eliminated by the immune system.

However, if the immune system is overwhelmed or over-worked, then these complexes can accumulate in places such as joints or the digestive tract resulting in the production of inflammatory cytokines, which lead to the manifestation of symptoms of food intolerance.

2. Increased intestinal permeability. This is linked to the promotion of low grade inflammation as a result of lipolysaccharides moving across the

disturbed gut mucosa. Disturbance of the tight junction proteins which maintain the gut membrane also allows the migration of large peptides into the circulation which would otherwise be blocked.

These peptides can induce an adverse immune response. Studies have found increased intestinal permeability in patients with food intolerances (Dupont et al 1989, Schrander et al 1990).

The "Leaky Gut"

One major theory as to how delayed food sensitivities develop revolves around the concept of a "leaky gut."

Ordinarily, the digestive tract will efficiently break down and absorb consumed food as small molecules, amino acids, simple carbohydrates, etc., which are, in general, non-antigenic.

The efficiency of the digestive system today with all the additional stressors that it has to deal with results in digestion becoming less efficient and the intestinal lining becoming more permeable to large molecules. It is assumed that this "leaky gut" condition allows macro-molecular food fragments into the circulation, where they can stimulate a typical immune response where IgG is the primary antibody produced to defend the body against perceived non-self-invaders.

Inadequate digestion of food products due to hypochlorhydria (insufficient secretion of hydrochloric acid by the stomach) and pancreatic enzyme deficiency is also thought to be a significant cause of food allergies.

Insufficient brush border enzymes such as lactase and sucrase also affect the body's ability to breakdown food to an elemental form.

When proteins are not digested to amino acids, dipeptides, or short chain polypeptides, they retain their antigenic properties. These antigenic molecules may then be absorbed through a damaged mucosal barrier or "leaky gut" and become exposed to the immune system.

This in turn can create a state of chronic immune hypersensitivity and inflammation.

In general, foods with a higher protein content (>20%) are more likely to be allergenic.

The following factors can all put stress on a person's health and can lead to increased gut permeability or leaky gut:

157

❖ **Low levels of secretory IgA**. Secretory IgA is an immune marker and is the first line of defence in the gut against bacteria, food residue, fungus, parasites and viruses (Walker & Bloch 1983).

❖ **Stress** can deplete the body of secretory IgA and hence reduce the body's defence system against foreign bodies. Also, stress depletes the gut of good bacteria, and therefore allows an overgrowth of bad bacteria and yeast such as Candida.

❖ **Imbalanced gut flora**. An overgrowth of bad gut bacteria (dysbiosis) can exacerbate intestinal permeability through inhibition of genes which regulate tight junction proteins protecting the gut mucosal barrier (Kennedy et al 2002).

❖ **Mucosal injury** due to infection or certain medical drugs. Non-steroidal anti-Inflammatory Drugs (NSAIDS) e.g. Aspirin, damage the intestinal wall causing inflammation resulting with an increase in permeability (Bjarnson et al 1987).

❖ **Parasites** also damage the intestinal wall causing inflammation, eventually resulting in an increase in permeability.

❖ **Low stomach acid** can arise due to lack of digestive enzymes caused by nutritional deficiencies or as a result of H. Pylori infection. Low stomach acid results in incomplete breakdown of protein leading to large peptides in the small intestine which can potentially cross the gut wall if there is increased intestinal permeability, pass into the bloodstream, stimulate antibody response and cause further inflammation (Gardner ML 1984).

❖ **Low pancreatic enzymes**. When the intestinal lining is damaged, the microvilli are also damaged thus reducing absorption of nutrients vital for the manufacture of digestive enzymes. Consequently, foods are not fully digested, pass into blood stream and stimulate antibody response.

❖ **Poor nutrient status**. Damage to the intestinal lining reduces nutrient absorption with the consequence of impaired gut repair, and therefore further impaired digestion and absorption.

❖ **A high fat diet** has been closely linked with increased intestinal permeability and the formation of chylomicrons, which transport inflammatory lipopolysaccharides across the gut wall and into the circulation. This results in systemic inflammation in tissues. It is possible they also promote intestinal absorption and systemic dissemination of dietary antigens (Wang et al 2010).

Leaky gut can be healed by taking supplements such as L-GLUTAMINE and BUTYRIC ACID to heal the mucosa of the gut, along with VITAMIN D3.

Have GMOs Contributed to the Rise in Allergies?

There is some discussion about the role that genetically modified (GM or GMO) food might play in the escalating incidence of food allergy, food intolerance, and digestive illnesses. Genetically modified food is the result of scientists inserting DNA from another species into the plant - typically corn, soybeans, canola, cotton (the source of cottonseed oil), and sugar beets - to make the plant resistant to insect damage, viral infections, and certain herbicides.

The FDA says that the GMO foods that have been evaluated through its voluntary consultation process are not more likely to cause an allergic or toxic reaction than foods from traditionally bred plants. When new genetic traits are introduced into plants, the developer evaluates whether any new material could be allergenic or toxic.

Yet some consumer groups are questioning whether there's a link between the dramatic rise in allergies in the past two decades and the introduction of GMO soybeans into the U.S. food supply in 1996.

GMO soy is now ubiquitous in many processed foods. While the timing does not prove any causal link between GMO food and allergies, these groups say it merits research. However, there is currently a lack of long-term independent scientific studies published in peer-reviewed journals that examine how ingesting GMO foods affects humans.

How Do These Foods Damage My Body?

It has been reported that while individuals may sometimes have adverse reactions to particular foods, these reactions are not always consistent. This is because the response to food involves not only the immune system or a sensitivity to some of the molecules in foods, but is also the health of the entire digestive tract and whether it is providing a good barrier for your body.

Therefore, when the health of your digestive system is compromised you may have a sensitivity to foods which otherwise would not affect you adversely, like in times of extreme stress. Thus, it is very important when dealing with any inflammatory disease of the bowel to make certain that all stressors that may be playing a role are eradicated concomitantly within a holistic model. This is the only way of succeeding.

The role of your gastrointestinal tract, which includes your oesophageal area, stomach, and your upper and lower intestinal tracts, is to take in the food you eat, break it down to molecule-size pieces, and allow it to be absorbed into your body in a controlled way.

Your gastrointestinal tract provides a protective barrier between the food you eat and the inside of your body. When it is healthy and functioning efficiently, it lets in specific food molecules in specific places at specific times. Many things can affect this barrier and, when it is compromised in any way, it can let in food molecules that are not properly digested. This can cause a reaction to a certain food, not because you are sensitive to it, but because it is in the wrong place at the wrong time.

Food Sensitivities, Oesophageal Reflux and Your Stomach

The beginning of food digestion occurs in the stomach at the upper end of the gastrointestinal (GI) tract. The stomach has a protective mucosal layer called the stomach lining which protects it from the strong acid that is produced by specialized stomach cells called parietal cells. The acid in the stomach is a vital component in breaking down food particles.

As already mentioned, the stomach lining contains specialized cells for producing hydrochloric acid called PARIETAL CELLS (Diagram 4) along with CHIEF CELLS that produce Pepsinogen. The pepsinogen is activated once it reaches the stomach, so it doesn't harm the cells that produce it.

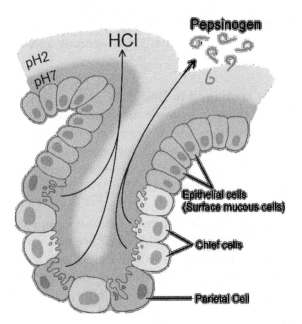

Diagram 4: Parietal and Chief Cells of Stomach

An allergic response in the stomach can produce inflammation in the stomach wall. This can cause lesions or sores as well as potentially destroy the parietal cells. The reduced number of parietal cells results in less acid production, ultimately inhibiting the proper breakdown of food in the stomach.

160

When food is improperly broken down in the stomach, large undigested particles are transported to the intestines where they cause additional inflammation and allergic responses as well as increasing the severity of symptoms that are already being experienced.

Along with toxic foods, alcohol consumption and non-steroidal anti-inflammatories (NSAIDs) can also destroy the stomach lining causing stomach inflammation and inadequate digestion of food. Medications that decrease stomach acid production also decrease the ability to digest food properly.

One specific type of food allergy in the stomach is called, allergic eosinophilic gastroenteritis. This condition is characterized by symptoms of acid reflux, severe abdominal pain after eating, vomiting, and diarrhoea. With allergic eosinophilic gastroenteritis, the oesophageal area, stomach and upper intestinal tract can become inflamed, compromising proper function.

Oftentimes, people who have serious acid reflux problems that are not responsive to medications have this condition. Although this condition is caused by an allergic reaction to food, food allergy tests reveal positive results in only about half of all cases. If left untreated, the inflammation in the stomach can result in ulceration and degeneration of the stomach lining, leading to additional problems.

Gentle foods that can support healing of an inflamed stomach include:
* ❖ Rice
* ❖ Lamb
* ❖ Vegetables such as cabbage in juices

These foods can be used with an Allergy Avoidance Diet to support healing of the stomach. Also, avoiding alcohol and the most commonly allergenic foods would also prove to be beneficial. These foods are:

* ❖ Cow's Milk
* ❖ Tomato
* ❖ Wheat
* ❖ Chocolate
* ❖ Peanuts
* ❖ Shellfish

Food Sensitivities and Systemic Responses

The travel of toxic food particles via the bloodstream to other parts of the body can account for a rash on your arms or legs as a result of an allergic response. Many scientists and clinicians have looked at the role of food allergy in a number of systemic (whole body) diseases and conditions.

Most notably, conditions associated with inflammation, such as red, inflamed patches of skin called dermatitis, asthma and joint pain all have been related to toxic food responses. Several studies have been published on the beneficial effects of using allergy-avoidance (elimination) diets to help decrease the symptoms of rheumatoid arthritis. It has also been observed that the symptoms of asthma become worse in some individuals after consuming certain foods.

Avoidance of these foods has helped decrease the number and severity of symptoms in these individuals.

Food Sensitivities and Processed Foods

Reports suggest the incidence of conditions such as asthma, allergic rhinitis, and atopic dermatitis has increased during the past decade. While the increase in damaging pollutants - particularly in large cities - is most often attributed for this increase, many scientists believe the consumption of processed foods and the increased level of stress in our daily lives are also major contributors to the rise in the frequency of these conditions.

As mentioned above, processed foods contain higher levels of additives such as preservatives (benzoate-containing substances like sodium benzoate, sulphites, hydroxytoluene-containing substances like BHT), flavouring agents (salicylates), and dyes. Processed, non-organically grown foods may also contain pesticides which can also promote toxic responses in the body. Candies like chocolates, also contain many colourings, additives and preservatives as well as simple sugars.

Processed foods can also contain small amounts of residue of foods that are not listed on the label. Most manufacturing plants produce several types of food products and although regulations exist to assure these companies manufacture products under clean conditions, they do not require sterile conditions that would prevent any cross-contamination from the production of other food products.

For example, a manufacturer may use the same equipment to produce wheat and non-wheat bread. It is possible that a small amount of wheat residue could inadvertently end up in a non-wheat product. However, these residues would not be listed as an ingredient on its label.

This is of concern with peanut residue which can cause a severe allergic reaction from amounts so small that they are undetectable by all tests used to determine the cleanliness of equipment. Government agencies are responding by requiring manufacturers that use the same equipment to produce peanut products and non-peanut products to label their non-peanut products as 'possibly containing peanut residue'.

Processed foods also add colours and flavourings which raise additional concerns. Colours, and particularly flavourings, are usually produced with "carrier" ingredients. In the past, manufacturers have been required to only list the main ingredients in the products, so carrier ingredients were not included on this list.

This practice has recently come under scrutiny by the FDA and other food industry organizations as reports of food intolerance or allergic reactions from allergens that were present in foods but were not listed on the labels continue to grow. The FDA is starting to require labels that list all ingredients, including carrier ingredients. However, it may be many years before all the processed food on our grocery shelves will have all the ingredients clearly labelled.

Whole, organically grown foods do not contain colourings, flavourings, preservatives or other hidden ingredients which may cause food sensitive reactions. This is a particularly important consideration for individuals with any type of food sensitivity.

Why Do I Crave Foods to Which I am Sensitive?
It is not clear why we often crave foods to which we are sensitive, but several theories have been proposed to help explain why this may occur.

Some researchers suggest that our bodies can become addicted to the chemical messengers, such as histamine or cortisol, which are secreted by immune cells in response to allergens in the body. It is hypothesized that while eating foods to which you are allergic can cause a rash or sneezing, the body also may experience a soothing response from the presence of the chemical messengers, increasing the desire to eat more of that food.

Another theory proposed by a well-known immunologist is based on the science of how antibodies and antigens connect (bind) to each other. Antibodies can bind to more than one site on an allergen in the food. Therefore, when there is very little antigen but many antibodies present, the antibodies will become cross-linked and make large complexes.

It is theorized that these large complexes can cause an increase in symptoms. In this theory, symptoms are related to the number of antibodies in relation to antigens, rather than being caused by the number of antigens themselves. In fact, it is suggested that if you eat more of the antigen, you can decrease the number of antibody complexes by allowing each antibody to bind to an antigen rather than forming the large complexes, thereby *reducing* the number of symptoms.

Normal metabolism works to remove the food antigens and as the ratio of antibodies to antigens begins to rise, symptoms will begin to increase. Cravings and addiction to food may be the result of the body's attempt to increase the number of antigens present in order to prevent the formation of the large antibody complexes that are associated with an increased number of symptoms (Diagram 5).

The Cycle of Addiction

Diagram 5. Antigen excess and antibody excess Marinkovich model

Succumbing to food cravings to help alleviate symptoms is the beginning of a cycle of short term relief from symptoms, then craving the food as symptoms increase again. This yo-yo effect is believed by some allergy specialists to be the reason why people who stop eating the foods to which they are allergic (go on elimination or avoidance diets) first go through several days when they feel worse before they start feeling much better.

An allergy avoidance diet (also called the Elimination Diet) is instrumental in avoiding allergic reactions to food and is the way to break the cycle of addiction. An allergy avoidance diet allows the body to completely remove the antigen, providing no reason for the formation of antibodies which will then also disappear. Clinicians suggest that this is the reason why some people can actually go back to eating a food to which they were once allergic after a year or two of avoiding the food.

In my clinical experience, however, having tested many thousands of patients over the years for food intolerances, I have found that patients who have food intolerances will always have them, unless they are treated using Bioresonance therapy. It appears that there is an *immune memory* that never forgets the food molecules that it reacts to, however many years go by.

Occasionally, a person will experience more symptoms for the first several days to a week when beginning an allergy avoidance diet. While some clinicians believe this is caused by the cross-linking of antibodies as explained in the model above, others believe it is because the body is starting to mobilize toxins that have been stored in fat tissue and other storage sites in the body. Whatever the reason, it is important to remain on the allergy avoidance diet, even though symptoms may appear to be worsening. After staying on the diet for several weeks, you should begin to feel relief from symptoms and generally feel much better.

Other Treatments of Food Intolerances
Perhaps one of the simplest and most effective ways of actually treating food intolerances (not allergies) is to use Bioresonance therapy. At the Da Vinci Holistic Health Center (www.naturaltherapycenter.com) where I work, we use the BICOM device for treating food intolerances.

It generally requires 3 treatments per food group. It is a fairly simple procedure where the patient lies on a couch and holds an electrode in each hand. The foods being tested are placed into the INPUT pot of the device.

The patient's body signals are conducted from the right hand into the input of the device using a BICOM electrode. In the BICOM device the disharmonious frequencies are filtered out and inverted. These inverted therapeutic oscillations are now given back to the patient via the left hand using another electrode.

BRT has been tested and approved throughout Europe and Canada, and it is in use in 85 countries worldwide. In Germany, where it was developed by Regumed, BRT has been in use for over 25 years.

Developing a Healthy Diet

1. *Avoid foods which you are intolerant and/or allergic to.* First and foremost, you must know your own body and what foods are toxic to you. Food sensitivities are very individual. You can be sensitive to a food that no one else in your family or groups of friends finds problematic. It's part of why we are all individuals, and you should determine for yourself what foods may be causing damage to your body. Many healthcare practitioners are knowledgeable about food sensitivities and, especially if you are experiencing significant symptoms, you should consider talking with your healthcare practitioner about your diet and suspected food sensitivities.

2. *Eat organically-grown foods whenever possible.* Especially if you suspect food sensitivities, you should avoid foods with pesticides, artificial colourings and preservatives. These synthetic food additives can cause food sensitivities and may intensify other symptoms you are experiencing. Avoiding these artificial additives is essential in determining the foods to which you are sensitive and in developing a diet that promotes your optimal health.

3. *Support healthy digestion.* One way you can support healthy digestion is to ensure you have adequate amounts of digestive factors. After chewing, the food's next stop is the stomach, where an adequate amount of stomach acid (hydrochloric acid) is the next necessity. Stomach acid is required for adequate breakdown of proteins, and without proper breakdown, all proteins are potential antigens and toxic food molecules.

Low stomach acid (hypochlorhydria) is common, especially in older people since as we age, we make less stomach acid. Research suggests that as many as half of people over 60 years old have hypochlorhydria. A variety of factors can inhibit sufficient stomach acid production, including the pathogenic bacteria, *Helicobacter pylori*, and frequent use of antacids.

Hypochlorhydria is also associated with many diseases, such as asthma, celiac disease, hepatitis, rheumatoid arthritis, osteoporosis, and diabetes mellitus. Signs of hypochlorhydria include a sense of fullness after eating, bloating, excessive belching, indigestion, multiple food allergies, undigested food in the stool, and peeling and cracked fingernails.

In addition to hydrochloric acid, the production of pancreatic enzymes and bicarbonate is also compromised in some people. If necessary, these digestive factors can be replaced with appropriate supplementation.

Digestive enzyme support can also be obtained from fresh pineapple or papaya, both of which contain the enzyme bromelain, as well as other fresh vegetables and herbs. Processed foods like canned pineapple contain little enzyme activity since digestive enzymes are proteins, which are destroyed by heating which occurs in the sterilization process.

4. *Support the gastrointestinal barrier.* The gastrointestinal cell wall is the barrier between potentially toxic food molecules and the inside of your body. Therefore, the integrity of this barrier is vital to your health. Support for the mucus that covers the cells in the gastrointestinal tract is very important, especially in the stomach.

The mucus layer is one way the stomach and upper small intestine protect themselves against the damaging effects of stomach acid. Alcohol, over-the-counter anti-inflammatory drugs called NSAIDS (e.g., aspirin), and the pathogenic bacteria, *Helicobacter pylori* can all reduce the mucous layer, leading to lesions in the stomach and small intestinal tract walls.

Choline provides nutritional support for a healthy mucous layer and is found in vegetables such as cauliflower and lettuce. Choline can be obtained from lecithin (phosphatidylcholine) as well, which is high in eggs and soybeans. Some foods also help combat or protect against the damage of *Helicobacter pylori*; these include catechins found in green tea, some spices such as cinnamon, carotenoids found in vegetables, and vitamin C, found in many fruits and vegetables.

Given that many food intolerances are acquired, the best advice to anyone is to ROTATE foods and never eat foods continuously, day-in, day-out. This is most certainly the best way to acquire food intolerances. It is very important that we DO NOT eat the same foods every day, even though our fast pace of life often entraps us into modes of convenience that are often difficult to break.

167

References

Ahmed T, Fuchs GJ. Gastrointestinal allergy to food: A review. *J Diarrhoeal Dis Res.* 1997;15(4):211-223.

Amre DK, D'Souza S, Morgan K, Seidman G, Lambrette P, Grimard G, Israel D, Mack D, Ghadirian P, Deslandres C, Chotard V, Budai B, Law L, Levy E, Seidman EG: Imbalances in dietary consumption of fatty acids, vegetables, and fruits are associated with risk for Crohn's disease in children. Am J Gastroenterol 2007; 102: 2016–2025.

Andre F, Andre C, Feknous M, Colin L, Cavagna S. Digestive permeability to different-sized molecules and to sodium cromoglycate in food allergy. *Allergy Proc.* 1991;12(5):293-298.

Bateman B, Warner JO, Hutchinson E, et al. The effects of a double-blind, placebo controlled artificial food colourings and benzoate preservative challenge on hyperactivity in a general population sample of preschool children. Arch Dis Child 2004; 89:506–11.

Breakey J. The role of diet and behaviour in childhood. J Paediatr Child Health1997; 33:190–4.

Cooney R, Jewell D: The genetic basis of inflammatory bowel disease. Dig Dis 2009; 27: 428–442.

David TJ. Adverse reactions and intolerance to foods. Br Med Bull 2000; 56:34–50.

Di Lorenzo G, Pacor ML, Mansueto P, et al. Food-additive-induced urticaria: A survey of 838 patients with recurrent chronic idiopathic urticaria. Int Arch Allergy Immunol 2005; 138:235–42.

Dominus S. *The Allergy Prison.* New York Times. June 10, 2001.

Edwards CRW. Lessons from licorice. N Engl J Med 1991, 325: 1242-3

Farrell RJ, Kelly CP. Celiac Sprue.*N Eng J Med.* 2002;346(3):180-188.

Fuglsang G, Madsen C, Halken S, et al. Adverse reactions to food additives in children with atopic symptoms. Allergy 1994; 49:31–7.

Gitzelman R, Steinmann B, Van den Berghe G Disorders of fructose metabolism. In: Scnver CR, Beaudet AL, Sly WS, Valle D (Eds) The Metabolic and Molecular Bases of Inherited Disease, 7th edtn New York: McGraw-Hill, 1995; 905-34

Hafstrom I, Ringertz B, Spangberg A, et al. A vegan diet free of gluten improves signs and symptoms of rheumatoid arthritis: the effects of arthritis correlate with a reduction in antibodies to food antigens. *Rheumatology.* 2001; 40:1175-1179.

Halmos, EP, Power VA, Shepherd SJ, et al. A Diet Low in FODMAPs Reduces Symptoms of Irritable Bowel Syndrome. Gastroenterology 2014; 146(1)67-75

Helm RM, Burks AW. Mechanisms of food allergy. *Current Opin Immunol.* 2000; 12:647-653.

Henderson WK, Raskin NH. 'Hog-dog' headache: individual susceptibility to nitnte. Lancet 972; u. 1162-3

Johnson JD, Kretchmer N, Simoons FJ Lactose malabsorpnon. its biology and history. Adv Pedtatr 1974; 21: 197-237

Jones VA, McLaughlan P, Shorthouse, Workman E, Hunter JO. Food intolerance: A major factor in the pathogenesis of irritable bowel syndrome. Lancet 1982; 8308:1115–7.

Kweon M-N, Takahashi I, Kiyono H. New insights into mechanism of inflammatory and allergic diseases in mucosal tissues. *Digestion.* 2001;63 (Suppl 1):1-11.

Lebenthal E, Rossi TM. Lactose malabsorpnon and intolerance. In Lebenthal E (Ed) Textbook of Gastroenterology and Nutrition in Infancy New York Raven, 1981; 673-88

Lichtenstein LM. Allergy and the immune system. *Sci Am.* 1993;269(3):117-124.
Loblay RH, Swain AR. Food intolerance. Rec Adv Clin Nutr 1986; 2:169–77.

Malone MH, Metcalfe DD. Histamine in foods: its possible role in non-allergic adverse reactions to ingestants. N E R Allergy Proc 1986; 7: 241-5

McCann D, Barrett A, Cooper A, et al. Food additives and hyperactive behaviour in 3-year-old and 8/9-year-old children in the community: A randomized, double-blinded, placebo-controlled trial. Lancet 2007; 370:1560–7.

Moneret-Vautrin DA, Einhorn C, Tisserand J. Le role du nitnte de sodium dans les urticaires histaminiques d'ongine ahmentaire. Ann Nutr Alim 1980; 34: 1125-32

Nanda R, James R, Smith H, et al. Food intolerance and irritable bowel syndrome. Gut 1983; 30:1099–104.

Nossal GJV. Life, death and the immune system. *Sci Am.* 1993;269(3):53-62.

Nsouli TM, Nsouli SM, Linde RE, O'Mara F, Scanlon RT, Bellanti JA. Role of food allergy in serous otitis media. *Annals Allergy.* 1994; 73:215-219.

Ong DK, Mitchell SB, Barrett JS, Shepherd SJ, Irving PI, Biesiekierski JR, Smith S, Gibson PR, Muir JG. Manipulation of dietary short chain carbohydrates alters the pattern of hydrogen and methane gas production and genesis of symptoms in patients with irritable bowel syndrome. J Gastroenterol. Hepatol. 2010 Aug ;25(8):1366-73

Paul G, Khare V, Gasche C: Inflamed gut mucosa: downstream of interleukin-10. Eur J Clin Invest 2012; 42: 95–109.

Pelsser LMJ, Frankena K, Toorman J, et al. A randomized controlled trial into the effects of food and ADHD. Eur Child Adolesc Psychiatry 2008; DOI 10.1007/s00787–008–0695–7.

Perry CA, Dwyer BA, Gelfand JA, et al. Health effects of salicylates in foods and drugs. Nutr Rev 1996; 54:225–40.

Perry CA, Dwyer J, Gelfand JA, Couris RR, McCloskey WW. Health effects of salicylates in foods adnd drugs. *Nutr Rev.* 1996;54(8):225-240.

Prenner BM, Stevens JJ. Anaphylaxis after ingestion of sodium bisulfite. Case report. Ann Allergy 1976; 37:180–2.

Sakamoto N, Kono S, Wakai K, Fukuda Y, Satomi M, Shimoyama T, Inaba Y, Miyake Y, Sasaki S, Okamoto K, Kobashi G, Washio M, Yokoyama T, Date C, Tanaka H: Dietary risk factors for inflammatory bowel disease: a multicenter case-control study in Japan. Inflamm Bowel Dis 2005; 11: 154–163.

Samartin S, Marcos A, Chandra RK. Food hypersensitivity. *Nutr Res.* 2001; 21:473-497.

Sampson HA. Food anaphylaxis. *Br Med Bull.* 2000;56(4):925-935.
Sampson HA. Food hypersensitivity: Manifestations, diagnosis, and natural history. *Food Tech.* 1992; May:141-144.

169

Sensenig J, Marrongelle J, Johnson M, Staverosky T. Treatment of migraine with targeted nutrition focused on improved assimilation and elimination. *Alt Med Rev.* 2001;6(5):488-494.

Shepherd SJ, Parker FJ, Muir JG and Gibson, PR Dietary triggers of abdominal symptoms in patients with irritable bowel syndrome- randomised placebo-controlled evidence Clin. Gastroenterol. Hepatol. 2008;6(7):765-771

Sicherer SH, Sampson HA. Food hypersensitivity and atopic dermatitis: Pathophysiology, epidemiology, diagnosis and management. *J Allergy Clin Immunol.* 1999; 104: S114-S122.

Sicherer SH. Manifestations of food allergy: evaluation and management. *Am Fam Phys.* 1999;59(2):415-24, 429-430.

Sinclair S. Migraine Headaches: nutritional, botanical and other alternative approaches. *Alt Med Rev.* 1999;4(2):86-95.

Soderholm JD, Perdue MH. Stress and the gastrointestinal tract II. Stress and intestinal barrier function. *Am J Physiol Gastrointest Liver Physiol.* 2001; G7-G13.

Swain A, Soutter V, Loblay R, Truswell AS. Salicylates, oligoantigenic diets and behaviour. Lancet 1985; 2:41–2.

Taylor SL, Hefle SL. Food allergies and other food sensitivities: A publication of the Institute of Food Technologists' Expert Panel on Food Safety and Nutrition. *Food Tech.* 2001; 55(9):68-83.

Taylor SL, Leatherwood M, Lieber ER. A survey of histamine levels in sausages. / Food Protect 1978; 41 634-7

Walker WA, Sanderson IR. Epithelial barrier function to antigens. *Neuro-Immuno-Physiology Gastrointestinal Mucosa.* 1992; 664:10-17.

Walker-Smith J. Food sensitivity enteropathy: Overview and update. *Acta Paediatrica Japonica.* 1994; 36:545-549.

Wuthrich B. Adverse reactions to food additives. Ann Allergy 1993; 71:379–84.

Xavier RJ, Podolsky DK: Unravelling the pathogenesis of inflammatory bowel disease. Nature 2007; 448: 427–434.

Chapter 5

The Optimal Diet: The Axis of Health and Wellbeing

When a patient with a chronic disease walks into my office at the Da Vinci Center in Larnaca, Cyprus, after taking a health history I explain that one of the most important lifestyle changes that they must make is to change their diet. Modern science now concurs that among all lifestyle factors, no single factor is more important to our health than the food we eat.

There are many scientific studies on the benefits of eating health-promoting, nutrient-dense foods, full of vitamins, minerals, trace elements, antioxidants and phytonutrients. These can both help cure chronic diseases, as well as prevent them.

There are some general guidelines regarding what foods are generally good for us, against those that should certainly not be on our plate or in our kitchens.

However, before we look at specific foods, let us examine an expression that you have all probably heard before: *"One man's meat is another man's poison."*

Eating According to Your Metabolic Type

For many years, people have been overwhelmed and confused with the complex and often sharply contradictory information about what to eat in order to stay healthy and fit.

There are many experts who argue about how much protein, carbohydrates and fats people should be eating. Off course, this is an important topic because this is the "octane" of fuel that our body needs. But we are genetically programmed from birth to be different, and we all require different octanes of fuel.

The primary problem for health consumers is this: since the market is flooded with so many dietary options, and so much conflicting advice and opinion, people are left feeling confused, not knowing how to make sense of it all. Since people have no way to make rational dietary choices, they're forced into a process of endless experimentation, forced to play a never-ending game of "dietary roulette."

171

In other words, the most profound limitation of virtually all diet and nutrition books is that they're based on a system of chance. Since these books offer generic rather than customized dietary advice - the programs they describe work fairly well for some people, some of the time. That's why most nutritional books offer up a decent range of positive case histories.

The Metabolic Typing Diet

This confusion has abounded for many years, but it was not until Bill Wolcott, a world-leading authority on Metabolic Typing, wrote his first book entitled, *The Metabolic Typing Diet*, a revolutionary dietary technology, that enabled people to optimize their health and fitness by identifying their own highly individualized nutritional needs, and were able to tailor their diets accordingly.

The Metabolic Typing Diet is a truly revolutionary book that provides what has long been desperately needed: a systematic, testable, repeatable, verifiable means for each of us to find an answer to the question, *"What's right for me?"*

As far back as the 1930s, scientists and researchers began to identify specific ways in which human beings differ from one another on a biochemical or metabolic level, due largely to genetic inheritance. Based on this information, researchers also began to discover that many kinds of chronic ailments could be resolved when people adopted dietary and nutritional regimes compatible with their own unique body chemistry. They began to differentiate people from one another on the basis of their "Metabolic   Type".

Over the course of the 20th century, many leading scientists and clinicians contributed to the field that has come to be known as "Metabolic Typing." It is actually the culmination of 70 years of pioneering research on the part of many of the 20th century's most significant nutritional researchers, including Francis Pottenger, M.D., Weston Price, D.D.S., Royal Lee, D.D.S., Emmanuel Revici, M.D., William Donald Kelley, D.D.S., George Watson, Ph.D., and Roger Williams, Ph.D.

Practitioners throughout the world use Bill's nutritional profiles as the basis of tailor-made therapeutic regimes for people with many different types of chronic health problems. Over the years, these customized metabolic protocols have proven to be remarkably effective in helping to prevent and reverse all kinds of chronic ailments.

Metabolic typing takes the guesswork out of nutritional science, and it doesn't leave anyone behind. It's an advanced but very easy and accessible methodology that anyone can use to rapidly cut through the information glut of confusing fact and opinion and accurately assess their own unique nutritional requirements.

You now have the opportunity to test your own <u>METABOLIC TYPING</u> and receive a full report with dietary guideline based on what type you are.

This Intermediate Metabolic Typing assessment will provide you with the following:

❖ **Metabolic Type® Report** — your personalized report describing the results of your own Metabolic Typing Assessment. This report not only describes your personal Metabolic Type, but also shows the relative balances between the various systems that determine your type of metabolism. This allows you to compare future test results and chart your progress as you achieve better health through improved metabolic balance.

❖ **Personalized Metabolic Type Eating Plan** — the heart of your Metabolic Typing recommendations. Your food list details exactly the right foods for your specific Metabolic Type and identifies all the foods you should avoid.

❖ **Starter Meal Plans** — to assist you in getting started right. Metabolic Typing is unique because there is <u>NO food weighing or measuring required!</u> With our Starter Meal Plans, you will quickly learn how relative food proportions are what really matters. Learn why you do not need to weigh food quantities or count calories to lose weight or improve your health.

❖ **Individualized Metabolic Type Supplement List** — the right nutritional supplements specifically created and combined only for your unique Metabolic Type. These supplements are unlike any others – they utilize the exact forms and balances of the vitamins, minerals, amino acids, fatty acids, herbs and enzymes shown to be supportive of your particular kind of metabolism.

When you identify your Metabolic Typing and fine-tune your diet, you'll learn two primary things:

1. Exactly what foods are compatible with your body chemistry.
2. How to combine proteins, carbohydrates and fats in a ratio that is just right for you.

In the Metabolic Typing Diet report that you will receive, you'll find very comprehensive lists of foods that are compatible with your metabolic type, including specific types of meat, poultry, fish, dairy products, grains, legumes, vegetables, fruits and nuts.

Three general Metabolic Types

The list below gives you a brief preview of the three general metabolic type categories and the diets that correspond to each category. But please remember that these three categories are just a starting point! Within each category, there is plenty of variation.

Once you identify your basic category, the report will guide you through fine-tuning techniques to customize a diet to your own highly individualized needs.

You'll know when you've identified the diet that's just right for you because your meals will leave you feeling full and satisfied, and free of the hunger pangs and food cravings that many people experience shortly after eating.

When you eat according to your metabolic type, you'll be able to last 4 to 5 hours between meals and snacks without feeling hungry. You'll also have lots of physical energy and mental clarity, and be free of fatigue, irritability and other problems that commonly occur when you fail to eat according to your genetically-based needs.

Needless to say, you'll experience plenty of longer-term benefits as well, including the ability to lose weight and keep it off, strengthened immunity and stamina, and the ability to prevent, reverse or greatly alleviate many kinds of common health disorders.

Below are brief highlights of the three basic Metabolic Type diets; your starting point on the road to truly effective, customized nutrition…

The Protein Type Diet

In general or simplistic terms, if you are a protein type it means one of two things: either your cells tend to burn carbohydrates too quickly (meaning you're a fast oxidizer), or the parasympathetic branch of your autonomic nervous system is stronger and more dominant than the sympathetic branch. This means you need a high-protein intake in order to strengthen your sympathetic system, and in turn acidify your too-alkaline metabolism. Or you need protein to slow down your overly rapid cellular oxidation rate, thereby alkalinizing your too-acid metabolism.

Protein types do very well on a diet that includes plenty of high-density, high-fat proteins known as "high-purine" proteins. These include foods like red meat, dark meat chicken and turkey, and various kinds of seafood such as salmon, tuna, herring, sardines, mussels, caviar and anchovies. Most protein types can also eat freely of whole fat foods, like cheese, eggs, cream and milk. It's especially important for protein types to include a significant amount of protein at every meal, and to moderate their intake of carbohydrates (grains, vegetables and fruits), especially the carbohydrates that are high in sugar and starch.

The Carbo Type Diet

Generally speaking, if you're a carbo type you need a higher percentage of carbohydrates in your diet in order to strengthen the parasympathetic branch of your nervous system, which is weaker than your sympathetic system, and thereby alkalinize your too-acid metabolism. Or you need more carbohydrates to speed up your naturally slow cellular oxidation rate, thereby bringing it into balance by acidifying your too-alkaline metabolism.

Carbo types typically do well on a low-fat, relatively low-protein diet; one that includes liberal amounts of carbohydrates in the form of vegetables, fruits and whole grains. However, carbo types need to remember that a "low-protein" diet does not mean a "no-protein" diet. In fact, most carbo types will find that they need to include protein at most meals, but they need to focus on leaner, lighter meats, seafood and poultry protein types. They should restrict their consumption of red meat in favour of light meat chicken and turkey and lighter seafood such as haddock, cod, perch, sole, catfish and flounder.

If you're a carbo type, you should stick to low-fat dairy products, but you can eat a very wide selection of vegetables, fruits, and grains. However, many carbo types, like protein types, do best by focusing on vegetables that contain low or moderate levels of sugar and starch.

The Mixed Type Diet

If you're a mixed type, it means you're somewhere in the middle of the other two types, which have more pronounced or clear-cut metabolic imbalances. You actually need to eat a mixture of protein and carbo type foods. This will accomplish two things:

1. It will support both sides of your autonomic nervous system, both the sympathetic branch and the parasympathetic branch.
2. It will keep your cellular oxidation rate, which is neither too fast or too slow, in balance.

Mixed types need to consume relatively equal ratios of proteins, fats and carbohydrates. They also need to eat a mixture of high-fat, high-purine proteins and low-fat, low-purine proteins. The same applies to all other foods contained on the protein type and carbo type diets - including grains, legumes, vegetables and fruits.

Now that we have covered these basic tenets of individualized nutrition based on your metabolic typing, what will follow will be generic and generalized as we cannot go into detail about everyone's type until you discover what type you are.

Metabolic Typing is available at www.worldwidehealthcenter.net.

Changing Lifestyles Saves Lives

Reducing identified, modifiable dietary and lifestyle risk factors could prevent most cases of CAD, stroke, diabetes, and many cancers among high-income populations (Willett 2002). These findings are profoundly important, because they indicate that these diseases are not inevitable consequences of a modern society (Fig 1).

Furthermore, low rates of these diseases can be attained without drugs or expensive medical facilities. An outcome that is not surprising because their rates have historically been extremely low in developing countries with few medical facilities. However, preventing these diseases will require changes in behaviours related to smoking, physical activity, and diet; investments in education, food policies, and urban physical infrastructure are needed to support and encourage these changes.

Dietary and lifestyle factors	CVD	Type 2 diabetes	Cancer	Dental disease	Fracture	Cataract	Birth defects	Obesity	Metabolic syndrome	Depression	Sexual dysfunction
Avoid smoking	↓	↓	↓	↓	↓	↓		↑			↓
Pursue physical activity	↓	↓	↓		↓			↓	↓	↓	↓
Avoid overweight	↓	↓	↓		↑	↓			↓		↓
Diet											
Consume healthy types of fats[a]	↓	↓							↓		
Eat plenty of fruits and vegetables	↓		↓		↓	↓	↓	↓			
Replace refined grains with whole grains	↓	↓						↓	↓		
Limit sugar intake[b]	↓	↓		↓				↓	↓		
Limit excessive calories								↓	↓		
Limit sodium intake	↓										

Fig 1. Convincing and Probable Relationships between Dietary and Lifestyle Factors and Chronic Diseases

Source: Authors' summary of a review by the WHO and FAO 2003; Bacon and others 2003; Fox 1999; IARC 2002.

Healthy Eating Plate & Healthy Eating Pyramid

Nutrition experts at Harvard School of Public Health have put together what they call the Healthy Eating Plate to provide detailed guidance, in a simple format, to help people make the best eating choices.

One of the emphasis is on eating quality foods; the *type* of food is more important than the *amount*. Let us look conceptually at what it means to eat healthily, and then we can discuss in more detail the quality of food families that would lead to an optimal diet. As we can see in Fig 1, the Healthy Eating Plate recommends the following:

❖ About half your plate should consist of vegetables and fruits.

❖ About one-quarter of your plate should consist of whole grains, such as whole wheat, barley, wheat berries, quinoa, oats, brown rice, and foods made with them, such as whole wheat pasta. White bread, white rice, and other refined grains should be avoided as they will have a negative effect on blood sugar levels and are generally deficient in nutrients.

❖ About one-quarter of your plate should be good-quality, clean protein. This could include organic meat, seawater fish (not farmed), beans and nuts. They can be mixed into salads, soups, stir fries or boiled, grilled, but frying should be avoided. Limit a lot of red meat, and avoid processed meats such as bacon and sausage.

❖ Use healthy, organic oils such as olive, coconut, avocado, pumpkin and even sunflower. Avoid partially hydrogenated oils, which contain unhealthy trans fats.

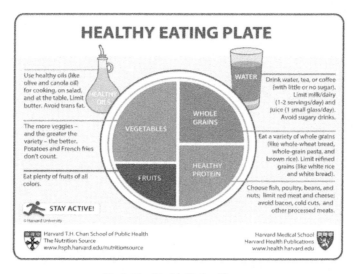

Fig 1. The Health Eating Plate

Drink plenty of clean mineral water, and having one or two organic coffees per day is healthy. Herbal teas are also beneficial.

Please note that one of the vegetables that we should add caution to is Potatoes. Even though potatoes do contain important nutrients such as vitamin C, potassium, and vitamin B6, to name a few, it is not the only source of these nutrients, nor is it the best. Cup for cup, for example, broccoli has nearly nine times as much vitamin C as a potato, and white beans have about double the potassium. Yet a cup of potatoes has a similar effect on blood sugar as a can of Coca Cola or a handful of jelly beans (Bazzano et al, 2008). That's a high metabolic price to pay for nutrients that children an easily get from other sources.

There are many similarities between the Health Eating Plate and the food pyramid design (Fig 2).

THE HEALTHY EATING PYRAMID

Department of Nutrition, Harvard School of Public Health

Fig 2. The Healthy Eating Pyramid

Consumers can think of the Healthy Eating Pyramid as a shopping guide. Vegetables, fruits, whole grains, healthy oils, and healthy proteins like nuts, beans, fish, and chicken should make it into the shopping cart every week, along with a little yogurt or milk if desired.

The Healthy Eating Pyramid also addresses other aspects of a healthy lifestyle. Exercise, weight control, vitamin D, and multivitamin supplements, as well as moderation of alcohol for people who drink. So, it's a useful tool for health professionals and health educators.

There are a number of studies that have been done to demonstrate the disease prevention benefits from following a diet similar to one based on the Healthy Eating Pyramid, here are a couple:

❖ A study that tracked 7,319 British civil servants for 18 years found that men and women with the highest scores on the Alternate Healthy Eating Index had a 25% lower risk of dying from any cause, and a 42% lower risk of dying from heart disease, than people with the lowest scores (McCullough et al, 2002).

❖ Another observational study of 93,676 post-menopausal women found that following a Healthy Eating Pyramid-style diet (as measured by adherence to the Alternative Healthy Eating Index), was superior to following a low-fat diet at lowering cardiovascular disease and heart failure risk (Akbaraly et al, 2011).

Now let us examine specific food families to see why they are healthy for the human body. Let's begin with a crucially important family - vegetables and fruits.

Vegetables and Fruits
It is important to realize that no single fruit or vegetable provides all of the nutrients you need to be healthy, so eating a variety is important.

A diet rich in vegetables and fruits can lower blood pressure, reduce risk of heart disease and stroke, prevent some types of cancer, lower risk of eye and digestive problems, and have a positive effect upon blood sugar which can help keep appetite in check.

Coloured vegetables and fruits are rich in many healthy antioxidants and phytonutrients, so try dark leafy greens; brightly coloured red, yellow and orange vegetables and fruits; and cooked tomatoes.

Protection Against Disease
There are many studies that have looked at how fruits and vegetables can help prevent many chronic diseases, here is a summary of some:

1. There is compelling evidence that a diet rich in fruits and vegetables can lower the risk of heart disease and stroke. The largest and longest study to date, done as part of the Harvard-based Nurses' Health Study and Health Professionals Follow-up Study, included almost 110,000 men and women whose health and dietary habits were followed for 14 years.

The higher the average daily intake of fruits and vegetables, the lower the chances of developing cardiovascular disease. Compared with those in the lowest category of fruit and vegetable intake (less than 1.5 servings a day), those who averaged 8 or more servings a day were 30 percent less likely to have had a heart attack or stroke (Hung et al, 2004).

Although all fruits and vegetables likely contribute to this benefit, green leafy vegetables such as lettuce, spinach, Swiss chard, and mustard greens; cruciferous vegetables such as broccoli, cauliflower, cabbage, Brussels sprouts, bok choy, and kale; and citrus fruits such as oranges, lemons, limes, and grapefruit (and their juices) make important contributions (Hung et al, 2004).

When researchers combined findings from the Harvard studies with several other long-term studies in the U.S. and Europe, they found a similar protective effect: Individuals who ate more than 5 servings of fruits and vegetables per day had roughly a 20 percent lower risk of coronary heart disease (He et al, 2007) and stroke (He et al, 2006), compared with individuals who ate less than 3 servings per day.

2. The Dietary Approaches to Stop Hypertension (DASH) Study (Appel et al, 1997) examined the effect on blood pressure of a diet that was rich in fruits, vegetables, and low-fat dairy products and that restricted the amount of saturated and total fat. The researchers found that people with high blood pressure who followed this diet reduced their systolic blood pressure (the upper number of a blood pressure reading) by about 11 mm Hg and their diastolic blood pressure (the lower number) by almost 6 mm Hg - as much as medications can achieve.

3. A randomized trial known as the Optimal Macronutrient Intake Trial for Heart Health (OmniHeart) showed that this fruit and vegetable-rich diet lowered blood pressure even more when some of the carbohydrate was replaced with healthy unsaturated fat or protein (Appel et al, 2005).

4. In 2014, a meta-analysis of clinical trials and observational studies found that consumption of a vegetarian diet was associated with lower blood pressure (Yokoyama et al, 2014).

Numerous early studies revealed what appeared to be a strong link between eating fruits and vegetables and protection against cancer. Unlike case-control studies, cohort studies, which follow large groups of initially healthy individuals for years, generally provide more reliable information than case-control studies because they don't rely on information from the past. And, in general, data from cohort studies have not consistently shown that a diet rich in fruits and vegetables prevents cancer.

For example, in the Nurses' Health Study and the Health Professionals Follow-up Study, over a 14-year period, men and women with the highest intake of fruits and vegetables (8+ servings a day) were just as likely to have developed cancer as those who ate the fewest daily servings (under 1.5). (Hung et al, 2004).

181

A more likely possibility is that some types of fruits and vegetables may protect against certain cancers.

A report by the World Cancer Research Fund and the American Institute for Cancer Research suggests that non-starchy vegetables—such as lettuce and other leafy greens, broccoli, bok choy, cabbage, as well as garlic, onions, and the like—and fruits "probably" protect against several types of cancers, including those of the mouth, throat, voice box, oesophagus, and stomach; fruit "probably" also protects against lung cancer (Wiseman et al, 2008).

Specific components of fruits and vegetables may also be protective against cancer. For example:

❖ Studies suggest that increased consumption of tomato-based products (especially cooked tomato products) and other lycopene-containing foods may reduce the occurrence of prostate cancer (Wiseman et al, 2008). Lycopene is one of several carotenoids (compounds that the body can turn into vitamin A) found in brightly coloured fruits and vegetables, and research suggests that foods containing carotenoids may protect against lung, mouth, and throat cancer.

Some research looks specifically at whether individual fruits are associated with risk of type 2 diabetes. While there isn't an abundance of research into this area yet, preliminary results are compelling.

❖ A study was conducted on over 66,000 women in the Nurses' Health Study, 85,104 women from the Nurses' Health Study II, and 36,173 men from the Health Professionals Follow-up Study who were free of major chronic diseases. Findings suggested that greater consumption of whole fruits – especially blueberries, grapes, and apples – was associated with a lower risk of type 2 diabetes.

❖ Another important finding: Greater consumption of fruit juice is associated with a *higher* risk of type 2 diabetes (Muraki et al, 2013).

❖ A study of over 2,300 Finnish men showed that fruit and vegetables, especially berries, may reduce the risk of Type 2 diabetes (Mursu et al, 2014).

Fruits and vegetables contain indigestible fibre, which absorbs water and expands as it passes through the digestive system. This can calm symptoms of an irritable bowel and, by triggering regular bowel movements, relieve or prevent constipation (Lembo et al, 2003). The bulking and softening action of insoluble fibre also decreases pressure inside the intestinal tract and may help prevent diverticulosis (Aldoori et al, 1998).

Eating fruits and vegetables can also keep your eyes healthy, and may help prevent two common aging-related eye diseases - cataracts and macular degeneration - which afflict millions of Americans over age 65 (Brown et al, 1999; Christen et al, 2005; Moeller et al, 2004). Lutein and zeaxanthin, in particular, seem protective against cataracts.

Whole Grains

Whole grains are far healthier than refined grains, which are stripped of valuable nutrients in the refining process.

- ❖ Whole grains contain bran and fibre, which slow the breakdown of starch into glucose - thus maintaining a steady blood sugar rather than causing sharp spikes.
- ❖ Fibre helps lower cholesterol as well as move waste through the digestive tract.
- ❖ Fibre may also help prevent the formation of small blood clots that can trigger heart attacks or strokes.
- ❖ Phytoestrogens (plant oestrogens) and essential minerals such as magnesium, selenium and copper found in whole grains may protect against some cancers.

The invention of industrialized roller mills in the late 19th century changed the way we process grains. Milling strips away the bran and germ, making the grain easier to chew and digest, but such highly processed grains are much lower in nutritional quality. Refining wheat creates fluffy flour that makes light, airy breads and pastries, but the process strips away more than half of wheat's B-vitamins, 90% of the vitamin E, and virtually *all* of the fibre.

A growing body of research shows that choosing whole grains and other less-processed, higher-quality sources of carbohydrates, and cutting back on refined grains, improves health in many ways.

Be careful when choosing whole grains: "Whole grain" doesn't always mean healthy. Consumers should steer towards whole grain breads that are high in fibre and that have few ingredients in addition to whole grain. In addition, eating whole grains in their *whole* forms, such as brown rice, barley, oats, corn, and rye are healthy choices because they pack in the nutritional benefits of whole grains without any additional ingredients.

Whole Grains and Disease

As researchers have begun to look more closely at carbohydrates and health, they are learning that the quality of the carbohydrates that you eat is equally as important as the quantity. Most studies, including some from several different Harvard teams, show a connection between whole grains and better health (Wu et al, 2015).

An intriguing report from the Iowa Women's Health Study linked whole-grain consumption with fewer deaths from non-cardiac, non-cancer causes. Compared with women who rarely or never ate whole-grain foods, those who had at least two or more servings a day were 30% less likely to have died from an inflammation-related condition over a 17-year period (Jacobs et al, 2007).

A meta-analysis combining results from studies conducted in the US, the United Kingdom, and Scandinavian countries (which included health information from over 786,000 individuals), found that people who ate 70 grams/day of whole grains - compared with those who ate little or no whole grains - had a 22% lower risk of total mortality, a 23% lower risk of cardiovascular disease mortality, and a 20% lower risk of cancer mortality (Zong et al, 2016).

Eating whole instead of refined grains substantially lowers total cholesterol, low-density lipoprotein (LDL, or bad) cholesterol, triglycerides, and insulin levels.

In the Harvard-based Nurses' Health Study, women who ate 2-3 servings of whole-grain products each day were 30% less likely to have a heart attack or die from heart disease over a 10-year period, compared to women who ate less than 1 serving per week (Liu et al, 1999).

A meta-analysis of seven major studies showed that cardiovascular disease (heart attack, stroke, or the need for a procedure to bypass or open a clogged artery), was 21% less likely in people who ate 2.5 or more servings of whole-grain foods a day compared with those who ate less than 2 servings a week (Mellen et al, 2008).

In a study of more than 160,000 women whose health and dietary habits were followed for up to 18 years, those who averaged 2-3 servings of whole grains a day were 30% less likely to have developed type 2 diabetes than those who rarely ate whole grains (de Munter et al, 2007).

When the researchers combined these results with those of several other large studies, they found that eating an extra 2 servings of whole grains a day decreased the risk of type 2 diabetes by 21%.

More recent findings from this study (the Nurses' Health Studies I and II) and the Health Professionals Follow-Up Study suggest that swapping white rice for whole grains could help lower diabetes risk. Researchers found that women and men who ate the most white rice - five or more servings a week - had a 17% higher risk of diabetes than those who ate white rice less than once a month. Those who ate the most brown rice - two or more servings a week - had an 11% lower risk of diabetes than those who rarely ate brown rice. Researchers estimate that swapping whole grains in place of even some white rice could lower diabetes risk by 36% (Sun et al, 2010).

A large, five-year study among nearly 500,000 men and women suggests that eating whole grains, but not dietary fibre, offers modest protection against colorectal cancer (Schatzkin et al, 2007; Strayer et al, 2007).

By keeping the stool soft and bulky, the fibre in whole grains helps prevent constipation, a common, costly and serious problem that greatly adds to the toxicity of the body. It also helps prevent diverticular disease (diverticulosis) by decreasing pressure in the intestines.

Fats and Cholesterol
When it comes to dietary fat, what matters most is the type of fat you eat. Contrary to past dietary advice promoting low-fat diets, newer research shows that healthy fats are necessary and beneficial for health.

When food manufacturers reduce fat, they often replace it with carbohydrates from sugar, refined grains, or other starches. Our bodies digest these refined carbohydrates and starches very quickly, affecting blood sugar and insulin levels, resulting in weight gain and disease.

Rather than adopting a low-fat diet, it's more important to focus on eating beneficial "good" fats and avoiding harmful "bad" fats. Fat is an important part of a healthy diet. Choose foods with "good" unsaturated fats, limit foods high in saturated fat, and avoid "bad" trans-fat.

* ❖ **"Good" unsaturated fats** (Monounsaturated and polyunsaturated fats) lower disease risk. Foods high in good fats include vegetable oils (such as organic olive, canola, sunflower, soy, and corn), nuts, seeds, and fish.

* ❖ **"Bad" fats** (trans-fats) increase disease risk, even when eaten in small quantities. Foods containing trans fats are primarily in processed foods made with trans-fat from partially hydrogenated oil. Fortunately, trans-fats have been eliminated from many of these foods.

❖ **Saturated fats**, while not as harmful as trans-fats, negatively impact health and are best consumed in moderation. Foods containing large amounts of saturated fat include red meat, butter, cheese, and ice cream.

Simply speaking, a fat is a combination of carbon molecules combined together to form a chain. Various combinations of the carbon molecules make different types of fats. There are saturated and unsaturated fats. Saturated fats can only have a straight structure, unsaturated fats on the other hand can be have a bent shape (like omega 3 and 6) or a straight shape (trans unsaturated fat). The reason trans-fats and saturated fats are considered bad is because their molecular structure is straight, and can clump together and clog arteries. Hydrogenated and trans-fats are artificial fats that have added hydrogen to make them straight in shape, increasing their melting point, and thus making them much more stable for increased shelf life.

When the fat is *Trans*, then it is straight in shape, with a kink in it, much like saturated fat.

Trans Fat   Unsaturated Fat   Saturated Fat

The walls of the cells in our bodies are made up of fats, mostly from the good essential fats like omega 3 (hemp, walnut, coconut, flaxseed) and omega 6 (soybean oil, corn oil, safflower oil, sunflower oil, peanut oil, cottonseed oil, rice bran oil) which combine together to form the cellular membrane.

Trans and hydrogenated fats are widely used in all sorts of processed foods; cookies, crackers, pastries, cakes, chips, fast food, margarine, popcorn, pretty much most of what is found on your grocery store shelves. These should all be avoided like the plague!

Vegetable oils are generally better than trans-fats but they also have some very negative effects on the body. Oils like canola, soybean, sunflower, safflower, and others contribute to major inflammation (the main cause of disease and aging) due to the upset in the ratio of omega 3 and omega 6 fatty acids.

186

Before the age of food processing, people had a good balance of fats, especially omega 3 and 6, with a ratio of about 2:1 or 3:1 (2 parts omega 6, to 1 part omega 3). The ratio now is about 20:1 or higher!

This high imbalance leads to inflammatory related diseases such as autoimmune, diabetes, cardiovascular and cancer. Consuming large amounts of vegetable oils damages our whole body, leading to irritability, learning disabilities, liver toxicity, decreased immune function, mental and physical growth problems and increased acidity. They have also been linked to mental disorders like Alzheimer's, dementia as well as accelerated aging - all signs of inflammation and acidity in the body.

A 1994 study appearing in a leading medical journal showed that almost three quarters of the fat clogged in arteries was unsaturated. This means it was not the "artery clogging" saturated fats, but vegetable oils!

Avoid Margarine, Shortening, and Spreads at all Costs!

There is a myriad of unhealthy components to margarine and other butter imposters, including:

- ❖ **Trans-fats:** These unnatural fats in margarine, shortenings and spreads are formed during the process of hydrogenation, which turns liquid vegetable oils into a solid fat. Trans-fats contribute to heart disease, cancer, bone problems, hormonal imbalance, skin disease, infertility, difficulties in pregnancy and problems with lactation, low birth weight, growth problems and learning disabilities in children. A U.S. government panel of scientists determined that man-made trans-fats are unsafe at any level (small amounts of *natural* trans-fats occur in butter and other animal fats, but these are not harmful).

- ❖ **Free radicals** and other toxic breakdown products are the result of high temperature industrial processing of vegetable oils. They contribute to numerous health problems, including cancer and heart disease.

- ❖ **Synthetic vitamins** are added to margarine and spreads. These often have an opposite (and detrimental) effect compared to the natural vitamins in butter.

- ❖ **Emulsifiers and preservatives.** Numerous additives of questionable safety are added to margarines and spreads. Most vegetable shortening is stabilized with preservatives like BHT.

- ❖ **Hexane and other solvents** are used in the extraction process. These industrial chemicals can have toxic effects.

187

❖ **Bleach.** The natural colour of partially hydrogenated vegetable oil is grey so manufacturers bleach it to make it white. Yellow colouring is then added to margarine and spreads.

❖ **Artificial flavours** help mask the terrible taste and odour of partially hydrogenated oils, and provide a fake butter taste.

❖ **Mono- and di-glycerides** contain trans-fats that manufacturers do not have to list on the label. They are used in high amounts in so-called "low-trans" spreads.

❖ **Soy protein isolate** is a highly-processed powder which is added to "low-trans" spreads to give them body. It can contribute to thyroid dysfunction, digestive disorders and many other health problems.

❖ **Sterols** are often added to spreads to give them cholesterol-lowering qualities, these estrogen compounds can cause endocrine problems; in animals, these sterols contribute to sexual inversion.

❖ **Sugary Drinks** are a major contributor to the obesity epidemic. The term "soft drink" refers to any beverage with added sugar or other sweetener, and includes soda, fruit punch, lemonade and other "-ades," sweetened powdered drinks, and sports and energy drinks.

People who drink sugary beverages do not feel as full as if they had eaten the same calories from solid food, and studies show that people consuming sugary beverages don't compensate for their high caloric content by eating less food.

Fruit juice is not a better option. Even though it has more nutrients, it contains as much sugar (though from naturally occurring fruit sugars rather than added sugar) and calories as soft drinks.

The more ounces of sugary beverages a person has each day, the more calories he or she takes in later in the day. This is the opposite of what happens with solid food, as people tend to compensate for a large meal by taking in fewer calories at a later meal. This compensatory effect doesn't seem to be present after consuming soft drinks, for several possible reasons:

❖ Fluids don't provide the same feeling of fullness or satisfaction as solid foods, as the body doesn't "register" liquid calories the same way it does calories from solid food. This may prompt a person to keep eating even after an intake of a high-calorie drink.

❖ It is possible that sweet-tasting soft drinks - regardless of whether they are sweetened with sugar or a calorie-free sugar substitute - might stimulate the appetite for other sweet, high-carbohydrate foods.

❖ Even though soda may contain more sugar than a cookie, because people think of soda as a drink and a cookie as a dessert, they are more likely to limit food than beverages.

The best-choice beverages are those that fall in the green category—drinks that have little or no sugar added to them, such as water, sparkling water, coffee, or tea.

There are some sugary drinks that have much more than 12 grams of sugar in a 12-ounce serving, and some have upwards of 40 grams of sugar (equivalent to about 10 teaspoons of sugar) and 200 or more calories in a 12-ounce serving.

There is now a lot of research to show that sugary drinks can cause a lot of health problems. Here is a summary of some of these studies:

❖ People who consume sugary drinks regularly - 1 to 2 cans a day or more - have a 26% greater risk of developing type-2 diabetes than people who rarely have such drinks (Piernas et al, 2014).

❖ A study that followed 40,000 men for two decades found that those who averaged one can of a sugary beverage per day had a 20% higher risk of having a heart attack or dying from a heart attack than men who rarely consumed sugary drinks. A related study in women found a similar sugary beverage/heart disease link.

❖ A 22-year-long study of 80,000 women found that those who consumed a can a day of sugary drink had a 75% higher risk of gout than women who rarely had such drinks. Researchers found a similarly elevated risk in men.

❖ Dr. Frank Hu, Professor of Nutrition and Epidemiology at Harvard School of Public Health, recently made a strong case that there is sufficient scientific evidence that decreasing sugar-sweetened beverage consumption will reduce the prevalence of obesity and obesity-related diseases.

Other Healthy Beverage Options

After water, coffee and tea are the two most commonly consumed beverages on the planet. They are brimming with antioxidants, flavonoids, and other biologically active substances that may be good for health.

Tea

Research suggests that drinking at least three cups of either black or green tea per day reduces the risk of stroke (Arab et al, 2009) and cancer (Lee et al, 2013; Nechuta et al, 2012).

Some teas taste sweet to the palate without added sugar. Try fruit-flavoured herbal teas, or teas with cinnamon or vanilla.

The Key to Tea: Antioxidants

Polyphenols are likely the key component to what makes tea a healthy drink. These chemical compounds act as antioxidants, which fight against free radicals in the body. Free radicals can alter DNA by stealing its electrons, and this mutated DNA can increase LDL cholesterol or alter cell membrane traffic – both harmful to our health. Though green tea is often considered higher in polyphenols than black or oolong (red) teas, studies show that – with the exception of decaffeinated tea – all teas have about the same levels of these chemicals, albeit in different proportions.

One study that analysed the effects of adding skimmed, semi-skimmed, and whole milk to tea concluded that skimmed milk significantly reduced the antioxidant capacity of tea. The fattier milks also reduced the antioxidant capacity of tea, but to a lesser degree (Ryan et al, 2010). Overall, it's important to keep in mind that tea – even tea with milk – is a healthy drink. To reap the full antioxidant benefits of tea, however, it may be best to skip the milk.

Three Big Benefits of Tea:

1. Reduced risk of cardiovascular disease

Polyphenols, the antioxidants abundant in tea, have been shown to reduce the risk of death due to cardiovascular disease (Kuriyama et al, 2006), including stroke (Holman et al, 2010; Larsson et al, 2013). In one study of 77,000 Japanese men and women, green tea and oolong tea consumption was linked with lower risk of death from cardiovascular disease (Mineharu et al, 2011).

Other large-scale studies show that black tea also contributes to heart health (Arab et al, 2009), with research suggesting that drinking at least three cups of either black or green tea per day appears to reduce the risk of stroke by 21%. The study also stated that drinking tea may be one of the most significant changes a person can make to reduce his or her risk of stroke (Arab et al, 2009).

2. Protection from cancer

Research shows benefits for a variety of types of cancer, including ovarian and digestive system cancers (Lee et al, 2013; Nechuta et al, 2012). Green tea might also have a positive effect in reducing risk of breast, prostate, and endometrial cancers (Johnson et al, 2012).

3. Reduced risk of high blood pressure
In a study of green and oolong tea consumption, regular consumption for one year reduced the risk of developing hypertension. Long-term regular consumption of black tea has also been shown to lower blood pressure.

Coffee
- ❖ 54% of American adults drink coffee every day, with an average of about 3 cups per day.
- ❖ It's considered safe to drink up to six cups of coffee per day. In fact, research suggests that drinking coffee may reduce some disease risks.
- ❖ Some people may want to consider avoiding coffee or switching to decaf, especially women who are pregnant, or people who have a hard time controlling their blood pressure or blood sugar.
- ❖ It's best to brew coffee with a paper filter to remove the substance that causes an increase in LDL cholesterol.

Four noted benefits of coffee:
1. Possible reduction in heart disease and stroke risk
Studies suggest that drinking coffee regularly decreases risk of heart disease or stroke.

- ❖ The Nurse's Health Study of 83,076 women showed that regular coffee consumption was associated with a modest reduction in stroke risk (Lopez-Garcia et al, 2009).
- ❖ Another study of 37,514 participants concluded that moderate coffee drinking was associated with a reduced risk of heart disease (Bhupathiraju et al, 2013).

2. Lower risk of developing type 2 diabetes
Research shows that caffeine raises blood sugar in the short term, but the antioxidants in coffee may improve insulin sensitivity and lower the risk of type 2 diabetes over many years.

- ❖ A study of over 125,000 participants tracked coffee consumption and new cases of type 2 diabetes for 18 years. This study showed that women who drink more than six cups of coffee per day reduced their risk for developing type 2 diabetes by almost 30% (Bhupathiraju et al, 2013).

- ❖ A study of 74,749 women analysed the intake of caffeinated and caffeine-free beverages with respect to the development of type 2 diabetes. The study

191

showed that caffeinated coffee reduced type 2 diabetes risk by 4% and decaffeinated reduced the risk by 7%. This suggests that a component of coffee independent of caffeine, perhaps antioxidants found in both regular coffee and decaf, is responsible for the decrease in type 2 diabetes risk (Bhupathiraju et al, 2013).

3. Protects against gallstones
A study of 46,008 men tracked their development of gallstone and their coffee consumption for 10 years. After adjusting for other factors known to cause gallstones, the study concluded that men who consistently drank coffee were significantly less likely to develop gallstones compared to men who did not (Leitzmann et al, 1999).

❖ A similar large study found the same result in women (Leitzmann et al, 2002).

4. Lower risk of developing Parkinson's Disease
The results of recent studies suggest that coffee consumed in moderate quantities may reduce the risk for developing Parkinson's Disease.

❖ A study tracked coffee consumption and Parkinson's Disease development of 6,710 men and women over 22 years. In that time, after adjusting for known risks of Parkinson's Disease, coffee drinkers had a significantly lower risk of developing the disease than non-drinkers (Saaksjarvi et al, 2008).

A plain "black" cup of coffee is a *very* low calorie drink; 8oz only contains 2 calories! However, adding sugar, cream, and milk can quickly bump up the calorie count. A tablespoon of cream contains 52 calories, and a tablespoon of whole milk contains 9 calories. While 9 calories doesn't seem like a lot, milk is often poured into coffee without measuring, so you may be getting several servings of milk or cream in your coffee. A tablespoon of sugar contains 48 calories, so if you take your coffee with cream and sugar, you're adding over 100 extra calories to your daily cup.

It's important to be aware of and account for these calories as part of your daily eats, or consider going with skimmed milk in your coffee (only 5 calories per tablespoon).

The real caloric danger occurs in specialty mochas, lattes, or blended ice coffee drinks. These drinks are often super-sized and can contain anywhere from 200-500 calories, as well as an extremely large amount of sugar. With these drinks, it's best to enjoy them as a treat or dessert, and stick with plain, minimally sweetened coffee on a regular basis.

Protein

Protein is found throughout the body in muscle, bone, skin, hair, and virtually every other body part or tissue. It makes up the enzymes that power many chemical reactions and the haemoglobin that carries oxygen in your blood. At least 10,000 different proteins make you what you are and keep you that way.

The Institute of Medicine recommends that adults get a minimum of 0.8 grams of protein for every kilogram of body weight per day (or 8 grams of protein for every 20 pounds of body weight) (Institute of Medicine, 2005). The Institute of Medicine also sets a wide range for acceptable protein intake; anywhere from 10 to 35% of calories each day. Beyond that, there's relatively little solid information on the ideal amount of protein in the diet or the healthiest target for calories contributed by protein.

In the United States, the recommended daily allowance of protein is 46 grams per day for women over 19 years of age, and 56 grams per day for men over 19 years of age.

All Protein Isn't Alike

Protein is built from building blocks called amino acids. Our bodies make amino acids in two different ways: either from scratch, or by modifying others. A few amino acids (known as the *essential* amino acids) must come from food.

Animal sources of protein tend to deliver all the amino acids we need.
Other protein sources, such as fruits, vegetables, grains, nuts and seeds, lack one or more essential amino acids.

Vegetarians need to be aware of this. People who don't eat meat, fish, poultry, eggs, or dairy products need to eat a variety of protein-containing foods each day in order to get all the amino acids needed to make new protein.

The Protein Package

Some high-protein foods are healthier than others because of what comes along with the protein: healthy fats or harmful ones; beneficial fibre or hidden salt. It's this protein *package* that's likely to make a difference for health.

For example, a 6-ounce broiled porterhouse steak is a great source of protein - about 40 grams worth. But it also delivers about 12 grams of saturated fat (Agriculture, 2005). For someone who eats a 2,000 calorie per day diet, that's more than *60%* of the recommended daily intake for saturated fat.

A 6-ounce ham steak has only about 2.5 grams of saturated fat, but it's loaded with sodium - 2,000 milligrams worth; about 500 milligrams more than the daily sodium max.

6-ounces of wild salmon has about 34 grams of protein, is naturally low in sodium, and contains only 1.7 grams of saturated fat (Agriculture, 2005). Salmon and other fatty fish are also excellent sources of omega-3 fats, a type of fat that's especially good for the heart. Alternatively, a cup of cooked lentils provides about 18 grams of protein and 15 grams of fibre, and it has virtually no saturated fat or sodium (Agriculture, 2005).

Protein and Chronic Diseases

Proteins in food and the environment are responsible for food allergies, which are overreactions of the immune system. Beyond that, relatively little evidence has been gathered regarding the effect of the *amount of dietary protein* on the development of chronic diseases in healthy people.

However, there's growing evidence that *high-protein food choices* do play a role in health and that eating healthy protein sources like fish, chicken, beans, or nuts in place of red meat (including processed red meat) can lower the risk of several diseases and premature death (Bernstein et al, 2010 and 2012; Aune et al, 2009; Pan et al, 2012; Song et al, 2016).

Calcium and Milk

Calcium is important. But milk isn't the only (*or even best*) source. It's not a news flash that calcium is key for healthy bones. Getting enough calcium from childhood through adulthood helps build bones up and then helps slow the loss of bone as we age. It's not clear, though, that we need as much calcium as is generally recommended, and it's also not clear that dairy products are really the best source of calcium for most people.

While calcium and dairy can lower the risk of osteoporosis and colon cancer, high intake can increase the risk of prostate cancer and possibly ovarian cancer.

Plus, dairy products can be high in saturated fat as well as retinol (vitamin A), which at high levels can paradoxically weaken bones.

Good, non-dairy sources of calcium include collards, bok choy, fortified soy milk, baked beans, and supplements that contain both calcium and vitamin D (a better choice than taking calcium alone).

Staying Active

In addition to eating high-quality foods, physical activity can help you reach and maintain a healthy weight.

Getting regular physical activity is one of the best things you can do for your health. It lowers the risk of heart disease, diabetes, stroke, high blood pressure, osteoporosis, and certain cancers. It can also help control stress, improve sleep, boost mood, keep weight in check, and reduce the risk of falling and improve cognitive function in older adults.

It doesn't take marathon training to see real health gains. A 30-minute brisk walk five days a week is all most people need. Getting any amount of exercise is better than none.

Being a "couch potato" may be harmful even for people who get regular exercise.

Regular physical activity helps the body function better – it keeps heart disease, diabetes, and a host of other diseases at bay, and is a key component for losing weight.

Sit Time

More recently, studies have found that people who spend more time each day watching television, sitting, or riding in cars have a greater chance of dying early than people who are more active (Dunstan et al, 2010; Patel et al, 2010).

Researchers speculate that sitting for many hours may change peoples' metabolism in ways that promote obesity, heart disease, diabetes, and other chronic conditions (Owen et al, 2010; Hu et al, 2003; Schmid et al, 2014; Chomistek et al, 2013). It is also possible that sitting is a marker for a broader sedentary lifestyle.

Furthermore, staying active does not mitigate the harmful effects of sit time. As you plan your daily activity routine, remember that cutting down on "sit time" may be just as important as increasing "fit time."

Conclusion

As we have mentioned in previous chapters, before you can optimize your diet, it is very important to remove food intolerances, which are one of the biggest sources of inflammation in the body. Given that many food intolerances are acquired, the best advice to anyone is to ROTATE foods and never eat foods continuously, day-in, day-out. This is most certainly the best way to acquire food intolerances.

It is therefore very important that we DO NOT eat the same foods every day, even though our fast pace of life often entraps us into modes of convenience that are often difficult to break.

Chapter 6

Candida: A Universal Cause of Many Diseases

One of the health challenges that I was facing many years ago was Candida. This is also known as Systemic Candidiasis; 'systemic' means "all body."

It took me over 11 years to finally rid myself of Candida after pursuing many different therapies from experts who had written books on the subject.

I will share with you the secrets that I discovered while formulating the Da Vinci Candida Protocol that has now been published in peer-reviewed journals[83, 84]. The protocol has been implemented with over *5,000* patients at the Da Vinci Holistic Health Centre that I founded and direct in Larnaca, Cyprus, with astounding success.

It was not until I began investigating the issue myself after completing a number of degree and diploma courses in natural medicine that I eventually managed to heal myself of Candida. Through trial and error I found that many practitioners that I had seen and read about where trying to kill off the pathogenic, mycelial form of Candida using natural substances, without converting the pleomorphic, pathogenic Candida back to the normal, budding type; this really is the key to success that I will share with you in this book.

---

83 Georgiou, G.J. (2008) British Naturopathic Journal, Vol. 25.,No. 1 & 2.
84 Georgiou, G.J. (2005) Explore! Volume 14, No. 6.

Another important element of success is to change the internal milieu using the detoxification protocols that I will talk about later below. Cleaning and adjusting the pH of the body are critical elements of success.

Pathogenic, Mycelial Candida albicans: Credit Wikipedia

Let's look at the topic of Candida in more detail. With the abuse of antibiotics and sugar-laden products, I find Candida in probably 30% – 35% of all patients that I see. This percentage exceeds 70% when the patient is suffering from chronic disease. I have never seen a cancer patient who does not have Candida, particularly if they have had chemotherapy and radiation treatments.

There have been a number of books written on Systemic Candidiasis that are considered classics, which you may want to read.[85,86,87,88]

According to various surveys, Candida may be present in up to 62% of healthy people. This was shown by more than 40 surveys published between 1960 and 1986. Indeed, as long ago as 1924, candida was found in the mouths of 54% of a large

---

85 Trowbridge JP and Walker M The Yeast Syndrome Bantam Books, New York, New York 1986.
86 Truss C: The Missing Diagnosis Birmingham Alabama (The author) 1983.
87 Crook, WG. The Yeast Connection and the Woman. Professional Books, Jackson TN 1987.
[88]88 Crook WG: The Yeast Connection, A Medical Breakthrough 2nd Addition Professional Books, Jackson, TN, 1984.
Odds FC. 1988. Candida and Candidosis, 2nd edn. Bailli`ere Tindall: London.
Al-Doory Y. 1969. The mycology of the freeliving baboon (Papio sp.). Mycopathologia et Mycologia Applicata 38: 7–15.
Hesseltine HC, Campbell LK. 1938. Diabetic or mycotic vulvovaginitis. American Journal of Obstetrics and Gynecology 35:
272–283.

number of infants aged 2–6 weeks; in 46% of those up to 1 year old; and in 39% of those aged 1–6 years (Al-Doory, 1969).

In 1938, experimental vulvitis was produced by applying glucose to healthy vaginal surfaces which carried candida; while controls, free from the yeast but treated similarly, produced no signs of the disorder (Hesseltine, 1938).

This organism is responsible for buccal (oral) thrush, a disease which has been recognized for over 2,000 years. The renowned Greek physician, Hippocrates (460–~370 BC), mentions oral thrush: aphthae in the mouth. Thrush usually refers to an infection by Candida within the mucous membranes of the mouth (particularly of babies), the throat or the vagina.

Many people have non-clinical infections of Candida, but its pathogenic effects are often experienced after treatment with antibiotics, which eliminates competing bacteria.

Those with an immune system which is suppressed (by the use of immune suppressants, or from infection such as AIDS), are also particularly subject to the pathogenic effects of Candida and other yeasts.

Modern Medicine Negates its Existence

Many researchers have spent decades studying Candida and its virulent properties, yet modern medicine still negates its existence and does not believe that "normal" people can be carriers of this virulent, disease-causing, pathogenic form.

Modern medicine believes that it exists, but only in seriously ill patients whose immune system has literally become destroyed, like AIDS patients, or those who have been given drugs to suppress their immune system. Modern medicine believes that this is the best way of dealing with auto-immune diseases such as Crohn's, Lupus, Ulcerative colitis and the like.

Given that fungal candida is associated with so many symptoms, conditions, and diseases, one would think that a medical doctor would be aware of well-documented, evidence-based, scientifically-backed research that demonstrates time and time again a common causative agent. Scientists have published more than 54,000 studies on Candida, just go to https://www.ncbi.nlm.nih.gov/pubmed/?term=candida where they are listed.

Ideally, medical doctors SHOULD be aware of the possible consequences that their prescription medication could have on the patient. Giving antibiotics time and time again, without also giving prebiotics in parallel, is a sure way for patients, even young children, to develop systemic Candidiasis.

I personally have gotten into debates with various medical doctors who simply did not want to understand the relationship between Candida and the internal milieu. It appeared that they could not understand that destroying the complex and highly sensitive microbiome of the patient would not have any dire consequences.

This ignorance needs to be transcended by medical doctors to serve their patients better. There is simply no justification for it. Hopefully this book will provide enough knowledge for all to be aware of the side effects of powerful drugs, one of which is the development of systemic Candidiasis.

The widespread use of antibiotics, which induce neutropenia (an abnormally low number of neutrophils or white blood cells) and immune system suppression, is commonly attributed by science to be the most consistent cause of systemic Candida – the scientific papers on this are too many to mention here.

Corticosteroids can also suppress the immune system and this too can lead to pathogenic candidiasis. Intestinal homeostasis is critical for human health and we should nurture it, not destroy it with powerful drugs.

The science of candida and how it affects the body goes far beyond what is written here. The ability of antibiotics to create systemic fungal candida is documented in thousands of studies dating back to the introduction of antibiotics in the 1940s. This gap between science and the practice of modern medicine is a major cause of sickness and illness today.

The consequences are often *dire* to many people's health. Only recently (July 2016) the National Geographic magazine published headlines such as: *"New and Deadly Drug-Resistant Yeast Emerges Globally."* The article goes on to say:

> *"One highly resistant form of yeast, called Candida auris, has been found in several hundred cases in nine countries since 2009: on the Pacific Rim, in South Asia, in the Middle East, in the United Kingdom, and in South America. The Centers for Disease Control and Prevention (CDC) is so concerned that it recently sent an alert to U.S. hospitals, even though only one possible case of the resistant fungus has been identified in the United States so far."*

Fatal Candida auris yeast. Credit: National Geographic

They continue:

"By themselves, fungal infections - even ones that invade the bloodstream or bones - aren't a new problem. Yeasts exist throughout our environment and move from there to our guts, where their growth is held in check by the complex interactions of all the bacteria that live there. But when some of those bacteria are killed off by antibiotics - especially the long courses of drugs given in intensive-care units - or when illness or infection disrupt the immune system, yeasts can surge out of control and cause a whole-body infection. These invasive infections can be deadly, killing maybe a third of patients who develop them."

Again, in June 2016, the Daily Mail reports:

"Thirteen cases of a sometimes deadly and often drug-resistant fungal infection, Candida auris, have been reported in the United States for the first time, health officials have confirmed.

The infection, which often spreads in hospitals and other health care settings, was identified by the US Centers for Disease Control and Prevention in June 2016 as an emerging global threat.

Four of the patients diagnosed with the infection have died, although the precise causes remain unclear, the CDC said."

This is a very serious issue. Indeed, Candida overgrowth can be fatal under varying circumstances, particularly anti-fungal resistant forms that are now appearing and spreading around the world.

This simply cannot be referred to as a gap in knowledge - it is a wide chasm that millions of people fall into while under modern medical care.

As modern medicine continues its decline, patients will search for the truths that lead them back to a state of health and a life of vitality. This is the premise of this book and I see hundreds of patients from all over the world who are on this search to be healed of their Candida and other related problems.

So, let's delve into this topic so that you can really understand what Candida is, how do you get it, and more importantly, how do you treat it.

What is Candida?

Every person lives in a virtual sea of microorganisms (bacteria, viruses, parasites, stealth organisms and fungi). These microbes can reside in the throat, mouth, nose, intestinal tract, almost anywhere; they are as much a part of our bodies as the food we eat. Usually, these microorganisms do not cause illness, unless our resistance becomes lowered.

Candida albicans is yeast that lives in the mouth, throat, intestines and genitourinary tract of most humans and is usually considered to be a normal part of the bowel flora (the organisms that coexist with us in our lower digestive tract). It is a member of a broader classification of organisms known as fungi.

Candida are unicellular yeasts, somewhat larger than bacteria, that divide mostly asexually, can switch between a yeast and a pseudohyphal or hyphal form and, like other yeasts, flourish in habitats where there is an abundance of sugar.

Pathogenic, mycelial Candida

Candida are normal human commensals, particularly in the mouth, skin, vagina and intestine. Candida can be cultured from faeces in up to 80% of healthy adults[89]. Candida numbers increase significantly following antibacterial therapy[90], but the numbers seem to be unaffected by a refined carbohydrate diet[91]. It seems likely that intestinal Candida numbers are regulated in a similar way to intestinal bacteria[92].

C. Albicans and C. glabrata are the two most common Candida species that cause Systemic Candidiasis. There are 81 different types of Candida species such as C. glabrata, krusei, lusitaniae, parapsilosis, tropicalis and more, but only half a dozen are commonly found in humans, with C. albicans dominating. More than 70% of Candida species found in humans are Candida albicans.

How Does Candida Behave?
Some strains of Candida produce gliotoxin which may impair neutrophil function[93]. However, it is a polyantigenic organism containing up to 178 different antigens[94], which might explain the number of cross-reactions to yeasts (Malassezia, bread/brewer's yeast) and moulds[95] and even human tissue[96].

It was shown recently that there is a potential cross reactivity with gluten. Such a mechanism might lead to wheat intolerance with its accompanying symptoms and even trigger celiac disease in genetically susceptible people[97]. Furthermore, a placebo controlled crossover study revealed that dietary yeast may affect the activity of Crohn's disease[98].

---

89 Bernhardt H, Knoke M. Mycological aspects of gastrointestinal microflora. Scand J Gastroenterol 1997; 32(suppl 222) :102–106.

90 Seelig MS. Mechanisms by which antibiotics increase the incidence and severity of candidiasis and alter the immunological defences. Bacteriol Rev 1 1966; 30 :4442–4459.

91 Weig M, Werner E, Frosh M, Kasper H. Limited effect of refined carbohydrate dietary supplementation on colonization of the gastrointestinal tract of healthy subjects by Candida albicans. Am J Clin Nutr 1999; 69 :1170–1173.

92 Fitzsimmons N, Berry DR. Inhibition of Candida albicans by Lactobacillus acidophilus: evidence for the involvement of a peroxidase system. Microbios 1994; 80 :125–133.

93 Shah DT, Jackman S, Engle J, Larsen B. Effect of gliotoxin on human polymorphonuclear neutrophils. Inf Dis Obster Gynecol 1998; 6 :168–175.

94 Poulain D, Hopwood V, Vernes A. Antigenic variability of candida albicans. CRC Crit Rev Microbiol 1985; 12:223-70.

95 Koivikko A, et al.. Allergenic cross-reactivity of yeasts. Allergy 1988; 43:192-200.

96 Vojdani A, Rahimian P, Kalhor H and Mordechai E. Immunological cross reactivity between candida albicans and human tissue. J Clin Lab Immunol 1996; 48:1-15.

97 Nieuwenhuizen WF, Pieters RH, Knippels LM, Jansen MC, Koppelman GJ. Is Candida albicans a trigger for the onset of coeliac disease? Lancet 2003; 361 :2152–2154.

98 Barclay GR, McKenzie H, Pennington J, Parratt D, Pennington CR. The effect of dietary yeast on the activity of stable chronic Crohn's disease. Scand J Gastroenterol 1992; 27 :196–200.

Candida produces alcohol and contains glycoproteins which have the potential to stimulate mast cells to release histamine and prostaglandin (PGE2), inflammatory substances which could cause IBS-like symptoms[99,100].

Secretory immunoglobulin A (SIgA) is front-line in the defence of mucous membranes, especially in the intestine where it is active against infectious agents and certain antigens[101]. At least three different Candida species are able to produce proteases[102]. This protease can induce inflammation. An infection of the intestinal mucosa with Candida might lead to inflammation in patients with IBS symptoms.

Candida is sensitive to a number of antifungal agents, such as nystatin, which is not absorbed from the gastrointestinal tract after oral administration.

Candida is a diploid organism which has eight sets of chromosome pairs. Interestingly, Candida is one of the few microorganisms that have a diploid gene controlling the same protein – this means that it is capable of pleomorphic activity, being able to mutate forms from the budding form to the mycelial, pathogenic form.

When Does Candida Become a Problem?
The problem begins when the normal, budding Candida species that we have in our gut, which 90% of babies are born with, actually changes form to the mycelial or hyphae form, which is pathogenic or disease-causing. This only happens when the internal milieu of the gut and other tissues becomes more acidic, either through taking a variety of drugs such as antibiotics that wipes out the friendly flora of the gut, or through eating very acidic foods such as sugar and other refined products.

---

[99] Romani L, Bistoni F, Puccetti P. Initiation of T-helper cell immunity to Candida albicans by IL-12: the role of neutrophils. Chem Immunol. 1997; 68:110-35.
100 Kanda N, Tani K, Enomoto U, Nakai K & Watanabe S. The skin fungus-induced Th1- and Th2-related cytokine, chemokine and prostaglandin E 2 production in peripheral blood mononuclear cells from patients with atopic dermatitis and psoriasis vulgaris. Clinical & Experimental Allergy; 32(8):1243-50.
[101] Brandtzaeg P. The mucosal B cell and its functions. In: Brostoff J, Challacombe S (eds): Food Allergy and Intolerance. London: Saunders; 2002:127-171.
[102] Reinholdt J, Krogh P, Holmstrup P. Degradation of IgA1, IgA2, and S-IgA by candida and torulopsis species. Acta Path Microbiol Immunol Scand, Sect C 1987; 95:65-74.

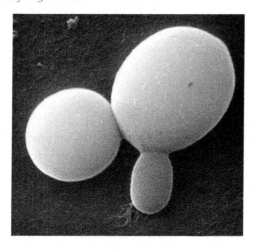

Normal, budding Candida

It appears that this change in pH can trigger genes in the Candida to begin a pleomorphic change into a stealth organism that is very virulent. If fed with sugar, it can increase itself from 1 to 100 cells in 24 hours. These 100 cells can then produce 100 each in the next 24 hours, and so on, so by the 4th day we will have 100 million Candida cells – this is really exponential, explosive growth!

Research has shown that it does not take longer than 1-2 days for this pathogenic form to get deep into the body tissues, inflaming them and damaging them in the process.

Normal, budding Candida on left; pathogenic on right

Fungus has many faces

A distinctive characteristic of Candida is its ability to grow with three distinct morphologies:

205

1. Yeast

2. Pseudohyphae

3. True hyphae

See Fig 1 below that illustrates the difference between these 3 forms. This is the same fungus, but it can change forms when given the right circumstances. This is typically known as PLEOMORPHISM, which is the Greek word for "many shapes or morphologies".

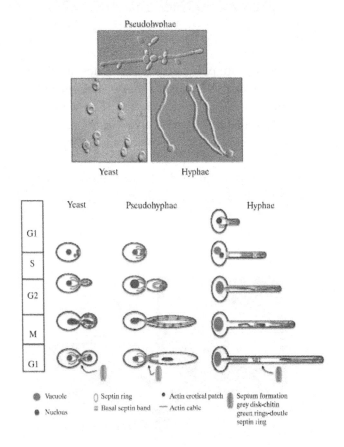

Fig 1. Different growth morphologies of Candida (reproduced from Sudbery et al., 2004).

Of all these forms, the Hyphal form is the worst. It can be aggressive and destroy tissues, causing disease. In other words, it is virulent or disease causing.

This form of virulent fungus is created when environmental conditions are conducive; 37°C growth temperature, the presence of serum, neutral pH, high CO2, growth in embedded conditions, and the presence N-acetylglucosamine.

Figure 3 shows this aggressive, hyphal form of Candida aggressively infiltrating the human small intestine.

Figure 2: Yeast, hyphal and pseudohyphal morphologies.

Fig 3. Candida albicans on human small intestine mucosa

The less virulent, yeast form of Candida favours a 30°C growth temperature and acidic pH (pH 4.0).

Pseudohyphal growth is an intermediate, transitional stage between the yeast form (less virulent) to the most virulent, hyphal form. This can occur in temperatures of 35°C or a pH of 5.5.

Biofilms

Have you ever picked up a rock from a nearby stream and wondered why it's slimy on the surface? That slimy layer is a group of microorganisms, collectively called a biofilm.

A biofilm is a community of bacteria that attach to a surface by excreting a sticky, sugary substance that encompasses the bacteria in a matrix. This might be the first time you've heard the term biofilm, but they're all around us, in streams, in drains, in fish tanks, even on our teeth.

A biofilm can be composed of a single species or a conglomerate of species. In many cases, biofilms are only bacteria, but they can also include other living things such as fungi and algae, creating a microbial stew of sorts. Biofilms are complex systems that are sometimes compared to multicellular organisms.

Biofilm of Candida

Candida is able to form a biofilm that basically protects it from being attacked by the immune system of the host (Blankenship and Mitchell, 2006; Nobile and Mitchell, 2006).

This biofilm of Candida is composed of protein polypeptides, polysaccharide carbohydrates, fibrinogen or fibrin and polynucleotides that contain RNA and DNA material. This structure is bound together with ligands that have stickiness properties.

As we will see later, the Enlyse™ enzymes present in one of the remedies used for treating Candida – Kandidaplex - can eradicate this biofilm, hence allowing the immune system to do its work.

How Does Candida Attack the Body?

When candida attacks the body, it does it in various stages. First is interaction with the host cells by adhesion. Candida acts bit like glue, binding to extracellular matrix proteins of mucosal or endothelial cells (Calderone, et al, 2001; Grubb et al, 2008).

The close association with cell surfaces stimulates the formation of biofilms that we have already mentioned above (Kumato et al, 2005). The biofilm surrounds the yeast cells like a protective cocoon and keeps out attacks from the environment, including the immune system.

These biofilms can also make the Candida more resistant to anti-fungal drugs by pushing out these drugs from the cells. It also reduces production of ergosterol in the cell membrane, which makes the yeast cells less sensitive to anti-fungals by a factor of 30 to 2000 (Douglas, L.J., 2003).

Candida is also able to rapidly change its cell surface structure, making it more difficult for the immune system to recognize it. This is known as "phenotypic switching" (Soll, D.R., 2002; Morita, E 1999; Pappas et al, 2004; Reinel et al, 2008).

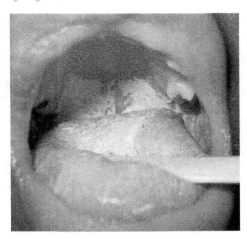

Candida attacking the mouth

As a consequence, the immune system can no longer recognize the fungi or initiate an immune reaction (Bastidas et al, 2009; Romani et al, 2003; Berman, J, 2006).

Some Candida strains avoid the attacks of the immune system by concealing themselves in host cells. They can survive unharmed in epithelial cells (Filler et al, 2006) or in non-activated white blood cells called macrophages (Raska et al, 2007; Dalkilic et al, 1991) and even replicate there.

In summary
Traditionally, fungi are considered plants, but they contain no chlorophyll and cannot make their own food. Fungi tend to inhabit cool to tropical climates.

The problem begins when the normal, budding yeast cell Candida that we have in our gut, which 90% of babies are born with, actually change forms to the mycelial or hyphae form which causes disease. This only happens when the internal milieu of the gut and other tissues change, either through taking a variety of drugs such as antibiotics that wipes out the friendly flora of the gut, or through eating acidic foods. Repressing the immune system certainly does not help matters either.

How is Candida Diagnosed?

Dr. Crook, an American trained medical doctor and lecturer, after repeated observations of his patients became interested in chronic health complaints related to yeast overgrowth and to nutritional and environmental factors.

Dr Crook was one of the modern-day pioneers who published, *The Yeast Connection* and brought the concept of yeast infections to the public eye, while also trying to teach his colleagues, which was not easy at the best of times. In his book, he developed a comprehensive questionnaire of many of the symptoms that are related to systemic Candidiasis.

Dr. Crook's Candida questionnaire (see Appendix) is very helpful because it enables the patient to score their symptoms and arrive at a number. Anything above 180 for women, and 140 for men is highly significant and represents the majority of symptoms that relate to Candida infestation.

There are also other testing procedures for picking up the Candida; the Vegetative Reflex Testing (VRT) biodermal screening, a form of Bioresonance testing initially invented by Dr Voll and later adapted by Dr Schimmel, is one.

The VRT testing is capable of highlighting the causes of illnesses by using homoeopathic biosonodes, this is usually a small portion of diseased tissue from a diseased organ that is ground up and made into a homoeopathic remedy.

When a particular biosonode that is placed on the honeycomb on the Bioresonance testing device induces a resonance reaction in the acupoint, then this infers a relationship between the diseased organ being tested and the related organ of the patient.

Even bacteria, viruses, fungi, stealth organisms and more can be tested for resonance with the patient and identified much quicker than any other type of biological testing.

In the case of identifying the pathological, hyphal form of Candida, as long as the practitioner has an ampoule of this form, then it is very easy to test whether the patient is resonating to it. In the hands of an experienced practitioner, this is an accurate and efficient way of testing, given that there are no real clinical tests for pathological Candida that have been developed yet.

There are a number of Bioresonance testing devices including the VEGA, the BICOM, the DETA PROFESSIONAL and more. The most cost effective device is the DETA PROFESSIONAL (http://www.deta-elis-uk.com).

I run 5-day intensive clinical workshops 3-4 times per year training practitioners to use VRT Bioresonance testing and treatment in Larnaca, Cyprus. There is also an online course to help practitioners understand the theory entitled, *Energy Medicine and Bioresonance* (http://www.collegenaturalmedicine.com).

Another method of testing for Candida is to use a form of kinesiological muscle testing called Autonomic Response Testing (ART), invented by a German neurologist, Dr. Dietrich Klinghardt, M.D. Ph.D. ART grew out of the importance of detecting and correct problems of the autonomic nervous system (ANS).

ART allows the practitioner to correct the problems of the ANS and to help restore the self-regulating mechanism of the body, allowing the patient to return to a state of health naturally.

To date, there is no conclusive blood or clinical test for diagnosing pathogenic Systemic Candidiasis. There are expensive genetic tests that can determine the genome of the mycelial, hyphal, pathogenic Candida, but these are not generally available on the open market as yet and are more used for research purposes. The other way is to examine tissue taken during a biopsy, as I have already mentioned above.

Conclusive laboratory tests have not yet been developed, even though there are a number of tests that can help in the diagnosis.

Other Factors Creating Pathogenesis
When other health conditions become involved, Candida becomes known as Candida-related complex (CRC). CRC, an excess of Candida in your system can cause a host of uncomfortable signs and symptoms which are syndromes within themselves, such as chronic fatigue syndrome, hypoglycemia, leaky gut syndrome, fibromyalgia, allergy or sensitivity, hormonal, thyroid, and adrenal dysfunction.

This syndrome isn't caused by Candida itself, but by the number of metabolites yeast colonies release inside the human colon when they exceed tolerable amounts.

Patients with CRC often have widespread symptoms affecting multiple organs systems such as:

❖ Gastrointestinal symptoms

❖ Chronic allergies

❖ Unexplained fatigue; always tired

❖ CNS fog, mood swings, depression

❖ Skin rashes, fungal infections

❖ Cravings for sugar, bread, beer

Toxicity in the colon affects the health of the whole body, particularly if one's elimination is slowed as in the case of constipation due to an imbalance in intestinal flora.

The delicate hormonal and chemical balance that orchestrates our emotional health can also be affected causing symptoms of mental illness.

Everyone can be Affected with Candida!

Anyone can be infected with Candida today! Women can be infected because of antibiotics, steroids, anti-inflammatory medications, hormones and birth-control pills. Men are also being infected with Candida from antibiotics, steroids, anti-inflammatory drugs, pain medications, and sexual relations with an infected partner (even though this often results in a topical infection, not a systemic spread).

Teenagers can get Candida from routine treatment with tetracycline or other antibiotics for acne. Babies have Candida from the birth canal or breast milk of the infected mother. That is why babies often have thrush (a white- coated tongue), which is a yeast infection.

Millions of people all over the world are infected with Candida. It is estimated that at least one out of three people in the Western world are affected. Because so many of the population can be infected and because so many factors can cause the condition, Candida is an enormous health problem today.

Candida coexists in our bodies with many species of bacteria in a competitive balance. Other bacteria act in part to keep Candida growth in check in our body ecology, when health is present, the immune system keeps Candida proliferation under control. But when the immune response is weakened, Candida growth can proceed unchecked.

What is the role of Candida?

Candida has two parasitic functions:

1. Gobble up any putrefied food matter in our digestive system (mostly caused by improper digestion due to low stomach acid).

2. After we die, Candida acts to decompose the body, feeding off our corpse and returning us to Mother Earth!

When conditions are right, they transform their yeast form into the hyphal, mycelial state, where filament-like roots invade deep into the mucosa in search of nourishment. The mycelia release enzymes such as phospholipase that attacks cell membranes of the mucosa, splitting fatty acids, generating free radicals, and causing inflammation in the intestine and other tissues.

Wherever the yeast colonizes they cause symptoms, whether an itchy anus or vagina, diarrhea, heartburn or sore throat. The mycelial forms release 79 different toxic by-products that damage specific tissues and organs and will determine which symptoms will occur.

These toxins, such as aldehyde, can also compete with hormone receptor sites and cause hypothyroidism, hypoestrogenism as well as binding cortisone, progesterone and other hormones for its own use and causing endocrine deficiency states.

How do you get it?

Candida albicans prefers people. Candida enters newborn infants during or shortly after birth. Usually, the growth of the yeast is kept in check by the infant's immune system and thus produces no overt symptoms. But, should the immune response weaken, the condition known as oral thrush can occur. By six months of age, 90% of all babies test positive for Candida and by adulthood, virtually all humans play host to Candida albicans and are thus engaged in a life-long relationship.

Unfortunately, there are many factors in our modern society that can upset the ecological balance of the body, weaken the immune system and allow the yeast to overgrow. The major risk factors, which may predispose one to the proliferation of Candida, are:

❖ **STEROID HORMONES, IMMUNOSUPPRESSANT DRUGS** such as cortisone, which treat severe allergic problems by paralyzing the immune system's ability to react.

❖ **PREGNANCY, MULTIPLE PREGNANCIES or BIRTH CONTROL PILLS** which upset the body's hormonal balance.

❖ **DIETS HIGH IN CARBOHYDRATE AND SUGAR INTAKE, YEAST AND YEAST PRODUCTS, AS WELL AS MOULDS AND FERMENTED FOODS.**

❖ **PROLONGED EXPOSURE TO ENVIRONMENTAL MOULDS.**

❖ **ANTIBIOTICS and SULPHA DRUGS** - probably the chief culprit of all. Antibiotics kill all bacteria. They do not distinguish good bacteria from bad. Antibiotics kill the "good" flora which normally keeps the Candida under control. This allows for the unchecked growth of Candida in the intestinal tract.

In the Kaiser Health News report in June 2016, this was what was said against antibiotics and the lethal fungus that can be created (a Candida species known as C. auris):

Hospitalized patients are at especially high risk from the fungus because many have had antibiotics, which can kill off healthy bacteria that help protect us from disease, said Peter Hotez, dean of the National School of Tropical Medicine at Baylor College of Medicine in Houston.

It's a warning or wake-up against the indiscriminate use of antibiotics, especially in hospital settings," Hotez said.

Hospitals have been testing for the fungus more frequently due to outbreaks in Asia and the United Kingdom, said Amesh Adalja, senior associate at the UPMC Center for Health Security in Baltimore.

In earlier outbreaks, the fungus has killed 59 percent of patients, including 68 percent of patients whose infection spread to the bloodstream, said Adalja, who published a brief report on the infection Friday. Previous patients have had a median age of 54, Adalja said. The most common underlying medical problem was diabetes, and half of the patients had undergone surgery within 90 days. Nearly 80 percent of patients had a catheter placed in a major vein in the chest and 61 percent had a urinary catheter.

"Candida auris is a major threat that carries a high mortality," Adalja said. "Candida fungal species are ubiquitous. ... As we learn more about this species, it will be essential to understand how it spreads in health care facilities and what the best infection control and treatment strategies are."

Antibiotic Abuse and Inappropriate Prescribing

The prevalence today of Candida may be most directly related to the widespread societal exposure to antibiotics - from prescriptions for colds, infections, acne, and from additional consumption of antibiotic-treated foods such as meats, dairy, poultry and eggs.

Notably, antibiotics do not kill viruses; they destroy bacteria. Yet, they are universally prescribed for all colds, flus and other viral problems. Such indiscriminate and extensive use of antibiotics is not only considered a primary cause of Candida overgrowth, but is recently being found to be responsible for the unbridled development of "killer bacteria."

The rapid and direct proliferation of the yeast following antibiotic use strongly suggests that the problem of Candida is one which stems from an inner state of imbalance, rather than from an outside attack by a microbe or disease. This is a very important point to understand if one wishes to get rid of an overgrowth problem, suggesting that Candida is not so much a problem as is the body's own failure to control it!

- ❖ Incorrectly prescribed antibiotics also contribute to the promotion of resistant bacteria (Center for Disease Control and Prevention).

- ❖ Studies have shown that treatment indication, choice of agent, or duration of antibiotic therapy is incorrect in 30% to 50% of cases (Luyt, C.E, 2014).

- ❖ One U.S. study reported that a pathogen was defined in only 7.6% of 17,435 patients hospitalized with community-acquired pneumonia (CAP) (Barlett, J.G., 2013).

- ❖ In comparison, investigators at the Karolinska Institute in Sweden were able to identify the probable pathogen in 89% of patients with CAP through use of molecular diagnostic techniques (polymerase chain reaction [PCR] and semiquantitative PCR), therefore prescribing the correct antibiotics for this particular health problem, as opposed to experimenting with many different types, to the detriment of the patient.

- ❖ In addition, 30% to 60% of the antibiotics prescribed in intensive care units (ICUs) have been found to be unnecessary, inappropriate, or suboptimal (Luyt, C.E., 2014).

- ❖ Incorrectly prescribed antibiotics have questionable therapeutic benefit and expose patients to potential complications of antibiotic therapy (Lushniak, B.D., 2014).

- ❖ Sub-inhibitory and sub-therapeutic antibiotic concentrations can promote the development of antibiotic resistance by supporting genetic alterations, such as changes in gene expression, HGT, and mutagenesis (Viswanathan, V.K.,2014).

- ❖ Changes in antibiotic-induced gene expression can increase virulence, while increased mutagenesis and HGT promote antibiotic resistance and spread.

- ❖ Low levels of antibiotics have been shown to contribute to strain diversification in organisms such as *Pseudomonas aeruginosa*. Sub-inhibitory concentrations of piperacillin and/or tazobactam have also been shown to induce broad proteomic alterations in *Bacteroides fragilis*.

Symptoms Related to Candida

There are many symptoms that can be caused by Candida – the following list is Dr. Jeff McComb's, D.C., a chiropractor working in the U.S. who has also created a

Candida Library with hundreds of research papers on Candida – see http://www.candidalibrary.org/cand_lib/.

This is a list of 100 Common Candida Symptoms associated with systemic fungal candida from his website:

ADD	ADHD	Acid reflux	Acne	Allergies
Anxiety	Arthritis	Asthma	Athlete's foot	Autism
Autoimmune conditions	Bladder infections	Blisters in mouth	Bloating	Blood sugar imbalances
Body odour	BPH	Brain fog	Bronchitis	Burping
Cancer	Chemical sensitivities	Chronic Fatigue Syndrome	Colitis	Concentration difficulty
Confusion	Congestion	Constipation	Crohn's Disease	Cough
Cystitis	Depression	Dermatitis	Diabetes	Diarrhoea
Eczema	Endometriosis	Excess mucous	Fibromyalgia	Flatulence
Fluid retention	Food allergies	Food cravings	Frequent colds	Frequent infections
Fungal infections	Gas	Gastritis	Genital rashes	Headaches
Heartburn	Hormonal imbalances	Hypoglycaemia	Hypothyroidism	Irritability
Inflammatory Bowel Disease	Immune system dysfunction	Impotence	Indigestion	Infertility
Irregular menstruation	Itchy skin	Joint pain	Lack of mental clarity	Leaky gut

Lethargy	Lupus	Migraines	Memory problems	Mood swings
Muscle pain	Nail fungus	Osteoarthritis	Penile itching	PMS
Poor concentratio n	Poor memory	Prostatitis	Prostate enlargement	Psoriasis
Rashes	Rectal itching	Rheumatoid arthrit is	Rhinitis	Scleroderma
Sexual dysfunction	Sinus problems	Sores	Sore throat	Sugar cravings
Swollen joints	Thrush	Urethritis	Vaginitis	
Weakness	Weight gain	White coating on tongue		

Why is it a serious problem?

Once begun, if not recognized and treated appropriately, Candida overgrowth can result in a self-perpetuating, negative cycle. Large numbers of yeast germs can weaken the immune system, which normally protects the body from harmful invaders. Even though Candida is part of the ecological balance in the body since birth, it is still recognized by the immune system as a foreign body that needs to be controlled.

So, when overgrowth occurs, a chronic stimulation to the immune system results - every second, every minute, every hour, every day, every month, every year - in an attempt by the immune system to regain control. In time, it is believed that this can exhaust the immune system, predisposing one to more serious degenerative processes. Many believe chronic drains on the immune system such as Candida and parasites can play a direct role in the development of cancer and AIDS. Seen in this light, Candida overgrowth should not be taken lightly.

Candida produces its effects by two routes. Firstly, there is a direct route initially by invasion of the gut and the vagina; Candida is capable of spreading along the entire length of the gut. The presence of chronic vaginitis can often indicate wide-spread Candidiasis. Secondly, there can be indirect effects caused by spread of mycotoxins through the bloodstream to other sites.

In the gut, Candida can alter its form from a simple yeast organism to a "mycelial fungal form" with a network of root-like fibres called rhizoids. These can penetrate and damage the gut lining, allowing foreign food proteins to be absorbed into the bloodstream and to challenge the immune system so that multiple food allergies or intolerances may result.

Electron micrograph of Candida

Toxic waste from Candida infestations can also be absorbed into the bloodstream causing "Yeast Toxin Hypersensitivity" leading to many symptoms such as anxiety, depression and impaired intellectual functioning. The main toxin implicated here is acetaldehyde, which is a normal by-product of metabolism, produced in small amounts and rendered harmless by the liver.

If, however, there is excess production of this by Candida, particularly in low-oxygen environments, and a lack of the appropriate liver enzymes which tend to be deficient in 5% of the general population, the acetaldehyde will bind strongly to human tissue. This may cause impaired neuro-transmission in the brain, resulting in anxiety, depression, defective memory and cloudy thinking.

Electron micrograph of Rhizoid penetrating tissue

Acetaldehyde, one of the mycotoxins secreted by Candida, mediates a good part of the cellular damage that occurs. Acetaldehyde in the intestinal wall and liver will disrupt intestinal absorptive processes, as well as impairing the function of lymphocytes and red blood cells. Acetaldehyde is damaging to host cells by free radical and peroxidative mechanisms. When yeast cells are limited in oxygen, they are also more resistant to immune defenses. Patient hypoxia is a major contributing factor to yeast susceptibility, for these two reasons.

Adequate amounts of glutamine, selenium, niacin, folic acid, B6, B12, iron, and molybdenum will allow the aldehydes to be metabolized into acetic acid, which can be excreted, or converted further into acetyl coenzyme A. Certainly, patients exhibiting toxic syndrome while treating Candida are highly recommended to take these food supplements for their own protection.

Effects on Immunity

Some 40 to 60% of all the immune cells in our body are in the gut. The immune system may concurrently be adversely affected by poor nutrition, heavy exposure to moulds in the air, as well as an increasing number of chemicals in our food, water and air, including petrochemicals, formaldehyde, perfumes, cleaning fluids, insecticides, tobacco and other indoor and outdoor pollutants.

Over 10,000 chemicals have been added to our food supplies alone that were not there just 100 years ago! We do not have the genetic recognition of these substances as foods or as useful additions to our bodies.

Specifically, yeast tend to secrete a toxin called Gliotoxin[103], which can disrupt the immune system by inactivating enzyme systems, producing free radicals, interfering with the DNA of leukocytes and being cytotoxic.

Resulting lowered resistance may not only cause an overall sense of ill health, but also may allow for the development of respiratory, digestive and other systemic symptoms. One may also become predisposed to developing sensitivities to foods and chemicals in the environment. Such "allergies" may in turn cause the membranes of the nose, throat, ear, bladder and intestinal tract to swell and develop infection.

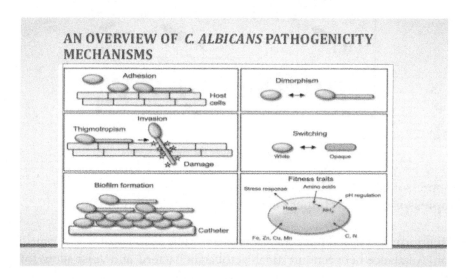

Such conditions may lead the physician to prescribe a "broad spectrum" antibiotic which may then further promote the overgrowth of Candida and strengthen the existing negative chain of events, leading to further stress on the immune system and increased Candida-related problems.

I have seen this happen in clinical practice many times. If only physicians could think laterally for a minute, many hundreds of thousands of superfluous antibiotic prescriptions could be done away with to the benefit of the patient as opposed to the pharmaceutical industry. Physicians talk about evidence-based medicine, but often drugs such as antibiotics are prescribed for the wrong infections because testing was not done in the first place.

---

[103] Iwata, K.; Yamamoto, Y "Glycoprotein Toxins Produced by Candida albicans." Proceedings of the Fourth International Conference on the Mycoses, PAHO Scientific Publication #356, June 1977.

Candida overgrowth results in production of the highly toxic canditoxin and ethanol which are known to cause fatigue, toxicity, and depressive symptoms. Another study found such impairment of neutrophils decreases the body's ability to combat viruses such as those that cause heart damage, resulting in more inflammatory damage.

The diagram below (Fig 5) clearly shows how Candida is known to impair immune functioning by directly and negatively impacting the helper-suppresser ratio of T lymphocytes.

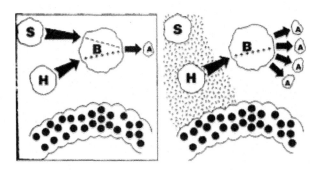

Fig 5: How Yeast Toxins Injure the Immune System

S = Suppressor cell; H = Helper cell; B = B-cell
S=Suppressor cell; H=Helper cell; B=B-cell; A=Antibodies

First diagram: Yeast and intestinal lactobacilli bacteria in balance = normal immune function. A balance between intestinal lactobacilli bacteria and yeast allow for normal immune lymphocyte function. Helper cells stimulate the B-cells to make antibodies, whereas suppressor cells appropriately oppose B-cell antibody production. Antibody production is in balance.

Second diagram: Overgrowth of intestinal yeast, release of toxins into the bloodstream, and altered immune function. Intestinal yeast overgrowth and yeast toxins released into the bloodstream inhibit suppressor cell function. Stimulation of antibody production by helper cells is now unopposed, and inappropriate antibody production occurs. Here we have a heightened state of allergy, as well as an increased susceptibility to autoimmune conditions.

The main components of the immune system are:

1. <u>B-lymphocytes</u>; these produce proteins called immunoglobulins, which bind antigenic substances and render them harmless. An antigen is a substance which the body recognizes as being alien and therefore potentially harmful. An immunoglobulin is a particular kind of protein which coats the antigen;

by being made harmless the antigens can then be digested by other cells.

2. <u>T-lymphocytes</u>; there are three types:

   a. The killer cells; these attack and destroy substances with enzymes and hormones.

   b. The helper cells; these help B cells to make the immunoglobulins.

   c. The suppressor cells; these protect the body from the excesses of the body's defence system.

T-cell efficiency can be influenced to a useful extent by nutrition. It is largely the suppressors which are involved in fighting the Candida challenge, partly because Candida's adaptability allows it to produce disguising antigens which deter the immune system from recognizing it as foreign and harmful. In this way, the immune system may eventually become non-responsive to the presence of Candida albicans. Candida toxins will then circulate virtually unchallenged, and Candida will grow in a range of tissues either as a yeast or a mycelial fungus.

This apparent tolerance of Candida by the immune system can only be reversed in the long term by ending exposure of the body to yeast antigens and toxins. A high percentage of serum from symptomless people has been found to contain yeast toxin immunoglobulins. This indicates that the B-cell immune defenses must be constantly counteracting Candida toxin.

When alive, yeasts are able to invade the immune system to a certain degree. When they are killed, proteins making up the yeast cell wall are absorbed through the lining of the intestine and can cause heightened allergy reactions, resulting in a phenomenon called 'Die off' or the 'Herxheimer reaction'. This may in fact signal a good response to treatment.

What are the signs of Candida infection?

Basically, the characteristics of Candida overgrowth fall under three categories, those affecting:

1. The gastrointestinal and genitourinary tracts
2. Allergic responses
3. Mental/emotional manifestations

Initially, the signs will show near the sights of the original yeast colonies. Most often the first signs are seen in conditions such as nasal congestion and discharge, nasal itching, blisters in the mouth, sore or dry throat, abdominal pain, belching, bloating, heartburn, constipation, diarrhea, rectal burning or itching, vaginal discharge, vaginal itching or burning, increasingly worsening symptoms of PMS, prostatitis, impotence, frequent urination, burning on urination, and bladder infections.

White blood cell killing Candida

But, if the immune system remains weak for long enough, Candida can spread to all parts of the body causing an additional plethora of problems such as fatigue, drowsiness, incoordination, lack of concentration, mood swings, dizziness, headaches, bad breath, coughing, wheezing, joint swelling, arthritis, failing vision, spots in front of the eyes, ear pain, deafness, burning or tearing eyes, muscle aches, depression, irritability, sweet cravings, increasing food and chemical sensitivities, numbness and tingling, cold hands and feet, asthma, hay fever, multiple allergies, hives and rashes, eczema, psoriasis, chronic fungal infections like athlete's foot, ringworm and fingernail/toenail infections.

In addition, *79 different toxic products* are released by Candida, which in itself places a considerable burden on the immune system. These get into the bloodstream and travel to all parts of the body where they may give rise to a host of adverse symptoms. Yeasts in the body produce a by-product called acetaldehyde, a toxic substance resulting in several health consequences. In fact, acetaldehyde is the compound that produces the symptoms in an alcohol "hang-over."

Molybdenum plays a role as a cofactor in helping break down acetaldehyde to a form that actually provides the body with energy. Molybdenum plays a large role in the detoxification pathway for acetaldehyde in the human body. There are dozens of

224

known toxins released by yeast in the body. This damages and overworks both the liver and the immune system as the body tries to detoxify these poisons.

In Candida overgrowth, the yeast colonies can dig deep into intestinal walls, damaging the bowel wall in their colonization. The invasive Candida filaments produce disease affecting the entire body in a number of ways:

Destruction of the intestinal membrane, allowing for:

❖ Severe leaks of toxins from activity of undesirable microorganisms within the layers of encrusted fecal matter into the bloodstream causing a variety of symptoms and aggravating many pre-existing conditions.

❖ Absorption of incompletely digested dietary proteins. These are extremely allergenic and may produce a large spectrum of allergic reactions. Food allergies are very common with Candidiasis, as is environmental hypersensitivity (to smoke, auto exhaust, natural gas, perfumes, air pollutants), probably due to Candida filaments infiltrating lung and sinus membranes.

❖ Migration of Candida itself into the bloodstream. Once in the blood, it has access to all body tissues and may cause various gland or organ dysfunctions, weakening the entire system and further lowering resistance to other diseases.

Candida can also attack the immune system, causing suppressor cell disease, in which the immune system produces antibodies to everything at the slightest provocation, resulting in extreme sensitivities.

Women are more likely to get Candida overgrowth than are men. This is related to the female sex hormone progesterone which is elevated in the last half of the menstrual cycle. Progesterone increases the amount of glycogen (animal starch, easily converted to sugar) in the vaginal tissues which provide an ideal growth medium for Candida. Progesterone levels also elevate during pregnancy. Men are affected less frequently but are by no means invulnerable.

The Relationship Between Candida and Chronic Diseases
A number of natural medicine practitioners have long been supporting the notion that intestinal fungi can contribute to chronic diseases.

However, the allopathic medical fraternity has been downplaying the role of intestinal fungi. This is largely due to the fact that little research has been done; it's difficult to diagnose and it can't be treated properly with pharmaceuticals.

New research at Cedars-Sinai Medical Center looked at the connection between fungi and Ulcerative Colitis.

Dr. David M. Underhill and his team at the Inflammatory Bowel and Immunobiology Research Institute have been studying the interaction between Commensal Fungi and the C-Type Lectin Receptor, Dectin-1. In healthy animals Dectin-1 is produced and works as the body's immune response against fungi.

The risk of developing Ulcerative Colitis increases significantly in mice with a defective form of Dectin-1. Dr. Underhill and his team treated these animals with an antifungal drug called Fluconazole and observed that their symptoms moderated.

In humans, a mutated form of Dectin-1 is closely related to Ulcerative Colitis that doesn't respond to medical therapy. When this important receptor isn't working properly, our protection against intestinal fungi is decreased and we are more prone to developing Candidiasis.

It's already known that gut flora in patients with UC differs significantly from healthy individuals. The fungal colonization of the colon may influence the activation of UC, and antifungal treatment causes clinical improvement in most individuals. Patients with Crohn's disease and their healthy relatives are colonized with Candida more commonly than control families.

30 years after, *The Missing Diagnosis* by Orian Truss and, *The Yeast Connection* by William Crook were released, there's growing research in the medical community on the importance of gut flora and intestinal fungi.

Candida has also been correlated with chronic inflammatory diseases such as arthritis and multiple sclerosis. That was the implication of a 2012 study in the prestigious journal *Nature*, conducted by researchers from Charite – Universitatsmedizin, Berlin and the Institute for Research in Biomedicine, Bellinzona, Switzerland.

The study found that cells of Candida seemed to trigger the immune system to produce more inflammation.
The findings are particularly significant because the immune cells being studied play a key role in autoimmune diseases such as multiple sclerosis, rheumatoid arthritis and psoriasis.

"This not only demonstrates that the composition of our microflora has a decisive role in the development of chronic illnesses, but also that the key cells causing illness can develop an anti-inflammatory 'twin'," first author Dr. Christina Zielinski said.

Scientific Research on Candida

The recent research indicates that yeast overgrowth in the intestines does occur and is associated with a variety of symptoms and other health conditions which improve with antifungal treatment. I will quote the scientific references of this research for those that want to look deeper into the topic, at least they will be able to find the research papers.

For example, Candida overgrowth of the GI tract was found in recent studies to:

- ❖ Promote the development of food allergies by increasing intestinal permeability and affecting immune function (Gut. 2006 Jul;55(7):954-60; Biosci Microbiota Food Health. 2012;31(4):77-84).
- ❖ Aggravate inflammation not only in the gut but in tissues all throughout the body, increasing the risk of allergies and autoimmune diseases. (Med Mycol. 2011 Apr;49(3):237-47; Curr Opin Microbiol. 2011 Aug;14(4):386-91).
- ❖ Directly correlate with the amount of inflammation and severity of symptoms in patients with ulcers, Crohn's disease, and ulcerative colitis (J Clin Gastroenterol. 2014 Jul;48(6):513-23; J Physiol Pharmacol. 2009 Mar;60(1):107-18; Curr Opin Microbiol. 2011 Aug;14(4):386-91.
- ❖ Increase with the use of antibiotics, especially when there is already inflammation in the intestines (Curr Opin Microbiol. 2011 Aug;14(4):386-91).
- ❖ Increase with the use of proton pump inhibitors, otherwise known as anti-acids – drugs that block the production of hydrochloric acid in the stomach (Aliment Pharmacol Ther. 2013 Jun;37(11):1103-11).
- ❖ Cause the same symptoms as small intestinal bacterial overgrowth (SIBO) when it occurs in the small intestine (Aliment Pharmacol Ther. 2013 Jun;37(11):1103-11). SIBO symptoms include abdominal pain, chest pain, belching, bloating, fullness, indigestion, nausea, diarrhoea, vomiting, gas, malabsorption, and vitamin deficiencies.
- ❖ Promote inflammation in the lungs (Cell Host Microbe. 2014 Jan 15;15(1):95-102).
- ❖ Occur more commonly in people with psoriasis and other inflammatory skin disorders (Int J Dermatol. 2014 Dec;53(12):e555-60.).
- ❖ Occur more commonly in people with chronic fatigue syndrome (Scan J Gastro. 2007;42(12):1514-1515.).
- ❖ Furthermore, people with irritable bowel syndrome (IBS) have more antibodies in their blood to Candida. The severity of IBS symptoms is directly associated with levels of those antibodies (BMC Gastroenterol. 2012; 12: 166).
- ❖ People with "medically unexplained symptoms" who also score high on a standardized Candida questionnaire (called the Fungus Related Disease Questionnaire-7) also have higher levels of antibodies against Candida. These

people often have a history of frequent or long-term antibiotic use along with symptoms like frequent yeast infections, sugar cravings, and fatigue (J Altern Complement Med. 2007 Dec;13(10):1129-33).

❖ Higher levels of antibodies against Candida albicans indicates the immune system is hypersensitive to the yeast or may simply reflect greater exposure to it (due to Candida yeast overgrowth) (BMC Gastroenterol. 2012; 12: 166.).

Curing My Own Candida

Before we begin discussing the details of the Candida protocol that I invented some years ago, let me take you on a health odyssey of what motivated me to spend many hundreds of hours investigating Candida and its related problems.

Despite all my knowledge in biology and the workings of the human body, after completing an initial degree in the Biological Sciences in the UK, by the time I had reached the age of 30 my health was a shamble.

I could just about manage to crawl out of bed with excruciating pain in my body and band-type headaches that would last most of the day. I would have a painful breakfast with many digestive issues, drag myself to my office, see patients for a couple of hours then back to bed for 2-3 hours before seeing a few more patients in the afternoon. Painkillers and anti-inflammatories were my main support to get through the day.

At the time, I was working as a Clinical Psychologist and Clinical Sexologist, as apart from the biology degree, I also had qualified in these too. I had not discovered the wonderful world of natural medicine now, but this was all going to change in the next few years.

By evening I was too tired to do anything and it required a concerted effort just to hold a conversation. I tended to avoid company for this reason and became a recluse – living life close to my devoted family and trying to enjoy the small moments of watching my children develop. I absolutely hated the way I was; by nature, I am a "Type A" personality who loves to be on the go, researching new things. I generally have a very inquisitive mind and like people.

After many months of these persistent symptoms, including chronic headaches that would last for days, accompanied by an unexplainable fatigue, I eventually went to the local G.P. who took some X-rays and found that my frontal sinuses were loaded with fluid – he immediately prescribed antibiotics. Less than two months later I was back there again for more antibiotics as my sinuses were again blocked and causing headaches and pain, not to mention the tiredness, apathy, and on occasions depression. I was quite incapacitated and this was certainly enough to cause an active person to fall into a depression; otherwise I loved my work. There is nothing more frustrating than waking every morning with band-type headaches that prevented me from concentrating on my work.

The Da Vinci Candida Treatment Protocol

This is a treatment protocol that I developed over many years of study, as well as trial and error with many patients that agreed to experiment – I continue to bow to these patients who helped my learning experience.

I had spent over 11 years trying to treat my systemic Candidiasis which was causing me many health problems and symptoms including chronic fatigue, brain fog, severe digestive disturbances, fibromyalgia, achlorhydria, pancreatic enzyme deficiencies, concentration and mood disturbances.

We have successfully treated over *5,000 patients* with Candida to date at the Da Vinci Center in Larnaca, Cyprus.

Preparing for the Da Vinci Candida Treatment Protocol

Before implementing the Da Vinci Candida Protocol with my patients, I make certain that the rest of the body's physiological systems are as optimized as possible.

I generally check for:

1. Food intolerances – these foods are probably one of the biggest sources of internal inflammation and can be a big burden when eradicating the Candida, so it is important to make certain that the patient avoids these foods. I used VRT Bioresonance testing to test over 100 different foods. We will talk more about the mechanisms of food intolerances a little later.

2. Nutritional deficiencies and heavy metals using a Tissue Hair Mineral Analysis test – this involves taking a small sample of hair and sending it to a laboratory abroad.

3. Using Kinesiology, Autonomic Response Testing, Bioresonance Testing, or any other similar test, the status of the stomach and pancreas – usually you will find many patients will not be secreting enough hydrochloric acid from the stomach and enough pancreatic enzymes from the pancreas.

Here is a table summarizing these preparatory steps:

PREPARATION STEPS BEFORE CANDIDA PROTOCOL

TASK	Supplements needed	Comments
Food Intolerance test		See a Bioresonance practitioner
Hair test for Mineral deficiencies/Heavy metal profile	Supplement what is needed with HMD™ heavy metal detox	Visit: www.worldwideahealthcenter.net
Heavy metal detox	Take HMD™, LAVAGE, CHLORELLA	www.worldwidehealthcenter.net
Constipated?	Take CONSTFORM and OXYGUT, COLFORM	Visit: www.worldwidehealthcenter.net
Digestive issues?	Take DIGESTIZYME & GASTRIC AID	Visit: www.worldwidehealthcenter.net
Bioresonance devices	DEVITA AP, DEVITA RITM, DEINFO USB	Visit: www.deta-elis-uk.com
Begin Candida protocol	KANDIDAPLEX, KOLOREX, CAPRYLIC ACID, ACIDOPHILUS & BIFIDUS, CANDIDA 30C	Visit: www.worldwidehealthcenter.net

Testing for heavy metals and mineral deficiencies

In clinical work, I have found one test that I use often, and find to be invaluable – is the Hair Tissue Mineral Analysis (HTMA) (104) that we have already mentioned in a previous chapter. This involves taking a small sample of hair by cutting the first inch-and-a-half of growth closest to the scalp at the nape of the neck, or even pubic hair if someone is completely bald. It is then sent to a licensed clinical laboratory where the hair is prepared through a series of chemical and high temperature digestive procedures and is finally analysed for levels of minerals and toxic metals, using sophisticated measuring devices called spectrometers.

Hair is considered an ideal tissue for sampling and testing (105). Firstly, it can be cut easily and painlessly and can be sent to the lab without special handling requirements. Secondly, clinical results have shown that a correctly obtained sample can give an indication of mineral status and toxic metal accumulation following long-term or even acute exposure. Hair is used as one of the tissues of choice by the US Environmental Protection Agency in determining toxic metal exposure. Indeed, several studies have concluded that human hair may be a more appropriate tissue than blood or urine for studying a community's exposure to harmful trace elements.

Although our aim is to rid the body of harmful toxic metals, conversely trace minerals are essential in countless metabolic functions in all phases of the life process (106). For example, zinc is involved in the production, storage, and secretion of insulin and is necessary for growth hormones. Magnesium is required for normal muscular function, especially the heart. A deficiency in magnesium has been associated with an increased incidence of heart attacks; anxiety and nervousness. Potassium is critical for normal nutrient transport into the cell – deficiency can result in muscular weakness, depression and lethargy. Excess sodium is associated with hypertension, but adequate amounts are required for normal health. Even vitamin status can be indirectly assessed from HTMA.

HTMA can detect recent exposure (from the last couple of months) of toxic metals in your blood that ultimately end up in the hair tissues as well. The way I use the test is to take an initial baseline sample to see the levels of minerals and toxic metals that are actively circulating in the blood during the last couple of months – this is basically the time it takes to grow the inch-and-a-half of hair that is taken.

---

104 Bland, J. Hair tissue mineral analysis. an emergent diagnostic technique. Thorsons Publishers, USA, 1983.

105 Watts, DL. Trace Elements and Other Essential Nutrients: Clinical Application of Tissue Mineral Analysis.

106 Wilson, LD. Nutritional Balancing and Hair Mineral Analysis: A Comprehensive Guide. LD Wilson Consultants, Inc., 1993.

I then put my patients on a natural chelator which I researched and invented – it is a natural chelator that has undergone double-blind, placebo controlled trials with 350 people and is called HMD™. A further HTMA is taken after 2 months to see how many metals have been mobilized from storage sites in the body. Usually we find a percentage increase of metals in the second test.

HTMA results two months apart after using HMD®

The two reports above are from the same patient, taken two months apart. On the left is the baseline sample before any natural chelator or minerals were given.

Generally, there is a low level of minerals with a little Cadmium and Aluminium burden. This is what has been circulating in the blood over the last couple of months, but is not a reflection of what is stored in the body tissues and organs. On the right are the results of the second hair test, taken two months after the first, while on the HMD™ protocol. Notice that there is a huge increase in the levels of aluminium with some arsenic also appearing – these are the heavy metals that were in the storage organs that were mobilized by the HMD™ (107).

Preparing by Detoxifying
It is very important for the success of the Candida protocol that the internal milieu is balanced and clean. One of the quickest, cheapest and most efficient ways of

---

107 This protocol using a pre-post hair sample can be found at
http://www.worldwidehealthcenter.net/product-category/hair-mineral-analysis/

achieving this is to undergo a 15-day alkaline detox programme using only fresh fruits, vegetables, vegetable juices and soups, steamed vegetables with olive oil and herbs, as well as herbal teas.

Below is a summary table of the steps required to prepare for detoxifying. It is highly recommended that you take the supplements recommended as they are doctor-formulated and have been tried and tested in clinical practice by myself personally. These are high quality and pure, but if you can find alternatives then this is fine.

STEPS IN DETOXIFICATION PROTOCOL

TASK	TIME TAKEN	Supplements needed	Comments
Alkaline Detoxification	15 days	HMD MULTIS, KRILL OIL, HEPATO PLUS, VITAMIN C	www.worldwidehealthcenter.net
Parasite detox	15-30 days	PARAFORM PLUS ONE, BLACK WALNUT TINCTURE	www.worldwidehealthcenter.net
Liver/GB cleanse	1 day	MAGNESIUM MALATE, EPSOM SALTS	www.worldwidehealthcenter.net
Heavy Metal Detox	2 months	HMD™, LAVAGE, CHLORELLA	www.worldwidehealthcenter.net

There are toxins in the food you eat, the water you drink and the air you breathe. Even your own body produces toxins as a result of its many metabolic processes that keep you alive.

There are a number of benefits of detoxification:

❖ The digestive tract is cleansed of accumulated waste and fermenting bacteria.

❖ Liver, kidney and blood purification can take place, which is not possible during regular eating patterns.

❖ Mental clarity is enhanced as chemical and food additive overload is reduced.

❖ Reduced dependency on habit forming substances such as sugar, caffeine, nicotine, alcohol and drugs.

❖ The stomach size is returned to normal as bad eating habits can be stopped.

❖ The hormonal system is enhanced which is especially true for growth hormones.

❖ The immune system is stimulated.

After detoxifying on an alkaline diet for 15 days, patients report higher energy levels, clear and glowing skin, weight loss of several pounds, clear-headedness, reduced cellulite, good body tone and a great feeling of being relaxed.

Before we look at the details, here is a summary table that will help you under the various steps that you need to follow.

Some of these supplements I give to all patients as part of a repair and rejuvenation process; these would include a high-potency multivitamin/mineral formula such as HMD MULTIS, KRILL PLUS, which is a good source of omega 3 fatty acids, but with a lower probability of being high in mercury.

I encounter almost 80% or more of my patient having digestive issues – bloating and distension in the stomach and the intestines - so I will give DIGESTIZYME which are pancreatic enzymes that will help gut digestion, and GASTRIC AID which contains hydrochloric acid for digesting concentrated proteins in the stomach.

For those that are doing the liver and gallbladder cleanse, MAGNESIUM MALATE is important in order to soften the stones before the cleanse as drinking apple juice which contains malic acid is too sweet and will feed the Candida.

TYPICAL DETOXIFICATION & REJUVENTATION SUPPLEMENT SHEET
The Da Vinci Centre Detoxification Diet

REMEDY	MORNING	LUNCH	DINNER	COMMENTS
HMD MULTIS Multivitamin/mineral	2	2	0	With food
KRILL OIL Fatty acids – omega 3	1	0	1	With food
DIGESTIZYME Pancreatic enzymes – gut digestion	1	1	1	With main meals only
GASTRIC AID Hydrochloric acid – stomach digestion	1	1	1	With main meals only
HEPATO PLUS Liver detox herbal formula	1	1	1	With food 15 – 30 days only
PARAFORM PLUS ONE Parasite detox herbal formula	1	1	1	Away from food
MAGNESIUM MALATE Softens gallbladder stones	1	1	1	With food, for 15 days only
HMD Heavy metal detox chelator	45 drops	45 drops	45 drops	In a little water or juice
LAVAGE Herbal drainage remedy	25 drops	25 drops	25 drops	Away from food
LUGOL'S IODINE Feeds the thyroid	2 drops	0	2 drops	
WALNUT TINCTURE Parasite detox herbal formula	2 tsp	0	0	
CHLORELLA Clears toxic metals from matrix and gut	2	0	2	With food
Alpha Lipoic acid Water & Fat soluble antioxidant	1	0	1	With food
IF CONSTIPATED:				
CONSFORM Herbal formula for constipation	1	1	1	With food

These are the foods that are allowed during the detoxification phase, no other family of foods is allowed. You may eat as many of the following foods as you wish, but it is best to eat only when you feel hungry. Wash all fruit and vegetables in a bowl of water with 4-5 tablespoons of grape vinegar added to help wash away any pesticide/ herbicide residues. Rinse afterwards with clean water. Here are the foods that you can eat in plenty:

1. **Salads** – use any type of fresh vegetables you like, in any combination. Use organic vegetables when available, and include bean sprouts when in season. Salad dressings should be kept simple - a little virgin olive oil with fresh lemon, or cider vinegar. Add plenty of fresh onion and garlic - these are very detoxifying.

2. **Steamed vegetables** – eat any variety you like, including broccoli, cauliflower, potatoes, beetroot, carrots etc. Steam as opposed to boil, and eat with a little herbal salt, lemon and a little virgin olive oil, with plenty of garlic.

3. **Vegetable soups** - of all kinds, but broccoli, leak and vegetable soups are fine.

4. **Stir-Fried Vegetables** – again, any type of vegetables are fine, cooked in their own juices using a Wok.

5. **Vegetable juices** - drink a minimum of 1-3 per day, and try to include one cocktail comprising one-third of a glass of raw green juice (spinach, parsley,

cabbage and any other green vegetables), with a small beetroot, topped up with carrot juice. Carrot juice has a strong effect on the digestive system, provides energy, serves as an important source of minerals, promotes normal elimination, has diuretic properties and helps to build healthy tissue, skin and teeth.

6. **Fresh Fruit** - choose the fruit of your choice and eat as much as you like, whenever you like. You could begin the day with 2-3 pieces of fruit, which are gentle on the digestive system. Make a tasty fruit salad. Try to avoid too many juicy fruits as this may overly feed the Candida, and certainly avoid all forms of fruit juices as this will give sugar to the body quickly, again feeding the Candida. Avocados provides a good source of protein. There is tremendous benefit in adding fruit during the detox due to their living enzymes and phytonutrients which are very cleansing to the body. Remember, we are not treating the Candida yet, only helping the body to cleanse and prepare for the 3-month Candida protocol.

7. **Fresh Nuts** – it is generally OK to have some fresh nuts such as almonds and walnuts.

8. **Herbal teas** - any of your choice. Chamomile is a good relaxant; aniseed and mint are good for the digestive system; Kombucha, dandelion tea is excellent for purifying the blood and detoxifying and stimulating liver function; sage tea is a blood cleanser; nettle tea is excellent for driving away excess fluid out of the tissues and is a wonderful cleanser for all the detoxification organs. Drink as many as you like, with a little honey on the tip of a teaspoon if you like.

The purpose of this diet is to detoxify – to remove the toxins from the fat cells and tissues as well as the organs, so that the body can return to its optimum level of functionality.

You will also need to drink at least 8-10 glasses per day of still mineral water to flush out the toxins – this is VERY IMPORTANT, so please take note!

When the 15 days are over, you should carry on eating the above for a couple more days while gently adding a little protein such as fresh steamed or grilled fish, organic chicken, pulses, a soft-boiled organic egg or a little cheese. Go gently on the protein for a couple of days before you begin eating normally again so that you do not overload your digestive system.

Parasites, Heavy Metals and Other Toxins

As part of the detoxification process, the Da Vinci Center also attempts to detoxify heavy metals that can easily be detected using a hair analysis, as already mentioned above.

One of the most researched natural chelators in the world that has undergone double-blind, placebo controlled trials with 350 people is called HMD™. It has been shown to safely chelate many different types of heavy metals, including uranium, a difficult metal to chelate. It was invented by myself and there are a number of scientific papers written in peer-reviewed journals – Natural Heavy Metal Chelators: Do They Work? and A Natural Heavy Metal Chelator is Born.

Dr. Hulda Clark, Ph.D., N.D., a naturopathic physician, has brought the issue of parasitically-caused diseases and other types of toxicity back into the spotlight in recent years, dealing with this subject at length in her book, *The Cure for all Diseases*. Dr. Hulda describes various methodologies and procedures to cleanse the body from these nasty creatures. Check out the questionnaire in the Appendix to see whether you are likely to have a parasite load.

The Herbal Parasitic Cleanse

There are some good herbal formulas that are designed to eradicate parasites.
One such formula that I use and formulated is called PARAFORM PLUS ONE (one capsule, three times daily, away from food). It contains a number of powerful anti-parasitic herbs that are suitable for vegetarians, such as:

Magnesium caprylate
Cinnamon powder
Cloves powder
Shiitake mushroom powder
Garlic powder extract (10000mg/g)
Glucomannan (95%)
Pumpkin seed P E 4:1 (40%) (equivalent to 200mg pumpkin seed powder)
Chicory root P.E 4:1 (equivalent to 120mg chicory root powder)
Grapefruit seed P.E 5:1 (equivalent to 100mg grapefruit seed powder)
Cayenne extract 7:1 (equivalent to 100mg cayenne powder)
Fenugreek seed P.E 4:1 (equivalent to 48mg fenugreek seed powder)
Olive leaf extract 15:1, 6% Oleurpein (equivalent to 50mg olive leaf powder)

It is a powerful formula that we have been using with good results in clinical practice, and goes well when combined with **PARAFORM TINCTURE**, another powerful anti-parasitic herb – 2 teaspoons in the morning in a little water, away from food.

Bioresonance Devices

As well as using herbal formulas to eradicate parasites, I recently have added other protocols using Bioresonance devices, researched by Russian scientists who developed a powerful, portable, programmable Bioresonance device called the DEVITA AP. This has undergone considerable trials from the Russians who purport its success in eradicating a number of parasites and microorganisms.

I have been using Bioresonance devices for many years now, but the innovation of the Russian devices is that they are portable, no larger than a mobile phone, and can be programmed to resonate with individual parasites and other microorganisms. There is also the DEVITA RITM that is for upregulating the organ systems.

If we take a crystal wine glass as an example, this has its own resonant frequency, of around 500 Hertz. If we can produce a sound at the same frequency and stand the glass in front of a speaker, then the glass will absorb this frequency and break. This is the phenomenon of RESONANCE.

In the same way, microbes also have their own resonant frequencies. If we can match these frequencies, the microbes will absorb this energy and burst.

Treatment with the devices is based on the principles of Bioresonance. They are as close as we can get to the Hippocratic Oath that says: *"Do no harm"* when treating people. These gentle devices achieve exactly this – they can heal without being invasive and causing side-effects.

Checkout a presentation at an international conference on YouTube talking about "Alternatives to Antibiotics" https://youtu.be/bYcvs4blUq8

The devices also have the approval of the Ministry of Health of Russia, as well as Israel and Germany where they are presently manufactured with CE approval as wellness devices. These devices also have patents in 73 different countries as well as more than 117 scientific research studies backing it in the last 20 years – see www.deta-elis-uk.com

The Secrets to Success
It is my opinion, if one wants to be successful at eradicating Candida, then you must eradicate the pathogen using natural anti-fungal remedies, while at the same time cleaning up your internal milieu.

One further key to success is the important step of converting the pathogenic, mycelial Candida back to the normal budding yeasts – this is a **crucially important step** often missed by many practitioners of natural medicine. The only remedies that can do this successfully are the Sanum isopathic fungal remedies that have been invented by Professor Enderlein after many years of experimentation using darkfield microscopy.

Many physicians now believe that an interim measure before embarking on any treatment should be a protocol for Candida overgrowth; this possesses such a minor risk and expense that it should be considered in any chronic illness.

One clinical trial a person may try is to avoid certain foods for five days that are known to facilitate the growth of yeast. Such foods include the following:

- ❖ **SUGAR and SIMPLE CARBOHYDRATES** such as those found in all sweetened food including honey, molasses, sorghum, maple syrup, sugar, fructose, maltose, dextrose, corn syrup, etc.

- ❖ **YEAST PRODUCTS** such as beer, wine, yeast leavened bread, natural B vitamins, brewer's yeast.

- ❖ **FERMENTED and MOULDY FOODS** such as mushrooms, cheese, vinegar, mustard, catsup, relish and other condiments made with vinegar.

After avoiding these foods for 5 days, try adding them back into the diet in large quantities. By observing how one feels while off these foods, in comparison to any adverse effects experienced when going back on the foods, one may get a clue as to any possible yeast involvement as a causative factor for any adverse symptoms.

If adverse symptoms are provoked by a return to the yeast enhancing foods, your physician may feel that there is at least a possible reason to suspect Candida overgrowth, which may then warrant more definitive action.

This may not be the best method and personally I do not use it as I will use VRT Bioresonance screening and ART to determine whether there is pathogenic Candidiasis, backed up by the signs and symptoms using Dr. Crook's Candida Questionnaire. However, if you are not a Bioresonance practitioner or use any other form of ANS testing, then this may be a good way to begin.

Detoxification Symptoms – "The Healing Crisis"
When the body detoxifies, it goes through various biochemical and physiological changes (108). Generally, on the first day of fasting, the blood sugar level is likely to drop below 65-70 mg/dl. The liver immediately compensates by converting glycogen to glucose and releasing it into the blood. After a few hours, the basal metabolic rate is likely to fall in order to conserve energy. This means that the heart, pulse and blood pressure will drop. More glycogen may be used from muscles, causing some weakness.

---

108 Salloum, TK. Fasting Signs and Symptoms: A Clinical Guide. USA: Buckeye Naturopathic Press, 1992.

As the body requires more energy, some fat and fatty acids are broken down to release glycerol from the glyceride molecules and are converted to glucose. You may notice the skin becoming quite oily as these fatty acids and glycerol increase in the blood. The skin is one of the largest detoxification organs, so you may get some skin problems such as pimples, acnes or a pussy boil – this is all part of the body trying to cleanse. The complexion may become pallid for a day or two as the wastes accumulate in the blood.

The incomplete oxidation of fats may result in the formation of Ketones, resulting in ketoacidosis. Combined with high levels of urea resulting from protein metabolism, this state can cause a number of symptoms which may suppress appetite, as they affect the satiety centre in the hypothalamus. Generally, this takes a few days to happen and you may notice your appetite dwindling. You may get pains in different joints, or organs such as the lungs. There may be a considerable amount of yellow mucus released from the throat and expelled. The sinuses may also begin clearing with more mucus secreted.

Given that the body is releasing these toxins quickly during the first few days of the detoxification process, it should not surprise us to experience some changes in our bodies that may cause certain symptoms. Initially, for the first 2-3 days, these symptoms can be a little unpleasant, SO BE WARNED! A fair number of people will have headaches, nervousness, diarrhea, upset stomach, energy loss, furry tongue, halitosis (bad breath), as well as acne or other skin rashes, a general feeling of malaise, frequent urination due to the toxins irritating the bladder, and some of their existing symptoms may be exacerbated. When the toxic residues enter the blood, they affect mind and body functions.

These may be unpleasant symptoms for the first couple of days, but they are a NORMAL part of the detoxification process, and in natural medicine we call this the HEALING CRISIS or HERXHEIMER REACTION. All these symptoms indicate that the DETOX IS WORKING! This is a temporary and transient crisis, it will pass – so hang on in there and don't worry that there is something wrong with you, apart from the fact that you are loaded with toxins.

There was always something wrong with you, and now you are doing something about it. You are reversing this toxic process that your body has adapted to, but that's not healthy. If you are a coffee drinker, then the symptoms will be more pronounced, as your body will be in a state of withdrawal. Yes, coffee is a drug, and when you come off it you go into withdrawal, meaning that your body will start asking for a dose of what it is addicted to. When it doesn't get it, then it screams for it louder and louder, usually in the form of headaches, migraines, muscle pains, general weakness and lack of concentration.

Enduring a cleansing crisis is the hardest part of the healing process. To stop feeling bad, most people want to eat - but do not eat during a cleansing crisis. The body is overloaded with the work of removing toxins. Digestion makes matters worse. Drinking one or two glasses of sodium bicarbonate (baking soda) – one teaspoon in each glass drunk twice daily - will help to neutralize the ketoacidosis.

Helter-Skelter rides are common. The 'downward slope' is when the body is vigorously cleansing and the blood gets swamped with toxins causing you to feel down, moody, depressed, achy – like having a bad cold. You feel weak and lethargic. The mind rationalizes: *'I feel horrible: this can't be working.'* You can maintain a normal routine of work on a dip but it requires willpower and determination. It also helps to know that the longer the down period, the greater the fasting high.

Clearing Toxic Metals

Clearing toxic metals, such as mercury that will further aggravate the Candida and cause free radical damage to many organs and tissues, is also a wise step to take.

There are many products on the market that purport to detoxify heavy metals from the body, but none of them are supported by scientific research using correct methodologies.

There is one natural product, however, that has been based on double blind, placebo controlled research with over 350 people. It has also been used clinically by many practitioners around the world in the last 8 years or so.

This is what I suggest can be used for most cases of heavy metal toxicity. I have called it the HMD ULTIMATE DETOX PROTOCOL and it consists of the following:

❖ HMD™ – 45 drops x 3 daily for adults (109) – sensitive adults who have chronic diseases or compensated detoxification organs, as well as people with neurological diseases such as multiple sclerosis and the like, as well as autistic people should begin with half this dose or less, and increase by one drop x 3 daily, every day until they reach a comfortable level.

❖ HMD LAVAGE – this is a herbal formula of wild-crafted and organic herbs such as Silybum marianum (Milk Thistle Seed), Taraxacum officinale (Dandelion Root), Arctium lappa (Burdock Root), Trifolium pratense (Red Clover Tops), Curcuma longa (Turmeric Root), Hydrangea arborescens

---

109 See http://www.worldwidehealthcenter.net/hmd-dosage-guidelines/ for full details

(Hydrangea Root) and Arctostaphylos uva ursi (Bearberry Leaf). This herbal formula is designed to facilitate detoxification of the liver, kidneys, lymphatics and skin, as well as cleanse the blood and act as a natural anti-inflammatory. Adult dosage: 25 drops x 3 daily for adults, or more as directed by a practitioner.

- ❖ NON-TOXIC CHLORELLA – there are many concerns about finding good quality, clean Chlorella that is void of heavy metals and xenobiotics. We have searched and travelled far and wide, and found an excellent source that is provided with a Certificate of Analysis with each pot. This chlorella comes from the western coast of Hai-Nan Island, China's southernmost island. Hai-Nan Island is a tropical island with an excellent climate and lies on the same latitude as Hawaii. The non-industrialized, pollution-free, tropical island offers favorable growth conditions for chlorella, including intense sunlight, pure water, and clean air. Available in 500mg tabs, adult dosage should be 2 tabs x 3 daily.

Chlorella is required in the gut to take it away toxic metals via the stools. If there is not enough chlorella, the neurotoxins are reabsorbed by the nerve endings in the gut wall, and are at risk of being redirected to the spinal cord, and the brain.

Good quality chlorella lines the gut wall, and mops up the free toxins found there. High toxicity and increasing symptoms need larger doses. This is very important, and differs from the usual advice to reduce supplements if detoxing intensifies symptoms.

- ❖ A-LIPOIC ACID – I believe that when metals and other xenobiotics are mobilized in the body, there should be some protection against free radical damage. Lipoic acid is that extraordinary antioxidant which is both water and fat soluble, able to penetrate the brain and other nervous tissues, and is therefore able to protect all parts of the body against free radical damage.

I will often fine-tune this protocol depending on the needs of the patient, but generally this works well for most cases as a basic protocol.

THE DA VINCI CANDIDA PROTOCOL (DCP)

Now that we have completed the preparation by detoxing on many different levels and preparing the internal milieu, we are now ready to begin the Candida protocol in order to eradicate the Candida.

Let's take a conceptual look at the components of the Da Vinci Candida Protocol before we look at the details.

Please note that we are aware that sourcing these products from different companies around the world is difficult and costly on freight charges. Rest assured, however, as you can purchase the complete package online from a one-stop shop at www.worldwidehealthcenter.net.

The Da Vinci Candida Protocol has five basic objectives:

1. Starve the Candida by eliminating the foods that feed it.

2. Kill the Candida using natural anti-Candida products that we will discuss below.

3. Repopulate the bowel flora with a high-potency Acidophilus and Bifidus probiotic that contains 60 billion live bacteria per capsule.

4. Regulate the dysbiosis and convert the pathological, mycelial form of Candida back to the normal form by the use of the SANUM remedies.

5. Restore biochemical balance to the body and strength to the immune system. This will allow the body to regain and maintain control over Candida growth by optimizing the diet. This would involve avoiding food intolerances and following the Metabolic Type Diet by Bill Wolcott. Also, eradicating parasites using herbal formulas that we discussed above as well as chelating heavy metals out of the system.

Here is a summary of the various steps that you need to follow to cure your Candida once and for all. Even though it may be quite detailed, I can guarantee that if you follow it you will succeed, as have more than 5,000 patients that I have treated in the last 15 years or so. The success rate of eliminating the Candida approaches 100%, and by the time you have read all this book you will understand why.

STEPS IN CANDIDA PROTOCOL

TASK	TIME TAKEN	Supplements needed	Comments
Starve the Candida	3 calendar months		Need to adhere to this religiously!
Killing the Candida	3 calendar months	KANDIDAPLEX, HOROPITO, CAPRYLIC ACID, ACIDOPHILUS & BIFIDUS, CANDIDA 30C	www.worldwidehealthcenter.net
Repopulating friendly bacteria in gut	1 day	ACIDOPHILUS & BIFIDUS	www.worldwidehealthcenter.net
Using SANUM remedies to convert pathogenic Candida	2 months	SANUM REMEDIES	www.worldwidehealthcenter.net
Balancing body chemistry		VITAMIN C, GASTRIC AID, DIGESTIZYME	www.worldwidehealthcenter.net

None of these objectives are mutually exclusive, nor can they be addressed in a serial way. They all need to be looked at concomitantly for the treatment protocol to be successful.

Let us now go through the various stages or phases of the Da Vinci Candida Protocol, beginning with a critically important stage – starving the Candida by not feeding it.

First Phase - Starving the Candida

I have found that it is literally impossible to treat Candida if one does not cut out ALL forms of sugar for a period of 3 months. This also includes natural fruit sugars or fructose. The foods that should be strictly AVOIDED for a 3-month period include:

1. **SUGAR** – and all foods that contain sugar. These include white and brown sugar, honey, syrups, liquors, lactose, fructose, all confectionary and sweet cakes, chocolates, ice-creams, home-made sweets and cakes, biscuits, fizzy beverages, all fruit drinks.

2. **YEAST** – all foods that contain yeast including breads, vinegar, ketchups, mayonnaise   and   pickles.

3. **MUSHROOMS** – all types, including Chinese mushrooms such as Shitake.

4. **REFINED FOODS** – all white flours, white rice, white pasta products, corn flour, custard and white cereal products, unless they are whole-meal or organic.

5. **FERMENTED PRODUCTS** – all alcoholic beverages, vinegar and all vinegar products such as ketchup, mayonnaise and pickles.

6. **NUTS** – all types of nuts that are cleaned and packaged without their shells – these have a tendency to collect fungal spores and molds from the atmosphere which will antagonize the Candida. Nuts that are fresh with their shells are OK.

7. **FRESH AND DRIED FRUIT** – all fresh fruit should be avoided for the initial **SIX WEEKS ONLY** as again, the fructose they contain will feed the Candida and make it extremely difficult to eliminate.

All other fruit that is not fresh such as cooked, tinned or dried and fruit juices should be avoided for the full 3 months – your health practitioner will advise you when to begin eating fruit again. Obviously, also avoiding fruit juices (vegetable juices are OK).

Second Phase – Killing the Candida

There are a number of herbal formulas, homeopathics and probiotics that are used in the Da Vinci Candida Protocol. They have been carefully selected after years of experimentation and the fact is they have worked time and time again with hundreds of people. The aim of using these supplements is to kill off the Candida. Here is a table of these supplements in order, taken from one of the handouts that we give our patients, with an explanation on why and how they work later on.

	REMEDY	MORNING	LUNCH	DINNER	COMMENTS
	MAIN PROTOCOL				
R	KandidaPlex	2	2	2	With meals
R	Horopito	1	0	1	With meals
R	Acidophilus and Bifidus	1	1	1	With meals
	Candida 30c	2 pillules	2 pillules	2 pillules	Dissolve in mouth Before meals
	Caprylic Acid	1	1	1	With meals
* *	Citricidal drops (Nail Fungus)	1 drop	0	1 drop	Under nails only
*	***Natural Antibiotics***				
	Liquid Silver 50	1 tsp	1 tsp	1 tsp	Before food in water
	Olive Leaf extract	1 tab	1 tab	1 tab	With meals
	Grapefruit Seed Extract	2 tabs	2 tabs	2 tabs	With meals
	Vitamin C Powder	1/3tsp - 1/2tsp	1/3tsp - 1/2tsp	1/3tsp - 1/2tsp	Before food in water
	PARAFORM PLUS TWO	1	1	1	With food
	Oregano Oil	1	1	1	With meals

NOTES:
R = Refrigerate

All the above-named products can be ordered from www.worldwidehealthcenter.net

* The **Natural Antibiotics** are only taken when there is an active infection such as a cold, flu or other infection. Take for 6 days **after** symptom withdrawal to make certain that all the bacteria have cleared from the body.
** Only taken if there is nail fungus

Now let us look at the specific remedies in a little more detail to understand why and how they work to eradicate the Candida:

1. <u>CANDIDA COMPLEX</u> **(was called KANDIDAPLEX)** - a doctor-formulated compound that contains:

❖ Biotin150 mcg;
❖ Calcium undecylenate;
❖ Pau d'arco (Tabebuia avellanedae) bark extract 100 mg;
❖ Enlyse™ enzyme blend (cellulase, chitosinase, hemicellulase, protease, serrapeptase, amylase and lipase) 100 mg;
❖ Berberine (as berberine sulfate) 50 mg;
❖ Sorbic Acid 25 mg;
❖ Trans-Resveratrol (from Japanese knotweed (Polygonum cuspidatum) root extract) 10 mg.

Dosage: 2 capsules 3 x daily

Each individual ingredient in CANDIDA COMPLEX has a specific function when it comes to eradicating Candida, as follows:

❖ Biotin negatively affects Candida because of its ability to prevent yeast from converting into its pathogenic or fungal form. Biotin does this by interfering with the growth of the Candida.

❖ Calcium undecylenate; undecanoic acid's ability to alter the composition of fatty acids in the cell membrane leading to an inability to sustain its fungal form.

❖ Pau D'Arco acts as a powerful antifungal agent. It contains several classes of compounds, lapachol, xyloidone and various napthaquinones. The most important of these is lapachol, which has been shown to inhibit the growth of Candida, similar to Amphotericin B.

❖ Enlyse™ destroys the BIOFILM of Candida that we previously talked about, which is composed of protein polypeptides, polysaccharide carbohydrates, fibrinogen or fibrin and polynucleotides that contain RNA and DNA material. This structure is bound together with ligands that have stickiness properties.

247

❖ Berberine exhibits a broad spectrum of antibiotic activity. Berberine has shown antimicrobial activity against bacteria, protozoa, and fungi and upregulates immunity.

❖ Sorbic acid inhibits fungi as well as molds often found together in the body.

❖ Trans-Resveratrol exhibited antifungal activity against Candida. It also inhibited the yeast-to-hyphae morphogenetic transition of C. albicans.

2. HOROPITO (practitioner-strength) – a New Zealand herbal product that contains two powerful anti-fungal agents that have been shown to kill Candida – Pseudowinterata colorata and the synergistic herb Aniseed that boosts effectiveness 6-fold.

Dosage: 1 cap twice daily

This natural herb, found mostly in New Zealand, has some amazing properties that have been scientifically researched.

Pseudowintera colorata, or mountain Horopito, is an evergreen shrub or small tree (1–2.5 m) commonly called pepperwood because its leaves have a hot taste.

Used by the indigenous Maori population of New Zealand. Infection due to Candida albicans is documented as once being a major cause of death of Maori babies, due to being fed an "unsatisfactory diet".

3. CAPRYLIC ACID (500 mg) – a derivative of coconut that stops the Candida reproducing as well as killing the Candida. Dosage: 1 tab x 3 daily

4. CANDIDA 30c - homeopathic – helps to eradicate the Candida, but using a different mechanism. Dosage: two pillules or one cap x 3 daily for 2 weeks only. These are stopped just as the Sanum remedies are begun.

Third phase – Repopulating the Friendly Bacteria

This phase runs parallel with phase 2 and uses good quality, human strain probiotics such as the high-potency ACIDOPHILUS and BIFIDUS probiotics by Custom Probiotics, an American company.

The Custom Probiotics formula that we use is a high count, multi strain Acidophilus and Bifidus probiotic dietary supplement containing 60 billion cfu's per capsule at the time of expiration; resistant to stomach acids, with a slow die-off with temperature.

The Ingredients include 5 different strains of probiotics such as L. Acidophilus, L. Rhamnosus, L. Plantarum, B. Lactis, and B. Bifidum.

There is considerable scientific evidence for activity of probiotics against a wide range of intestinal pathogens, including Candida species. Despite this, the mechanisms of effect have been poorly defined. However, it can be speculated that one or more of the following possible effects are in operation:

- competition for nutrients
- secretion of antimicrobial substances (e.g. bacteriocins, peroxides)
- reduction of gut pH
- blocking of adhesion sites (Kennedy et al, 1985)
- repression of virulence
- blocking of toxin receptor sites
- immune stimulation (local and systemic)
- suppression of toxin production

To these supplements, we add a good-quality multivitamin such as HMD MULTIS to provide all the vitamins and minerals that the immune system requires for optimal functioning. Also, taking KRILL PLUS is helpful as this acts as a natural anti-inflammatory.

Phase 4 – Using SANUM Isopathic Remedies to Normalize Pathogenic Candida

All of the above must be taken for the full 90 days of the protocol, with the exception of the Candida 30c. After two weeks of the anti-Candida diet, certain specialized isopathic remedies are introduced, known as SANUM remedies from Germany, after the work of the famous Prof. Enderlein.

SANUM therapy is widely recognized to positively influence the regulatory processes, the internal milieu, immune response capacity and the symbiotic bacterial ecology within the body.

Each of these isopathic remedies are only taken a couple of times per week, with the exception of the Albicansan remedy that is taken day by day. The reason that we have spaced them out in the table below is that they tend to clash and antagonize each other, and cannot all be taken at the same time. So, if you follow the sequence in the table below, beginning from the specific day that you begin taking them, whether this is Monday, or Tuesday or Wednesday and so forth:

	Mon A m	Mon p m	Tue a m	Tue p m	Wed a m	Wed pm	Thu a m	Thu p m	Fri a m	Fri p m	Sat a m	Sat p m	Sun a m	Sun p m
Albicansan Capsules or/& Suppositories		■		⊘		■		⊘		■		⊘		■
Mucokehl Tablets	■						■							
Pefrakehl Capsules				■				■						
Nigersan Tablets					■						■			
Fortakehl Tablets							■						■	
Notakehl Tablets			■								■			

Specifically, each of the 6 remedies is taken as follows:

- ✓ Albicansan ® (Candida albicans) – caps 4X - **1 cap every second day**.
- ✓ Fortakehl ® (Penicillium roquefortii) – tabs 4X - **1 tab twice weekly**.
- ✓ Mucokehl ® (Mucor racemosus) – tabs 5X - **1 tab twice weekly**.
- ✓ Nigersan ® (Aspergillus niger) – tabs 5X - **1 tab twice weekly**.
- ✓ Notakehl ® (Penicillium chrysogenum) – tabs 5X - **1 tab twice weekly**.
- ✓ Pefrakehl ® (Candida parapsilosis) – Caps 4X - **1 cap twice weekly**.

If there is vaginal discharge, or anal Candida, then vaginal or anal pessaries of Albicansan D3 must also be used to eliminate this topical infection. These can be used every second day last thing at night, after sex and are shown on the table above with the symbol ⊘.

The SANUM remedies are continued for 10 weeks until the end of the Candida protocol.

These remedies are taken BEFORE or AWAY from food. This is why it is best to store them in the bedroom, away from electrical equipment, and take them as soon as you wake in the morning and last thing at night.

There are both capsules and tablets. The capsules you need to open and pour the powder that they contain under the tongue and allow it to absorb for a few minutes. The tablets dissolve under the tongue for a few minutes. No water needs to be drunk, as they will absorb directly into the blood stream from the blood vessels under the tongue.

1. **ALBICANSAN** - European health practitioners report that this remedy may be useful as supportive therapy in:

    ✓ intestinal overgrowth of Candida
    ✓ mycosis
    ✓ resistant skin infections of mouth
    ✓ stomatitis
    ✓ gingivitis
    ✓ urogenital mycosis
    ✓ vaginitis
    ✓ urethritis with subsequent adnexitis
    ✓ cholecystitis
    ✓ colitis of fungal origin
    ✓ allergies

2. **FORTAKEHL** - European practitioners report that Fortakehl promotes normal bowel flora in the gastro-intestinal tract (especially after antibiotic therapy) which could be helpful for such conditions as gastritis, enteritis, colitis, gall bladder problems, pancreatitis, diarrhea, constipation, ulcers, yeast infections of the intestines, the vagina, and the skin.

3. **MUCOKEHL** - European health practitioners report that this remedy is useful as supportive therapy in chronic and acute disturbances of circulatory system, such as:

    ✓ thrombosis
    ✓ embolism
    ✓ angina pectoris
    ✓ post infarct
    ✓ varicosities
    ✓ hemorrhoids
    ✓ diabetic gangrene and neuropathy

✓ constipation.

4. **NIGERSAN** - European health practitioners report that this remedy is useful in disorders that have to do with disturbed calcium metabolism which could involve bone and tooth rehabilitation. European reports further indicate that Nigersan, also known as Pleo™ Nig, has been successfully used for urogenital tract problems in men and women such as prostate, ovaries, kidney and bladder complaints. It appears to be helpful for enhancing lymph circulation which in turn leads to increased detoxification, especially after illness.

5. **NOTAKEHL** - European practitioners report that Notakehl, otherwise known as Pleo™ Not, is very useful to enhance the immune system, and as a supportive therapy for infections of bacterial origin and inflammations such staph, strep, acne, ear infections, tonsil infections, sore throat, neuritis, neuralgia, urinary tract infections, prostate irritation, respiratory infections and neuropathy.

6. **PEFRAKEHL** - European health practitioners report that Pefrakehl, otherwise known as Pleo™ Pef, may be useful as a supportive therapy in relieving the symptoms of intestinal overgrowth of Candida, yeast infections, mycosis, fungal, bacterial and viral infections of the mouth and the teeth, ear infections, gingivitis, urogenital yeast infections, vaginal yeast infections, anal inflammations and irritations.

N.B. Please note that if you are allergic to PENICILLIN, you should not take the <u>NOTAKEHL</u> (Penicillium chrysogenum) and <u>FORTAKEHL</u> (Penicillium roquefortii) as these are likely to cause unpleasant symptoms such as lethargy, fatigue, brain fog, muscle pains and a general feeling of unwellness. The treatment will still work without these two SANUM remedies.

Phase 5 - Balancing Body Chemistry

It is a commonly recognized and accepted fact that immune system efficiency is highly dependent on the proper biochemical balance in the body. This of course, is dependent on proper and adequate nutrition to supply the body with all the required biochemical constituents (vitamins, minerals, enzymes, intrinsic factors, etc.).

Different people require different amounts of nutrients for optimum health. The criteria for the determination of these differing nutritional requirements lies within the definition of one's metabolic type, i.e. the genetically determined metabolic and nutritional parameters that define each person's individuality on every level.

It is precisely because different people have different metabolic types, and therefore different needs for nutrition, that the allopathic, symptom-treatment approach in nutrition is baseless and so often ineffective. This further explains why what (nutritionally) helps make one person better, may have little or no effect on another, or even make a third person worse.

I have not tried to modify this protocol as I have found it to be so successful in the treatment of over 5,000 patients to date, that I dare not juggle with it in case it loses its effectiveness. I'm sure that it can be improved upon, and would welcome comments from other practitioners working with Candida. It is only through sharing that we will grow and become better practitioners.[110, 111]

Package of all supplements required for the Da Vinci Candida Protocol

If you purchase the **DA VINCI CANDIDA PROTOCOL – COMPLETE PACKAGE** of supplements from www.worldwidehealthcenter.net you will receive the following products to last you throughout the complete treatment over 3 months:

- ❖ 6 containers of CANDIDA COMPLEX
- ❖ 3 containers of HOROPITO
- ❖ 6 containers of CAPRYLIC ACID
- ❖ 3 containers of ACIDOPHILUS AND BIFIDUS
- ❖ 1 jar of CANDIDA 30 C
- ❖ SANUM REMEDIES – complete set for 3 months (7 packs in total) containing Nigersan D5, Pefrekehl D4, 2 x Albicansan D4, Fortakehl D5, Notakehl D5, Mucokehl D5.
- ❖ All handouts required giving detailed instructions, written and used by Dr. Georgiou at the Da Vinci Center. Handouts include: "Da Vinci Candida Protocol"; "Sanum Remedies"; "Anti-Candida Diet"; "Candida Meal Plan". These can be downloaded as soon as you purchase the package.

Reintroducing Fruit

Fruit can be re-introduced back into the diet **FOUR WEEKS** after you begin taking the SANUM remedies, or 6 weeks after beginning the Candida protocol.

Stay with two SOLID portions of fruit daily for the remainder of the protocol. One medium apple would be considered as one portion, or ½ teacup of berries would be one portion, or 2 small plums would be one portion.

---

[110] Georgiou, G.J. Scourge of the 21st Century: Systemic Candidiasis – Part 1. British Naturopathic Journal, Vol. 25, No. 1, 2008.
[111] Georgiou, G.J. Treatment of Systemic Candidaisis – Part 2. British Naturopathic Journal, Vol. 25, No. 1, 2008.

All JUICY fruits such as watermelon, grapes, oranges, grapefruit, tangerines, mangos, pineapple and sweet figs should be avoided throughout the 3 months of the treatment as they give their sugars to the blood too quickly. Stick with apples, pears, plums, ½ cup of berries, kiwi, and paw paw. Have these in between meals as snacks, one mid-morning and one mid-afternoon.

Herxheimer Reactions

Depending on the severity of Candida overgrowth and the amount of the agents taken, the Candida can be killed off in vast numbers in a very short period of time. As the fungi are killed, they release substances that are toxic to the body called mycotoxins. If the elimination organs such as the kidneys, liver, lymphatics, gut and skin cannot clear these mycotoxins quickly and they accumulate in the tissues, then a temporary toxic or allergic-type reaction can occur. The technical name for this experience is a 'Herxheimer reaction'; it is more commonly referred to as "die off."

Usually die-off lasts about 12 – 24 hours, though on rare occasions it can last several days. It can usually be controlled by reducing the dosage of the remedies used to kill the Candida, as well as taking drainage herbs and homeopathics that your practitioner will advise you of.

Signs of Herxheimer reaction can be many and varied but generally involve such discomfort as aching, bloating, dizziness, nausea, and an overall "goopy sick" feeling, or a worsening of original symptoms. Fortunately, die off is generally short in duration, and although uncomfortable, is at least a confirmation of the presence of Candida and that something "good" is happening.

Exercise as well as ensuring proper, daily bowel evacuation has been reported as being helpful in countering the adversities of die off. Maintaining a high daily intake of pure water is also important to keep the channels of elimination open. Sometimes taking a teaspoon of baking soda (sodium bicarbonate) in a glass of water can help to quickly neutralize acidic reactions in the body that lead to inflammation and pain.

It may be possible to slow down these symptoms, many of which are caused by acetaldehyde, one of the main toxins produced by yeast. Taking Molybdenum – 10 drops x 2 times daily in water, away from food - can break down this toxin into something far less harmless. It may be worth considering adding these to the Candida protocol if Herxheimer reactions are bad.

The Blocking Factors of Recovery – Reasons for Failing

Many times, people who have Candidiasis don't follow the Candida protocol precisely, consistently, and for a long enough period of time. Often when people feel better while they are on the Candida diet, they tend to go off it too quickly.

When people have Candida or CRC, they usually have weakened immune systems. When the immune system is suppressed, it is prone to more infections and disease, making it impossible for a person to fully recover. This is why it is important to help boost the immune system by using a variety of supplements. One of the most powerful ones that is so simple to take is VITAMIN C. Taking a couple of grams, twice per day really helps to keep the immune system working well.

Some of the factors responsible for failure to achieve a total cure could be:

1. Lack of hydrochloric acid (HCL) in stomach

Hydrochloric acid is produced in the stomach to aid in activating digestion of foods and protection of the intestinal flora, but mostly to help digest proteins and help absorb nutrients such as vitamin B12, calcium, iron and intrinsic factor.

One of the most common causes of HCL imbalances is past antibiotic use. Antibiotics destroy the beneficial bacteria that synthesize B vitamins necessary for HCL production in the stomach. Proper HCL levels in the stomach kill off many pathogens that otherwise would enter into the intestinal tract and potentially create problems.

HCL's important functions include:

- ✓ Breaking down proteins into essential amino acids and nutrients
- ❖ Stimulating your pancreas and small intestines to produce the digestive enzymes and bile necessary to further breakdown the carbohydrates, proteins and fats
- ❖ Preventing disease by killing pathogenic bacteria and yeast normally present in foods
- ❖ Low stomach acid leads to a cascade of digestive problems such as bloating, gas and constipation.
- ❖ Low gastric acid causes a variety of intestinal problems such as bloating, flatulence and indigestion. So, if the patient suffers from hypochlorhydria or low production of hydrochloric acid from the stomach, then add GASTRIC AID.

It is only those very rare cases where we have a case of antifungal-resistant Candida that is a problem. This usually happens when the patient has been treated time and time again with medicinal anti-fungals and the Candida have now become a 'super Candida'. This again can be eliminated using this protocol but the time required will be stretched to 4-5 months.

I have never had an antifungal-resistant case that was not cured in a maximum of 5 months, but as I said earlier, these are very rare occurrences and personally I have not seen more than a handful of cases in my career.

Natural Antibiotics During the Candida Protocol
It is critical that anyone on the 3-month Candida protocol stock-up on NATURAL ANTIMICROBIAL PACK that they might require if they come down with a cold, flu, sore throat or any kind of infection while they are still on the Candida protocol.

These natural antibiotics have been tried and tested for many years and seem to work fine with most infections. However, it is very important to take these immediately when the first symptoms appear. If you leave the infection for a couple of days, the microbes will spread quickly and it will be more difficult to shift it with the natural antibiotics.

This is why it is critical to have these natural antibiotics in your medical dispensary BEFORE beginning the Candida protocol. They have an expiry date of between two and five years, so you will no doubt use them during this time.

The dosages mentioned below are for adults. For maximum effectiveness it is good to use at least four of the natural antibiotics mentioned below, all in combination together.

These natural antibiotics and herbal supplements include the following that have been used successfully in clinical practice, and in fact have been used by all my family for over 30 years, given that none of my 4 children have ever taken antibiotics in their lives!

1. GRAPEFRUIT SEED EXTRACT **(Citricidal™)**: Is a very effective anti-fungal, available in tablet form as well as liquid form which can be placed under nails with fungus. Take 2 tablets 3 times daily. For nails, one drop under each nail morning and evening.

2. OREGANO OIL: If one is citrus intolerant, then you can use Oregano oil gel capsules instead – 1 gel capsule 3 times daily.

3. SILVER LIQUID 50 ppm (colloidal silver) – You can take 1 teaspoon 3 times daily.

4. VITAMIN C – Take either 2 caps (1000 mg each) 3 times daily, or ½ teaspoon 3 times daily of the calcium ascorbate powder form.

5. PARAFORM PLUS TWO – this contains a broad spectrum of active herbals, probiotics and other natural cleansing and protective agents, which have anti-bacterial, anti-fungal, anti-microbial and anti-inflammatory actions. Take one cap x 3 times daily.

There is no reason why ALL these should not be combined together, but at least 4 of the 5 should be combined for maximum effectiveness. Please do not underestimate the importance and value of stocking up on these natural antimicrobials.

We have prepared a NATURAL ANTIMICROBIAL PACK in our one-stop shop for your convenience (www.worldwidehealthcenter.net).

On a few occasions I have seen patients that I was treating for Candida not stocking these natural antibiotics and they came down with a nasty bug that went deep into the lungs within days. By the time they could obtain all these remedies, their symptoms had reached a level where they had to see a medical practitioner, who rightly so, prescribed antibiotic drugs.

It is touch and go whether the Candida protocol will succeed or not when taking antibiotic drugs. The problem is that the antibiotics will inevitably kill off the good bacteria in the gut as well as the bad, and if this creates a severe enough dysbiosis, then the pathogenic, hyphal forms of Candida will begin to proliferate again.

This is very sad when you have to announce to the patient that they have to extend their Candida protocol for another month or longer – very frustrating!

My Own Case Studies from Patients Cured
There is still a lot of controversy around the topic of Candida, and I am the first to agree that we do not have all the answers. One thing that I have witnessed in clinical practice, however, is the astounding recovery that many of these so-called Candidiasis patients make when placed on the Da Vinci Candida Protocol (DCP).

Personally, I have seen many different skin problems clear when the systemic Candidiasis is treated including psoriasis, as well as chronic sinusitis, joint pains, cheloids or scar formations, splitting skin on hands, chronic coughs and sore throats of many years standing, chronic thrush and vaginal discharge, headaches and migraines, chronic fatigue or myalgic encephalomyelitis (ME) and many other rather atypical symptoms that were labeled as "Idiopathic" which basically means "unknown etiology." Here are a few case histories for your interest:

Case 1

This is a case of a woman who went in for a D&C scrape of the uterus and the gynecologist ruptured the uterus and she required emergency surgery due to heavy internal hemorrhage. She received a number of IV antibiotics and a couple of months after being discharged she suffered from splitting hands along with chronic thrush, fatigue and other skin rashes of unknown origin. She made a dramatic improvement in all these symptoms after completing the Da Vinci Candida Protocol.

Case 1: Bad case of splitting hands after IV antibiotics

Case 1: Two-months into the Da Vinci Candida Treatment

Case 2

This is a lady that had suffered from chronic psoriasis for over 20 years. This had spread to most of her torso as well as limbs. One of the underlying problems of the skin problem was systemic Candidiasis which cleared after three months of the Da Vinci Candida Protocol.

Case 2: Chronic psoriasis (left) and 3-months after completion of Da Vinci Candida Treatment

Case 3

A complex case of an idiopathic skin problem of 20 years' duration. Using the Candida Treatment Protocol resulted in over 75% improvement, but there was a bacterial element that needed further treatment to eliminate it.

Case 3: Idiopathic skin problems of 20-years duration (left) and after treatment (right)

Case 4

A young adult who had contracted herpes and Steven-Johnson Syndrome during blood infusions – when presented for treatment he was in excruciating pain, had lost 8 kg and was tube feeding. Treatment using the Candida Treatment Protocol eliminated this difficult problem.

Case 4: Complex case with underlying Candida (left) and one month into treatment (right)

Other Clinical Cases

Here are a few more cases that I have seen in clinical practice – each has different symptoms, yet one of the major underlying factors was Systemic Candidiasis.

Case No. 1: Mrs. A, Age 44

Mrs. A's presenting symptoms were somewhat unusual in that she continually complained that she frequently had the sense of a strong fishy odor in her nostrils over the last 7 years.

She remembers that this began when she had cleaned mold in her house with chlorine – the mold had appeared after a flood.

She also suffered from many allergies which included allergy to flowers, bananas and melon.

Her main symptoms apart from the annoying fishy odor was, constant intermittent coughing as well as a heavy pressure-type sensation in the chest and lungs. She had clear signs of nail fungus as well as frequent vaginal discharge.

She had consulted a number of medical doctors and dermatologists, but with no success. The dermatologist gave her antifungal cream for the nails. The condition remained as before.

She underwent Bioresonance diagnosis using the VEGA system and was found to have a number of food intolerances too such as: wheat, lactose and milk products, bananas, caffeine, sugar, chicken, pork, nightshade family of vegetables (potatoes, tomatoes, peppers, and aubergines), olive oil and olives.

The VEGA test also showed that she was resonating with pathological, mycelial forms of Candida albicans, indicating that she was suffering from systemic Candidiasis – mixed molds were also found during this testing protocol.

It was decided to help her body to detox and return back to an alkaline pH, as well as help eliminate inflammatory chemicals and other toxins. She followed an alkaline detoxification diet for 2 weeks based on alkaline foods such as fruit and vegetables. Her energy levels after the detox had tremendously increased and she reported clarity of mind. She began the Da Vinci Candida Protocol for 3 months – see main text for details.

The smell of fish had decreased by 30% in intensity and the frequency to cough had also decreased by 40% within the first 3 weeks of the protocol treatment. After two months of treatment, the cough had improved 60%.

Previously she would cough for one hour, now she coughs less than one minute. The smell of fish has improved by 70%.

After the completion of the Candida protocol (3 months), the Candida finally disappeared and the cough had improved by 100%. This was the first time that the cough had improved in the past 7 years. The smell of fish had also vanished as well as the nail fungus on her toes – this was also helped by adding grapefruit seed extract liquid – one drop per nail morning and evening. She was a very happy woman!

Case No. 2: Mr. M, Age 45

Mr. M presented with a chronic cough that he had for the past 7-8 years, accompanied by whitish phlegm. He was diagnosed with H. Pylori for which the medical doctor prescribed antibiotics which were taken on and off for a period of 2 years. The coughing however persisted even though he had consulted many doctors, including ENT (otolaryngologists) and pneumologists with no results.

Before coughing began he lived in a moldy apartment.

He underwent VEGA food intolerance testing that showed intolerance to a number of foods such as: wheat, soya, lactose and milk products, beans, caffeine, almonds and walnuts, pork, citrus (lemon, grapefruit, and oranges), olive oil and olives. He is a vegetarian but includes lactose and fish in his diet.

The VEGA testing also showed that he was suffering from systemic Candida albicans. He followed an alkaline detoxification diet for 15 days based on fruit and vegetables. During the detox the cough had decreased by 50% in frequency and 70% decrease in intensity. The white phlegm had stopped completely.

261

Immediately after the detox he began the Da Vinci Candida protocol for 3 months. During the Candida protocol his energy levels had massively increased and he had incredible clarity of mind.

After the Candida treatment, his cough had completely vanished and the phlegm decreased to minimum.

Case No. 3: Mrs. S, Age 49

Mrs. S complained that she had bronchial asthma and suffered from allergies. Medical doctors gave her cortisone sprays. She also suffered from obesity (147 kg) and whenever she tried to diet she suffered from hypoglycemia.

Other health issues included atrial fibrillation (cardiac arrhythmia) and GERD-gastroesophageal reflux disease. She was taking Warfarin, an anticoagulant, to prevent blood clots from forming. She was also taking medication to control her arrhythmia.

She had also removed her thyroid nodules and was taking thyroxine daily.
It was recommended that she begin with a compromised alkaline detoxification diet lasting 1 month. This means that the body will be detoxing slower than the 15-day alkaline detox diet by leaving in protein foods the first two weeks. This procedure is recommended when there are chronic degenerative diseases, in order to prevent any possible adverse reactions caused by the elimination of inflammatory chemicals.

So, the first week of detox she was allowed to eat fish and pulses along with fruit and vegetables. The second week the fish was eliminated and only the pulses remained along with the fruit and vegetables. During the final two weeks, she only ate fruit and vegetables.

During the detox her stomach digestion improved and she was feeling much better; edema had also disappeared after some heavy urination initially, and she had lost noticeable inches around her waist – to her delight as weight loss had been blocked for a long time.

During Bioresonance testing it was shown that she was intolerant to a number of foods such as: wheat, lactose and milk products, citrus (oranges, lemons, grapefruits), caffeine, sugar, hazelnut, walnuts, almonds, pork, chicken, and nightshade family of vegetables (potatoes, tomatoes, aubergines, peppers).

In addition, the Vega Bio-dermal testing also showed that she was suffering from systemic Candidiasis. She therefore began the Da Vinci Candida protocol for 3 months. During the Candida protocol, she had lost a total of 12 kg, her asthmatic symptoms had gone completely, and she could now climb steps without wheezing and panting, being much quicker on her feet. As an added gift, her chronic sinusitis had also completely cleared.

APPENDIX

If you would like to know if your health problems are yeast-related, take this comprehensive test. Questions in Section A focus on your medical history-factors that promote the growth of Candida and that are frequently found people with yeast-related health problems. In Section B, you will find a list of 23 symptoms that are often present in patients with yeast-related health problems. Section C consists of 33 other symptoms that are sometimes seen in people with yeast-related problems – yet they may also be found in people with other disorders.

Fill out and score the questionnaire should help you, and your physician, evaluate the possible role that candida plays in your health problems.

SECTION A: HISTORY

- Have you ever taken tetracycline, or other antibiotics, for acne for one month or longer? (points 35)
- Have you, at any time in your life, taken broad-spectrum antibiotics or other antibacterial medication for respiratory, urinary or other infections for two months or longer, or in shorter courses four or more times in a one-year period? (Points 35).
- Have you taken a broad-spectrum antibiotic drug even in a single dose? (points 6)
- Have you at any time in your life been bothered by persistent prostatitis, vaginitis or other problems affecting your reproductive organs? (points 25)
- Are you bothered by memory or concentration problems do you sometimes feel spaced out? (points 20)
- Do you feel "sick all over", yet despite visits to many different physicians the cause has not been found? (points 20)
- Have you been pregnant two or more times? (points 5)
- One time? (points 3)
- Have you taken birth control pills for more than two years? (points 15)
- For six months to two years? (points 8)
- Have you taken steroids orally, by injection or inhalation for more than two weeks? (points 15)
- For two weeks or less? (points 6)
- Does exposure to perfume, insecticides, fabric shop odours and other chemicals provoke symptoms? Moderate to severe (points 20) Mild (points 5)
- Does tobacco smoke really bother you? (points 10)

- Are your symptoms worse on damp, muggy days or in mouldy places? (points 20)
- Have you had athlete's foot, ring worm, jock itch or other chronic fun-gal infections of the skin or nails? Severe or persistent (points 20) Mild to moderate (points 10)
- Do you crave sugar? (points 10)

Total Score, Section A _____
SECTION B: MAJOR SYMPTOMS

For each of your symptoms, enter the appropriate figure in the pint score column.

1. If a symptom is occasional or mild   **3 points**
2. If a symptom is frequent and/ or moderately severe   **6 points**
3. If a symptom is severe and/ or disabling   **9 points**

Add total score and record it at the end of this section.

- Fatigue or lethargy   _____
- Feeling of being "drained"   _____
- Depression or manic depression   _____
- Numbness, burning or tingling   _____
- Headache   _____
- Muscle aches   _____
- Muscle weakness or paralysis   _____
- Paint and/ or swelling in joints   _____
- Abdominal pain   _____
- Constipation and/ or diarrhea   _____
- Bloating, belching or intestinal gas   _____
- Troublesome vaginal burning, itching or discharge   _____
- Prostatitis   _____
- Impotence   _____
- Loss of sexual desire or feeling   _____
- Endometriosis or infertility   _____
- Cramps and/ or other menstrual irregularities   _____
- Premenstrual tension   _____
- Attacks of anxiety or crying   _____
- Cold hands or feet, low bode temperature   _____

265

- Hypothyroidism   _____
- Shaking or irritable when hungry   _____
- Cystitis or interstitial cystitis   _____

TOTAL SCORE, SECTION B

_____

SECTION C: OTHER SYMPTOMS

For each of your symptoms, enter the appropriate figure in the point score column.

1. If a symptom is occasional or mild   **3 points**
2. If a symptom is frequent and/ or moderately severe   **6 points**
3. If a symptom is severe and/ or disabling   **9 points**

Add total score and record it at the end of his section.

- Drowsiness, including inappropriate drowsiness   _____
- Irritability   _____
- In coordination   _____
- Frequent mood swings   _____
- Insomnia   _____
- Dizziness/ loss of balance   _____
- Pressure above ears, tenderness of cheekbones or forehead_____
- Tendency to bruise easily   _____
- Eczema, itching eyes   _____
- Psoriasis   _____
- Chronic hives (urticaria)   _____
- Indigestion or heartburn   _____
- Sensitivity to milk, wheat, corn or other common foods _____
- Mucus in stools   _____
- Rectal itching   _____
- Dry mouth or throat   _____
- Mouth rashes, including "white" tongue   _____
- Bad breath   _____
- Foot, hair or body odour not relieved by washing   _____
- Nasal congestion or postnasal drip   _____
- Nasal itching   _____
- Sore throat   _____

- Laryngitis, loss of voice　　　　　　　　＿＿＿＿＿＿
- Cough or recurrent bronchitis　　　　　＿＿＿＿＿＿
- Pain or tightness in chest　　　　　　　＿＿＿＿＿＿
- Wheezing or shortness of breath　　　　＿＿＿＿＿＿
- Urinary frequency or urgency　　　　　　＿＿＿＿＿＿
- Burning on urination　　　　　　　　　　＿＿＿＿＿＿
- Spots in front of eyes or erratic vision　＿＿＿＿＿＿
- Burning or tearing eyes　　　　　　　　＿＿＿＿＿＿
- Recurrent infections or fluid in ears　　＿＿＿＿＿＿
- Ear pain or deafness　　　　　　　　　　＿＿＿＿＿＿

TOTAL SCORE, SECTION C

＿＿＿＿＿

GRAND TOTAL (SECTION A, B AND C)

＿＿＿＿＿

The **Grand Total Score** will help you and your physician decide if your health problems are yeast-connected. Scores in women will run higher, as seven items in the questionnaire apply to women, while only two apply exclusively to men.

- Yeast –connected health problems are almost certainly present in women with scores of **more than 180,** and in men with of **more than 140.**
- Yeast-connected health problems are probably present in women with scores of **more than 120,** and in men with scores **more than 90.**
- Yeast-connected health problems are possibly present in women with scores of **more than 60,** and in me of **more than 40.**
- With scores of less than 60 in women and 40 in men, yeasts are less apt ti be the cause of health problems.

> Score of **60-99** yeast a possible cause of health problems
> PA Score of **100-139** yeast a probable cause of health problems.
> Score of **140 or more** yeast **almost certainly** a cause of health problems.

These are many causes for each symptom listed below. Assign points to each symptom and see if a pattern develops.

A= Symptom never occur

B= Symptom occurs occasionally

C= Symptom occurs frequently

D= Symptom occurs regularly

Questions		A	B	C	D
	Restless sleep	0	1	2	3
	Skin problems, rashes, itches	0	1	2	3
	Increased appetite, hungry after meals	0	1	2	3
	Frequent diarrhea, loose stools	0	1	2	3
	Grinding of teeth when asleep	0	1	2	3
	Variable, changeable consistency of stools	0	1	2	3
	Picking of nose, boring nose with finger	0	1	2	3
	Abdominal pains	0	1	2	3
	Vertical wrinkles around mouth	0	1	2	3
	Rectal, anal itching	0	1	2	3
	Parallel lines (tracks) in soles of feet	0	1	2	3
	Intestinal cramps, burning	0	1	2	3
	Irritability (no apparent reason)	0	1	2	3
	Feeling bloated, gaseous	0	1	2	3
	Diarrhea alternating with constipation	0	1	2	3
	Bowel urgency, occasional accidents	0	1	2	3
	Hyperactive tendency (nervous)	0	1	2	3
	Dark circles under eyes	0	1	2	3
	Need for extra sleep, waking unrefreshed	0	1	2	3
	Allergies, food sensitivities	0	1	2	3
	Fevers of unknown origin	0	1	2	3
	Night sweats (not menopausal)	0	1	2	3
	Kissing pets, allowing them to lick your face	0	1	2	3

	Anaemia	0	1	2	3
	Frequent colds, flu, sore throats	0	1	2	3
	Going barefoot in parks, public streets	0	1	2	3
	Travelling in 3rd countries	0	1	2	3
	Eating lightly cooked pork products	0	1	2	3
	Eating sushi, sashimi	0	1	2	3
	Sleeping with pets on bed	0	1	2	3
	Bed wetting	0	1	2	3
	Men: sexual dysfunction	0	1	2	3
	Forgetfulness	0	1	2	3
	Slow reflexes	0	1	2	3
	Loss of appetite	0	1	2	3
	Yellowish face	0	1	2	3
	Heart beat rapid	0	1	2	3
	Heart pain	0	1	2	3
	Pain in the umbilicus	0	1	2	3
	Blurry, unclear face	0	1	2	3
	Pain: back, thighs, shoulders	0	1	2	3
	Lethargy, apathy	0	1	2	3
	Numbness, tingling in hands, feet	0	1	2	3
	Burning pains in the stomach, intestines	0	1	2	3
	Menstrual problems	0	1	2	3
	Dry lips during day, damp at night	0	1	2	3
	Drooling while asleep	0	1	2	3
	Occult blood in stool (shown from lab tests)	0	1	2	3
	History of giardia, pin worms, other worms	0	1	2	3
	Swimming in creeks, rivers, lakes	0	1	2	3

Total score

10-14 points = maybe parasite infestation

15- 20 points = suspect parasites

22-25 points = likely- (Further testing helpful)

25 or more = parasites involvement high likely

REFERENCES

Al-Doory Y. 1969. The mycology of the freeliving baboon (Papio sp.). Mycopathologia et Mycologia Applicata 38: 7–15.

Anderson KE, Kappas A. Dietary regulation of cytochrome P-450. Annu Rev Nutr. 11:141-167, 1991.

Ballie-Hamilton, P. The Detox diet. UK: Penguin, 2002.

Banerjee, M., D.S. Thompson, A. Lazzell, P.L. Carlisle, C. Pierce, C. Monteagudo, J.L. Lopez-Ribot, and D. Kadosh. 2008. UME6, a novel filament-specific regulator of Candida albicans hyphal extension and virulence. Mol. Biol. Cell 19, 1354-1365.

Barclay GR, McKenzie H, Pennington J, Parratt D, Pennington CR. The effect of dietary yeast on the activity of stable chronic Crohn's disease. Scand J Gastroenterol 1992; 27 :196–200.

Bartlett JG, Gilbert DN, Spellberg B. Seven ways to preserve the miracle of antibiotics. Clin Infect Dis. 2013;56(10):1445–1450.

Bartlett JG, Gilbert DN, Spellberg B. Seven ways to preserve the miracle of antibiotics. Clin Infect Dis. 2013;56(10):1445–1450.

Bastidas RJ, Heitman J: Trimorphic stepping stones pave the way to fungal virulence. PNAS 2009; 106: 351–2.

Bastidas RJ, Heitman J: Trimorphic stepping stones pave the way to fungal virulence. PNAS 2009; 106: 351–2.

Berman J: Morphogenesis and cell cycle progression in Candida albicans. Curr Opin Microbiol 2006; 9: 595–601.

Bernhardt H, Knoke M. Mycological aspects of gastrointestinal microflora. Scand J Gastroenterol 1997; 32(suppl 222) :102–106.

Bland JS, Bralley JA. Nutritoinal upregulation of hepatic detoxification enzymes. J Appl Nutr. 44(3&4):2-15, 1992.

Blankenship, J.R. and A.P. Mitchell. 2006. How to build a biofilm: a fungal perspective. Curr. Opin. Microbiol. 9, 588-594.

Brandtzaeg P. The mucosal B cell and its functions. In: Brostoff J, Challacombe S (eds): Food Allergy and Intolerance. London: Saunders; 2002:127-171.

Budtz- Jorgensen, E. Cellular immunity in acquired Candidiasis of the palate. Scand. J. Dent. Res. 81, 372, 1973

Cabot, S. Juice Fasting Detoxification. USA: The Sprout House, 1992.
Calderone RA, Fonzi WA: Virulence factors of Candida albicans. Trends Microbiol 2001; 9: 327–35.

Calderone, R.A., and R.L. Cihlar (e.d.). Fungal pathogenesis: principles and clinical applications. Marcel Dekker, Inc., New York, N.Y, 2002

Carlisle PL, Banerjee M, Lazzell A, Monteagudo C, Lopez-Ribot JL, Kadosh D: Expression levels of a filament-specific transcriptional regulator are sufficient to determine Candida albicans morphology and virulence. PNAS 2009; 106: 599–604.

Carlisle, P.L., M. Banerjee, A. Lazzell, C. Monteagudo, J.L. LopezRibot, and D. Kadosh. 2009. Expression levels of a filament-specific transcriptional regulator are sufficient to determine Candida albicans morphology and virulence. Proc. Natl. Acad. Sci. USA 106, 599-604.

Centers for Disease Control and Prevention, Office of Infectious Disease Antibiotic resistance threats in the United States, 2013. Apr, 2013. Available at: http://www.cdc.gov/drugresistance/threat-report-2013. Accessed January 28, 2015.

Crampin, H., K. Finley, M. Gerami-Nejad, H. Court, C. Gale, J. Berman, and P.E. Sudbery. 2005. Candida albicans hyphae have a Spitzenkorper that is distinct from the polarisome found in yeast and pseudohyphae. J. Cell. Sci. 118, 2935-2947.

Crandall M. The pathogenetic significance of Intestinal Candida Colonization, 2004

Crook WG: The yeast connection, A medical Breakthrough 2nd Addition Professional Books, Jackson, TN, 1984

Crook WG: The Yeast Connection, A Medical Breakthrough 2nd Addition Professional Books, Jackson, TN, 1984.

Crook, WG. The Yeast Connection and the Woman. Professional Books, Jackson TN 1987.

Dalkilic E, Aksebzeci T, Kocatürk I, Aydin N, Koculu B: The investigation of pathogenity and virulence of Candida. In: Tümbay E, Seeliger HPR, Ang Ö (eds.): Candida and Candidamycosis. New York: Plenum Press 1991; 50: 167–74

Davies MH, Gough A, Sorhi RS, Hassel A, Warning R, Emery P. Sulphoxidation and sulphation capacity in patients with primary biliary cirrhosis. J Hepatol. 22(5):551-560, May 1995.

Enderlein, G. (1925). Bakterien-Cyclogenie, Verlag de Gruyter & Co, Berlin.

Fitzsimmons N, Berry DR. Inhibition of Candida albicans by Lactobacillus acidophilus: evidence for the involvement of a peroxidase system. Microbios 1994; 80 :125–133.

Gail Burton. Candida - The Silent Epidemic, Candida Causative factors, 4-9, 2003

Georgiou, G.J. (2005) Explore! Volume 14, No. 6.

Georgiou, G.J. (2008) British Naturopathic Journal, Vol. 25., No. 1 & 2.

Grant DM. Detoxification pathways of the liver. J Inher Metab Dis. 14;421-430, 1991.

Grubb SEW, Murdoch C, Sudbery PE, Saville SP, Lopez-Ribot JL, Thornhill MH: Candida albicans-endothelial cell interactions: a key step in the pathogenesis of systemic candidiasis. Infect Immun 2008; 76: 4370–7.

Hesseltine HC, Campbell LK. 1938. Diabetic or mycotic vulvovaginitis. American Journal of Obstetrics and Gynecology 35:
272–283.

Hornby, J.M., E.C. Jensen, A.D. Lisec, J.J. Tasto, B. Jahnke, R. Shoemaker, P. Dussault, and K.W. Nickerson. 2001. Quorum sensing in the dimorphic fungus Candida albicans is mediated by farnesol. Appl. Environ. Microbiol. 67, 2982-2992

Hube B: From commensal to pathogen: stage- and tissue-specific gene expression of Candida albicans. Curr Opin Microbiol 2004; 7: 336–41.

Hulda Regehr Clark, Ph.D., N.D., The Cure for all Diseases 1995
Hussein, H.S., and J.M. Brasel. Toxicity, metabolism, and impact of mycotoxins on humans and animals. Toxicology 167, 2001

Iwata, K.; Yamamoto, Y "Glycoprotein Toxins Produced by Candida albicans." Proceedings of the Fourth International Conference on the Mycoses, PAHO Scientific Publication #356, June 1977.

John Parks Trowbridge, M.D., and Morton Walker, D.P.M., The yeast syndrome- Antibiotics Encourage Yeast Overgrowth, 45-46, 1986

Kanda N, Tani K, Enomoto U, Nakai K & Watanabe S. The skin fungus-induced Th1- and Th2-related cytokine, chemokine and prostaglandin E 2 production in peripheral blood mononuclear cells from patients with atopic dermatitis and psoriasis vulgaris. Clinical & Experimental Allergy; 32(8):1243-50.

Kennedy MJ, Volz PA. Ecology of Candida albicans gut colonisation: inhibition of Candida adhesion, colonisation and dissemination from the gastrointestnal tracy by bacterial antagonism. Infect Immun 1985; 49: 654–63.

Koivikko A, et al. Allergenic cross-reactivity of yeasts. Allergy 1988; 43:192-200.

Kubo I, Fujita K, Lee SH, Ha TJ. Antibacterial activity of polygodial. Phytother Res. 2005 Dec;19(12):1013-7.

Kumamoto CA, Vinces MD: Alternative Candida albicans lifestyles: growth on surfaces. Annu Rev Microbiol 2005; 59: 113–33.
Douglas LJ: Candida biofilms and their role in infection. Trends Microbiol 2003; 11: 30–6.

Kumamoto CA, Vinces MD: Alternative Candida albicans lifestyles: growth on surfaces. Annu Rev Microbiol 2005; 59: 113–33.

Lee SH, Lee JR, Lunde CS, Kubo I. In vitro antifungal susceptibilities of Candida albicans and other fungal pathogens to polygodial, a sesquiterpene dialdehyde. Planta Med. 1999 Apr;65(3):204-8.

Leon Chaitow N.D, D.O, Candida Albicans- Could yeast be your problem? How Candida gets out of hand. Chapter 3- Immune System Deficiency, 24-26, 1991

Lushniak BD. Antibiotic resistance: a public health crisis. Public Health Rep. 2014;129(4):314–316.

Luyt CE, Brechot N, Trouillet JL, Chastre J. Antibiotic stewardship in the intensive care unit. Crit Care. 2014;18(5):480.

Magee PT, Chibana H: The genomes of Candida albicans and other Candida species. In: Calderone RA (ed.): Candida and candi - diasis. Washington: ASM Press 2002; 293–304

Michael T. Murray, N.D., Chronic Candidiasis, Dietary factors, sugar and the yeast syndrome: 43,44, 1997

Morita E, Hide M, Yoneya Y, Kannbe M, Tanaka A, Yamamoto S: An assessment of the role of Candida albicans antigen in atopic dermatitis. J Dermatol 1999; 26: 282–7. 20. Pappas PG, Rex JH, Sobel JD, et al.: Guidelines for treatment of Candidiasis. CID 2004; 38: 161–89. 21.

Morschhäuser J, Köhler G, Ziebuhr W, Blum-Oehler G, Dobrindt U, Hacker J: Evolution of microbial pathogens. Phil Trans R Soc Lond 2000; 355: 695–704.

Netea MG, Brown GD, Kullberg BJ, Gow NAR: An integrated model of the recognition of Candida albicans by the innate immune system. Nat Rev Immunol 2008; 6: 67–78.

Nieuwenhuizen WF, Pieters RH, Knippels LM, Jansen MC, Koppelman GJ. Is Candida albicans a trigger for the onset of coeliac disease? Lancet 2003; 361 :2152–2154.

Nobile, C.J. and A.P. Mitchell. 2006. Genetics and genomics of Candida albicans biofilm formation. Cell. Microbiol. 8, 1382-1391

Noverr MC, Falkowski NR, McDonald RA, McKenzie AN, Huffnagle GB: Development of allergic airway disease in mice following antibiotic therapy and fungal microbiota increase: role of host genetics, antigen, and interleukin-13. Infect Immun 2005; 73: 30–8.

Noverr MC, Phare SM, Toews GB, Coffey MJ, Huffnagle GB: Path - ogenic yeasts Cryptococcus neoformans and Candida albicans produce immunomodulatory prostaglandins. Infect Immun 2001; 69: 2957–63.

Noverr MC, Noggle RM, Toews GB, Huffnagle GB: Role of antibiotics and fungal microbiota in driving pulmonary allergic responses. Infect Immun 2004; 72: 4996–5003.

Odds FC. 1988. Candida and Candidosis, 2nd edn. Bailli`ere Tindall: London.

Piddock LJ. The crisis of no new antibiotics—what is the way forward? Lancet Infect Dis. 2012;12(3):249–253.

Piispanen AE, Hogan DA: PEPped up: induction of Candida albicans virulence by bacterial cell wall fragments. Cell Host Microbe 2008; 4: 1–2

Polakova S, Blume C, Zarate JA, Mentel M, Jorck-Ramberg D, Stenderup J, et al.: Formation of new chromosomes as a virulence mechanism in yeast Candida glabrata. PNAS 2009; 106: 2688–93

Poulain D, Hopwood V, Vernes A. Antigenic variability of candida albicans. CRC Crit Rev Microbiol 1985; 12:223-70.

Raska M, Belakova J, Krupka M, Weigl E: Candidiasis – Do we need to fight or to tolerate the Candida fungus? Folia Microbiol 2007; 52: 297–312.

Reinel D, Plettenberg A, Seebacher C, et al.: Orale Candidose. Leitlinie der Deutschen Dermatologischen Gesellschaft und der Deutschsprachigen Mykologischen Gesellschaft. JDDG 2008; 7: 593–7.

Reinholdt J, Krogh P, Holmstrup P. Degradation of IgA1, IgA2, and S-IgA by candida and torulopsis species. Acta Path Microbiol Immunol Scand, Sect C 1987; 95:65-74.

Romani L, Bistoni F, Puccetti P. Initiation of T-helper cell immunity to Candida albicans by IL-12: the role of neutrophils. Chem Immunol. 1997; 68:110-35.

Romani L, Bistoni F, Puccetti P: Adaptation of Candida albicans to the host environment: the role of morphogenesis in virulence and survival in mammalian hosts. Curr Opin Microbiol 2003; 6: 338–43.

Salloum, TK. Fasting Signs and Symptoms: A Clinical Guide. USA: Buckeye Naturopathic Press, 1992.

Scrivner, J. Detox Yourself. UK: Judy Piatkus (Publishers) Ltd., 1998.

Seelig MS. Mechanisms by which antibiotics increase the incidence and severity of candidiasis and alter the immunological defences. Bacteriol Rev 1 1966; 30 :4442–4459.

Shah DT, Jackman S, Engle J, Larsen B. Effect of gliotoxin on human polymorphonuclear neutrophils. Inf Dis Obster Gynecol 1998; 6 :168–175.

Shen J, Cowen LE, Griffin AM, Chan L, Kohler JR: The Candida albicans pescadillo homolog is required for normal hypha-to-yeast morphogenesis and yeast proliferation. PNAS 2008; 105: 20918–23.

Soll DR: Phenotypic switching. In: Calderone RA (ed.): Candida and Candidiasis. Washington: ASM Press 2002; 123–42.

Sudbery, P.E., N.A.R. Gow, and J. Berman. 2004. The distinct morphogenic states of Candida albicans. Trends Microbiol. 12, 317- 324

The Chronic Candidiasis Syndrome: Intestinal Candida and its relation to chronic illness OAM 1996-1997, 16. Gutierrez, J.; Maroto, C. et al: Circulating Candida antigens and antibodies: useful markers of candidemia. Journal of Clinical Microbiology. 31(9):25502, 1993.

Thewes S, Kretschmar M, Park H, Schaller M, Filler SG, Hube B: In vivo and ex vivo comparative transcriptional profiling of invasive and noninvasive Candida albicans isolates identifies genes associated with tissue invasion. Mol Microbiol 2007; 63: 1606–28.

Trowbridge JP and Walker M The Yeast Syndrome Bantam Books, New York, New York 1986.

Trowbridge JP and Walker M. The yeast Syndrome Bantam Books, New York, N.Y, 1986
Truss C: The Missing Diagnosis Birmingham Alabama (The author) 1983.

Truss C: The missing Diagnosis Birmingham Alabama (The Author), 1983

Truss, CO. Metabolic abnormalities in patients with chronic Candidiasis - the acetaldehyde hypothesis, Journal of Orthomolecular Medicine, 13:63- 93, 1984

Viswanathan VK. Off-label abuse of antibiotics by bacteria. Gut Microbes. 2014;5(1):3–4.

Vojdani A, Rahimian P, Kalhor H and Mordechai E. Immunological cross reactivity between candida albicans and human tissue. J Clin Lab Immunol 1996; 48:1-15.

Wade, C. Inner Cleansing: How to Free Yourself from the Joint-Muscle-Artery-Circulation Sludge. New York: Parker Publishing Co., 1992.

Walsh, TJ.; Lee, JW.; et al: "Serum Darabinitol measured by automated quantitative enzymatic assay for detection and therapeutic monitoring of experimental disseminated candidiasis: correlation with tissue concentrations of Candida albicans." Journal of Medical & Veterinary Mycology. 32(3):20515, 1994.

Weig M, Werner E, Frosh M, Kasper H. Limited effect of refined carbohydrate dietary supplementation on colonization of the gastrointestinal tract of healthy subjects by Candida albicans. Am J Clin Nutr 1999; 69 :1170–1173.

William G. Crook, M.D., Chronic Fatigue Syndrome and the yeast connection, Probiotics: 260,261, 1992

William G. Crook, M.D., The yeast connection - Candida questionnaire and score sheet - Diagnosis of a yeast-Related disorder, 29-33, Food allergies: 122, 1986

Xu XL, Lee RTH, Fang HM, Wang YM, Li R, Zou H, et al.: Bacterial pepti doglycan triggers Candida albicans hyphal growth by directly activating the adenylyl cyclase cyr1p. Cell Host Microbe 2008; 4: 28–39

VIDEOS

If you wish to watch some webinars and videos that I have done on the subject of Candida and others, here they are (if you cannot see the link, just search on YouTube for "Dr. Georgiou and Candida"):

Candida Videos:

https://www.youtube.com/watch?v=nOYIFKrGbrM&t=620s

https://www.youtube.com/watch?v=VQnE8VQXEpc

Heavy Metals Video:

https://www.youtube.com/watch?v=lZNFPWPWNnc&index=7&list=PLXDVp62iaBwzezTyezZ4M8ZFhL5sz
J-hR

In the next chapter we will examine how teeth can be linked to a number of chronic diseases in the holistic model of health.

Chapter 7

Teeth Linked to Chronic Diseases

It is estimated that 70% of all medical illnesses are directly or indirectly caused by human intervention in the dental structures (teeth and jawbones). This includes impacted teeth, infected root canalled teeth, new and recurrent decay around old fillings, cysts, bone infections in areas of previously extracted teeth, granulomas and areas of bone condensation to osteitis.

Our mouths are full of bacteria. Bacteria in the mouth use the sugar in food to make acids. Over time, the acids can attack the tooth, creating decay leading to a cavity.

Diseased Tooth/Gum

Periodontal Pocket

Inflammation

Healthy Tooth/Gum

Gingivae (Gums)

These bacteria, along with mucus and other particles, constantly form a sticky, colourless film called "plaque" on teeth. Brushing and flossing help get rid of plaque. Plaque that is not removed can harden and form "tartar" that brushing doesn't clean.

Only professional cleaning by a dental health professional can remove tartar. The longer plaque and tartar are on teeth, the more harmful they become. Untreated decay can become so advanced that the tooth must be removed (extraction).

The bacteria cause inflammation of the gums called "gingivitis." In gingivitis, the gums become red, swollen and can bleed easily. Gingivitis is a mild form of gum disease that can usually be reversed with daily brushing and flossing, as well as regular cleaning by a dental health professional. This form of gum disease does not include any loss of bone and tissue that hold teeth in place.

Untreated gum disease can advance to periodontitis (meaning "inflammation around the tooth"). In periodontitis, gums pull away from the teeth and form spaces called "pockets" that become infected. The body's immune system fights the bacteria as the infection spreads and grows below the gum line. Bacterial toxins and the body's natural response to infection start to break down the bone and connective tissue that hold teeth in place. If not treated, the bones, gums, and tissue that support the teeth are destroyed.

Otherwise functional teeth may eventually become loose and must be removed. Overall, 70% of tooth loss is due to tooth decay, 20% due to periodontal diseases and 10% due to other causes (Brown LJ et al, 1989).

Periodontal disease is one of the most common diseases and if untreated becomes a serious and destructive chronic infection. However, this is not the only problem.

Oral health problems are also related to general health. This is an important connection in terms of preventing chronic disease and disability and reducing health care costs.

The World Oral Health Report (2003) stated clearly that the relationship between oral health and general health is proven by evidence. Since that report, new evidence has emerged further strengthening the case. Oral health and general health are related in four major ways:

1. Poor oral health is significantly associated with major chronic diseases.
2. Poor oral health causes disability.
3. Oral health issues and major diseases share common risk factors.
4. General health problems may cause or worsen oral health conditions.

Poor Oral Health Related to Major Chronic Diseases

A large prospective study of 7,674 subjects, with a long follow-up period (1976-2002), presents a linear relationship between number of teeth and death from CVD, indicating a direct link between oral health and CVD. It was shown that the number of teeth can be used to assess increased risk of CVD in adults.

Alman et al (2011) showed a significant positive association between loss of bone supporting teeth due to periodontal disease and CVD. This was found at even low levels of bone loss between 10% and 20%.

After conducting a systematic review in 2007 of studies examining the association between periodontal disease and CVD, Bahekar and colleagues concluded that the number of existing and new cases of coronary heart disease are both significantly increased in periodontal disease. Khader et al (2004) in a meta-analysis also reported similar relationships.

A new Korean study has identified a relationship between total tooth loss from any cause and diabetes. People with diabetes are more likely to have periodontal disease than people without diabetes, probably because diabetics are more susceptible to infection anywhere in the body.

A 2006 systematic review looked at the association between respiratory diseases and oral health. There was good evidence that improved oral hygiene and frequent professional oral health care reduces the progression or occurrence of respiratory diseases among high-risk elderly adults living in nursing homes, especially those in intensive care units (ICUs). There was evidence that the risk of pneumonia was related to level of oral health.

There is also an increasing number of well-designed studies providing evidence that periodontitis is associated with a steady increase in circulatory levels of pro-inflammatory cytokines, that will predispose the individual to chronic diseases (Figueredo et al, 2000; D'Aiuto et al, 2005, 2004; Fredriksonn et al, 1999; Montebugnoli et al, 2004).

279

There may also be a cancer connection. Dr. Robert Jones, a researcher, found an extremely high correlation between root canals and breast cancer. He claims to have found the following correlations in a five-year study of 300 breast cancer cases:

❖ 93% of women with breast cancer had root canals.
❖ 7% had other oral pathology.
❖ Tumours, in most cases, occurred on the same side of the body as the root canal(s) or other oral pathology.

Dr. Jones found that toxins from the bacteria in an infected tooth or jawbone can inhibit the specific proteins that suppress tumour development. His findings were confirmed by a University of Michigan study about protein suppression.

A German physician, Dr. Josef Issels, reported similar findings. Dr. Issels reported that, in his 40 years of treating "terminal" cancer patients, 97% of his cancer patients had root canals. If these physicians are correct, the cure for cancer may be as simple as having a tooth pulled, then rebuilding your immune system.

The Toxic Element Research Foundation (TERF) used DNA analysis to examine root-canaled teeth. They found bacterial contamination in 100% of the samples tested. They identified 42 different species of anaerobic bacteria in 43 root canal samples. In cavitation's, 67 different bacteria were identified among the 85 samples tested, with individual samples housing between 19 to 53 types of bacteria each. The bacteria they found included the following types:

❖ Capnocytophagaochracea (Hua-Kung Wang et al, 2007)
❖ Fusobacteriumnucleatum (Michael D et al, 2003)
❖ Gemellamorbillorum (Sanjeev, V et al, 1996)
❖ Leptotrichiabuccalis
❖ Porphyromonasgingivalis (Boston University Medical Center, 2011).

Are these just benign, ordinary mouth bugs? *Absolutely not!* Four can affect your heart, three can affect your nerves, two can affect your kidneys, two can affect your brain, and one can infect your sinus cavities... so they are anything but friendly!

Dental Mercury Poisoning in Focus
The World Health Organization has found the average individual can absorb as much as 120 micrograms of mercury per day from his or her amalgam fillings, a level which is considered a toxic dose.

Further research has shown a positive correlation between the concentration of mercury in mothers' breast milk and the number of dental amalgams in these women's mouths. The mean level of mercury in the milk of amalgam-free mothers was less than 0.2mcg/litre, while milk from mothers with one to four amalgam fillings contained 0.50 mcg/litre; with five to seven fillings at 0.57mcg/litre and more than seven fillings at 2.11 mcg/litre.

Dr Murray Vimy, clinical associate professor of the Department of Medicine, as well as several other medical researchers from the Departments of Radiology, Medicine and Medical Physiology at the University of Calgary in Canada, have spent more than a decade examining the effects of amalgam fillings on sheep, monkeys and humans.

Their published evidence conclusively proves that mercury from amalgam fillings migrates to tissues in the oral cavity, the lungs and the gastrointestinal (GI) tract, causing a 'time-released poisoning'.

New evidence on human health shows that mercury fillings in pregnant women may also affect the growing foetus. In 1989, the University of Calgary Medical School published evidence that showed that within three days of placing amalgam fillings in pregnant sheep, mercury showed up in the blood, pituitary glands, liver and kidneys of their lambs. By 33 days (around the time of birth), most foetal tissue had higher levels of mercury than that of the parent animals. During nursing, the mother sheep were found to have eight times more mercury in their milk as in their blood.

More recently, Professor Gustav Drasch, a forensic toxicologist and his colleagues at the Institut fur Rechtsmedicine in Munich, examined the brain, liver, and kidneys of dead human babies and foetuses that had been aborted for medical reasons. They found that the mercury levels correlated significantly with the number of amalgam fillings their mothers had.

Meanwhile, children were found to have accumulated mercury in their kidneys, apparently from the mothers' amalgams, to a similar extent that adults do from their own fillings. As most of the children weren't breastfed, or only for a short period, the researchers concluded that mercury must have passed through the placenta.

Current research suggests that mercury vapour from fillings may be a predominant underlying cause of a broad spectrum of conditions, ranging from gum disease, migraine, headaches, poor memory, depression, anxiety, mental lethargy, chronic fatigue, allergies such as eczema and asthma, sensitivity reactions to food and inhalants, rheumatism, arthritis, backache, kidney disease, Alzheimer's disease, Parkinson's disease, multiple sclerosis and other neurological disorders.

Considering the evidence for such wide-ranging mercury poisoning effects, many patients and dentists then began replacing amalgams with alternative materials, without realizing the risks involved in the amalgam removal process. The removal of toxic materials calls for specially-prepared, expert handling and many dentists are simply not trained or equipped for the job.

Dental amalgam fillings slowly leak mercury, tin, silver, copper and sometimes nickel. These metals have various degrees of toxicity. A large mercury filling contains enough mercury to kill a child if given as a single dose!

Mercury and tin are prime neuro-toxic substances. Mercury can destroy and or damage the transport fibres inside each nerve. The latest research from one of the top German toxicologists, Max Daunderer, MD, reveals that the entire jawbone (upper and lower) has become a toxic waste dump for the following substances:

- ❖ Pesticides
- ❖ Solvents (mostly present in lower jaw)
- ❖ Formaldehyde (mostly lower jaw)
- ❖ Amalgam (mercury, tin, copper and silver) – jawbone and maxillary sinus
- ❖ Palladium (from gold/palladium alloys) – mostly upper jawbone

Through biopsies, Daunderer found that virtually all inhaled toxins are stored in the jawbone in the areas adjacent to the root tips. Also of great interest is Daunderer's serial biopsies on malignant tumours in patients that had amalgam fillings. He found, predictably, mercury in the tumour. The concentration is highest in the centre of the tumour (malignant melanoma, brain cancer, bladder, stomach, colon and tongue cancer).

The most common symptoms caused by amalgam fillings are:

- ❖ Chronic fatigue
- ❖ Tendency to chronic inflammatory changes – rheumatoid arthritis, phlebitis fibromyalgia, irritable bowel syndrome
- ❖ Chronic neurologic illnesses, especially when numbness is one of the primary symptoms
- ❖ Lowering of pain threshold

Removing amalgams can seriously damage your health!

TAKE PRECAUTIONS BEFORE REMOVAL!

I have already mentioned in a previous chapter the dreadful health consequences that I had as a result of mercury amalgam removal, without taking safety precautions and being on a proper chelation protocol. Therefore, I must issue a strong warning here for all those who are thinking of removing their amalgams without the proper preparation – DO NOT DO IT!

Do not go to any dentist and begin to remove amalgam fillings without understanding the safety precautions that you need to take. I will outline some of these below so there will be no excuse for ignorance. I am quite categorical here, only because I had 10 amalgams removed many years ago and developed symptoms of mercury poisoining that took years to overcome. Being a victim of ignorance in those days was no fun!

Removing Amalgams Safely

A dental mercury detoxification protocol is a demanding task. If you intend to remove any metal fillings from your mouth, the following steps can help prevent plenty of grief and suffering. There are a few safety issues that you should have in mind:

1. The mercury in the filling is in the elemental form. It easily penetrates the rubber dam[112] and all mucous membranes (the oral cavity, GI tract and lungs).
2. Mercury is highly volatile when heated. The dental drill operating at 100,000rpms will generate much mercury vapour during the removal procedure.
3. It is estimated that 80% of the mercury vapour inhaled enters the body through the lungs and is distributed to various bodily tissues and organs, with the potential for causing severe illness.

Even though the very best precautions are taken to prevent mercury exposure during dental removal, some exposure still occurs. Therefore, the patient needs to take detoxification agents to chelate any mercury and prevent inadvertent absorption.

Patient Protection Protocol

Here are some guidelines for removing amalgams – most of these follow Dr. Huggins' protocol[113] but have been somewhat adapted based on my experience and research with mercury detoxification. He is one of the leading research dentists in

---

112 A rubber dam is used in the mouth to cover the back of throat so that less mercury vapour and debris from the amalgam removal is swallowed.
113 http://www.hugginsappliedhealing.com

this field of Holistic Dentistry and has written much based on his empirical knowledge.

Always prepare your body as best as you can before, during and after amalgam removal. It is always prudent to observe the heavy metal detoxification protocols already discussed before removing any amalgams. It may take three to six months to prepare your body to withstand the potential mercury intoxication from the removal process. Otherwise, you risk ending up with more health problems than when you started.

The good health of the human organism must be built up and maintained so it can withstand the risks of amalgam removal. Even if the removal is done at a modern dentistry office with a biological setup, accidents with hazardous materials can happen anywhere! I have seen too many patients who developed very serious chronic disease after mercury amalgam removal; heart disease, cancer, MS and other degenerative diseases.

While the detoxification protocols are crucial, there are other preparations to help optimize health, too, such as proper nutritional support. Optimizing nutrition will also help to strengthen your body. The stronger your body is, the more capable it will be to handle an accidental mercury overdose.

It is imperative to be on a safe chelation protocol using HMD®, HMD LAVAGE, HMD CHLORELLA[114] and a potent nutritional supplementation program before, during and after the amalgam removal. A rule of thumb is to use the chelation and the supplements protocols long BEFORE you start the amalgam removal – at least 2 months – to remove some of the toxic metal burden that you already have.

You should also continue the chelation protocol throughout the removal procedures, and for at least six months to a year thereafter. Only after all symptoms have subsided and Hair Mineral Analysis testing[115] has shown that you are low on toxins can you relax the protocol, but always be on guard regarding this issue. Observe and listen to your body. Tell your practitioner about your symptoms. He or she should correlate them with further testing to guide you.

Only once you are in good shape should you dare to have the mercury amalgams removed by a qualified, experienced, capable and fully-equipped biological dentist. While nearly any dentist is technically qualified to replace your amalgam fillings, less

---

114 See http://www.worldwidehealthcenter.net/product/hmd-ultimate-detox-pack-10-discount/ for more details of these protocols.
115 http://www.worldwidehealthcenter.net/product-category/hair-mineral-analysis/

than 1% of dentists have any clue on how to do it properly, so that your risk of mercury poisoning is minimized. Do it right the first time and you will save yourself the grief and expense associated with severe mercury poisoning-derived diseases.

Do not extract more than one amalgam every month. This will buy you time to detoxify your body slowly. Better safe than sorry. If you are not in a desperate hurry, allow even longer spacing between amalgam removals.

It is best if the dentist measures the electrical potential of each amalgam filling to determine the sequential order in which the restorations should be carried out. The most negatively charged tooth is the one that is removed first, followed by the next negatively charged and so on. Never work on both sides of the head in any one sitting.

Do not take Vitamin C the day of dental procedures. Vitamin C by mouth will shorten the effect of the dental anaesthetic to literally around 10 minutes – after that it gets painful! The IV form of Vitamin C does not do this for reasons unknown, but even 500 milligrams in the tablet form will detoxify the anaesthetic adequately to let you feel the pain of drilling or surgery.

It is wise to get a practitioner like myself who can perform VRT Bioresonance testing to determine whether the composite materials that will be used to fill the tooth after the amalgam is removed, is immune-compatible with you.

At the Da Vinci Holistic Health Centre we take a sample of the patient's hair from the nape of the neck and this is sent to a lab in the USA for mineral and toxic metal testing. This Hair Tissue Mineral Analysis provides a baseline of metals and minerals present in the blood over the previous two months and can then be compared with another hair test a couple of months later.

Observe the Patient Protection Protocol as closely as is possible during removal procedures. Complete protection includes the use of the rubber dam during amalgam removal and the use of a face flannel soaked in charcoal or chlorella powder placed over the face of the patient, to absorb any stray mercury. Moreover, the mouth can also be painted with a slurry mix of chlorella powder and water – the rubber dam can also be coated with this chlorella slurry.

A cotton roll can also be coated with chlorella and placed as a reservoir around the teeth to catch escaping mercury vapour. It is best for the holistic dentist to remove the filling in as large chunks as possible to minimize vaporisation of mercury during drilling.

285

A copious amount of water should be used to cool the drill and contain the amalgam dust, and reduce vapour formation. There should be a large high-power suction hose at the side of the patient's mouth leading to a special mercury filter outside the clinic premises.

It is best to use nasal oxygen during the whole procedure as this allows the patient's face to be covered with a flannel coated with chlorella or charcoal while they are still able to breathe in through the nose. The presence of a negative ion generator in the dental office will also facilitate the removal of mercury vapour. If your dentist does not have all these safety protocols in their office, then you need to assess what you could do without. A dentist that takes none of these precautions will only worsen your health, so it is best to search for another dentist, rather than risk your health further.

If surgery is done during the procedure, use ice packs immediately after the procedures are finished, as well as magnets if desired, to help the inflammation. Minimal travel after surgery is advisable (i.e. one or two miles) as the vibration in a car can release a blood clot, resulting in the famous, painful 'dry socket.' Smoking after surgery will almost guarantee the formation of a painful dry socket. Be forewarned.

If your dentist is using vitamin B12 in an IV, <u>then tell them not to</u>. Vitamin B12 in any form is a methylator, and methyl-mercury is extremely damaging to your nervous system.

The International Academy of Oral Medicine and Toxicology (IAOMT)[116] posts correct and incorrect protocols for amalgam removal for dentists. Read every word and discuss the issues raised with your dentist, as well as your holistic medicine practitioner. I would not necessarily adopt all their guidelines, like the possibility of removing two amalgams in one visit, but their overall recommendations are a good starting point. Bear in mind that judgment and discretion in dealing with individual cases is crucial. The IAOMT website also contains images of how a biological dentist goes about removing amalgams.

In December 2016, they updated their protocols which they now call the SMART protocol – The Safe Mercury Amalgam Removal Technique – see https://iaomt.org/safe-removal-amalgam-fillings/. In the reference section we have listed some good, professional videos to watch.

What to expect following the safe removal of amalgams

---

116 See http://www.iaomt.org

There is no doubt that the safe removal of amalgams can greatly facilitate the healing of many health issues that are related to mercury toxicity. However, the key words are 'safe removal.' The following published scientific references have been compiled by Bernie Windham, a chemical engineer who has spent years researching the hazardous health effects of mercury amalgam poisoning:

❖ For a period of one week following amalgam removal, the levels of mercury increase approximately 30%. Within 2 weeks, levels reduce significantly[117,118] (symptoms may initially increase before improving).

❖ Removal of amalgam fillings results in significant reduction in body burden and mercury in body waste.[119,120]

❖ Total reduction of mercury in blood and urine levels is often reduced by 80% within a few months following removal.[121]

❖ In a German study of Multiple Sclerosis patients whose amalgam dental fillings were removed, 85% recovered from illnesses.[122,123]

❖ In interviews of a large population of Swedish patients who had amalgams removed, it was found that virtually all reported significant permanent health.[124]

❖ A 17-year study of an even larger population had similar results[125,126] (i.e. 89% of those reporting allergies had significant improvement or total elimination. This would represent over 17 million people with allergies who would benefit).

---

117 Begerow, J et al, Long-term mercury excretion in urine after removal of amalgam fillings, *Int Arch Occup Health* 66:209-212, 1994.

118 Molin, M et al, Kinetics of mercury in blood and urine after amalgam removal, *J Dent Res* 74:420, IADR Abstract 159, 1995.

119 Katsunuma et al, Anaphylaxis improvement after removal of amalgam fillings, Annals of Allergy, 1990, 64(5):472-75 & Drouet, M et al, Is mercury a respiratory tract allergen?, *Allerg Immunol Paris*: 22(3):81, 1990.

120 Begerow, J et al, Long-term mercury excretion in urine after removal of amalgam fillings, *Int Arch Occup Health* 66:209-212, 1994.

121 Barregard, L et al, People with high mercury uptake from their own dental amalgam fillings, *Occup Envir Med* 52: 124-128, 1995.

122 Klinghardt, D. IAOMT Conference & tape, 1998; large study by M.Daunderer (Germany) of MS patients after amalgam removal. (over 200 cases)

123 Daunderer, M. Handbuch der Amalgamvergiftung, Ecomed Verlag, Landsberg, 1998.

124 Langworth, S et al, Amalgamnews and Amalgamkadefonden, 1997. (www.tf.nu) & Berglund, F, Bjerner/Helm, Klock, Ripa, Lindforss, Mornstad, Ostlin, Improved Health after Removal of dental amalgam fillings, *Swedish Assoc. Of Dental Mercury Patients*, 1998. (www.tf.nu) (over 1000 cases)

125 Foundation For Toxic-Free Dentistry. Compilation of health consequences resulting from amalgam removal of 1569 patients, (compiled by type of health problem and consequences after removal for 31 major types of health problems), *Bio-Probe* Home Page, 1997.

126 Press Release, Swedish Council for Planning and Coordinating Research (FRN), Stockholm, 19 February, 1998.

❖ Body mercury burden was found to play a role in resistant viral infections such as Chlamydia trachomatis and herpes. Many cases can be effectively treated by antibiotics only after removal of mercury.[127,128]

Thousands of documented cases are available supporting improved health and/or cure of serious chronic illnesses after removal of mercury amalgam fillings coupled with nutritional, antioxidant and detoxification treatment:

Allergies,[129] ALS,[130] Alzheimer's,[131] anxiety & neuropathy/paraesthesia, Parkinson's, oral keratosis,[132] rages and anger,[133] schizophrenia,[134] tachycardia and heart conditions.[135] mental confusion,[136,137] arthritis,[138] asthma,[139] Chronic Fatigue Syndrome,[140,141,142] Crohn's disease,[143] depression,[144] dizziness, endometriosis,[145]

127 Omura Y et al, Heart Disease Research Foundation, NY, Role of mercury in resistant infections and recovery after Hg detox with cilantro. *Acupuncture & Electro-Theraputics Research*, 20(3):195-229, 1995.
128 Eriksen, SE. et al, Effect of mercuric chloride on macrophage- mediated resistance mechanisms against infection, *Toxicology*, 93:269- 297, 1994.
129 Ziff, MF. Documented clinical side effects to dental amalgams, ADV. *Dent. Res*. 1(6):131-134, 1992; & Ziff, S., Dentistry without Mercury, 8th Edition, 1996, Bio-Probe, Inc., & Dental Mercury Detox, Bio-Probe, Inc. http://www.bioprobe.com. (cases: FDA Patient Adverse Reaction Reports - 762, Dr. Hanson, M - Swedish patients - 519, Dr. Lichtenberg, H - 100 Danish patients, Dr. Larose, P - 80 Canadian patients, Dr. Siblerud, R - 86 Colorado patients, Dr. Zamm, AV - 22 patients) (& over 1000 additional cases of significant improvement reported to FDA).
130 Merritt's Textbook of Neurology, 9th Ed., Williams and Wilkins, Baltimore, p668, 1995; & Redhe, O et al, Recovery from ALS after removal of dental amalgam fillings, *Int J Risk & Safety in Med* 4:229-236, 1994; & Vanacore, N et al, Dirparimento di Scienze Neurologiche, Univer. La Sapienza, Roma, Med Lav (Italy), 86(6): 522-533, Nov 1995.
131 Tom Warren, Beating Alzheimer's, Avery Publishing Group, 1991.
132 Skoglund, A. *Scand J Dent Res* 102(4): 216-222, 1994; and 99(4):320-9,1991; Ostman, PO et al, Clinical and histologic changes after removal of amalgam, *Oral Surgery, Oral Medicine, & Endodontics*, 81(4):459-465, 1996, (77 cases).
133 Malt, UF et al, Physical and mental problems attributed to dental amalgam fillings, *Psychosomatic medicine*, 59:32-41, 1997, (100 cases).
134 Huggins, H. It's All in Your Head: Diseases Caused by silver-mercury fillings, USA: Life Sciences Press, 1990; & Observations From The Metabolic Fringe, ICBM conf. Collarado,1988; & Center for Progressive Medicine, 1999, http://www.hugnet.com (Over 1000 cases).
135 Ziff, MF et al, A Persuasive New Look at Heart Disease As It Relates to Mercury, Bio-Probe, Inc., & J. of American College of Cardiology V33,#6, pp1578-1583, 1999.
136 Davis, M (ed), Defense Against Mystery Syndromes, Chek Printing Co., March, 1994 (case histories documented).
137 Malt, UF et al, Physical and mental problems attributed to dental amalgam fillings, *Psychosomatic medicine*, 59:32-41, 1997 (100 cases).
138 Tanchyk, AP. Amalgam Removal for Treatment of Arthritis, *Gen Dent*, v42,n4, p354, July 1994.
139 Seidler, A et al, Possible environmental factors for Parkinson's disease, *Neurology* 46(5):1275-1284, 1996; & Vroom, FO et al, Mercury vapour intoxication, 95: 305-318, 1972; Ohlson et all, Parkinsons Disease and Occupational Exposure to Mercury, *Scand J. Of Work Environment Health*, Vol 7, No.4: 252-256, 1981.
140 Huggins, H & Editors of Alternative Medicine Digest, Chronic Fatigue, Fibromyalgia & Environmental Illness, Future Medicine Publishing, Inc, p197, 1998.
141 Adolph Coors Foundation, Coors Amalgam Study: Effects of Placement and Removal of Amalgam fillings, 1995. Internations DAMS Newsletter, p17, Vol VII, Issue 2, Spring 1997, (31 cases).

epilepsy,[146] eczema,[147] gastro intestinal problems,[148] infertility,[149] leukemia,[150] (lupus, migraines, multiple chemical sensitivities, multiple sclerosis,[151]

Root Canals and Dental Foci

In recent years, there has been a reawakening of the dangers of oral infections and their potential disastrous effects on systemic health. Dead and infected teeth are often treated 'conservatively' in modern dentistry by performing a treatment called 'Root Canal Therapy'. The aim is to 'save' a tooth which has become infected or dead, to make it functional and pain free.

So, how is a root canal performed? First, the nerve in the large pulp chamber at the top of the tooth is cleaned out using a round bur on a slow speed drill. Then the canals are cleaned with a series of tiny files which look like flexible pins with

---

142 Malt UF et al, Physical and mental problems attributed to dental amalgam fillings, *Psychosomatic medicine*, 59:32-41, 1997, (100 cases).

143 Davis, M (ed), Defense Against Mystery Syndromes, Chek Printing Co., March, 1994 (case histories documented).

144 Do amalgam fillings influence manic depression? Journal of Orthomol. Medicine, 1998, http://www.depression.com/news/news_981116.htm

145 Ziff S. and Ziff M. Infertility and Birth Defects: Is Mercury from Dental Fillings a Hidden Cause? Bio-Probe, Inc., 1987.

146 Klinghardt, D, Migraines, Seizures and Mercury Toxicity, Future Medicine Publishing, 1997.

147 Dr. Kohdera, Faculty of Dentistry, Osaka Univ, International Congress of Allergology and Clinical Immunology, EAACI, Stockholm, June 1994; & Heavy Metal Bulletin, Vol 1, Issue 2, Oct 1994, (160 cases cured).

148 Langworth, S et al, Amalgam news and Amalgamkadefonden, 1997. (www.tf.nu) & Berglund, F, Bjerner/Helm, Klock, Ripa, Lindforss, Mornstad, Ostlin), Improved Health after Removal of dental amalgam fillings, Swedish Assoc. Of Dental Mercury Patients, 1998, (www.tf.nu) (over 1000 cases).

149 Dr. Gerhard, I and Dr. Roller, E et al, Tubingen Univ. Gynecological Clinic, Heidelberg, 1996; & Gerhard, I et al, Heavy Metals and Fertility, *J of Toxicology and Environmental Health*, Part A, 54:593-611, 1998.

150 Ziff S. and Ziff M. Infertility and Birth Defects: Is Mercury from Dental Fillings a Hidden Cause? Bio-Probe, Inc, 1987.

151 Davis, M. (ed), Defense Against Mystery Syndromes', Chek Printing Co., March, 1994 (case histories documented).

serrations along their lengths (see image above). The dentist will begin with a very thin burr followed by progressively thicker files until the entire mass of the nerve is removed and the sides of the root canals are made smooth and clean. As the filing progresses, the tooth is washed or irrigated with a dilute solution of laundry bleach (Clorox), or a 2% solution of chlorhexidine, to wash out the debris, and to sterilize and chemically neutralize any dead tissue that may be missed by the files.

When the root canal is completely clean, it is dried out with tiny paper points, and each canal is fitted with the appropriate diameter rubber cone that will entirely fill and block that canal. Each file is numbered to denote its diameter, and there is a corresponding rubber cone size to be used in canals finished to that size file. The rubber is a special form called 'Gutta Percha'. It is less refined than regular rubber and is somewhat gummy, sticking to the walls of the canal and thoroughly waterproofing them.

After scraping out the inside of the tooth the dentist will attempt to disinfect the tooth and the canals to eliminate any source of infection. The canal is then filled with a combination of cement and Gutta Percha to completely occlude these canals. This is supposedly to prevent any microorganisms from entering the tooth, either through the crown or the root.

If you consider pain control, mechanical function and aesthetics to be the limit of good dental treatment, then you will have 'SAVED' the tooth.

If systemic effects are included in your concept of dentistry, then you must understand that all that has happened is that you have kept dead, infected tissue, buried in the bone, within a couple of inches from your brain.

For some obscure reason, we are all conditioned to think that teeth are not a part of the body, but that they are inert calcified material; that they are sort of dead anyway. Dentistry is the only one of all the medical & para-medical professions that thinks it is a good idea to keep dead, gangrenous tissue in the body. The way to do this is to perform a root canal treatment.

One eminent Endodontist says:[152]

"It is wrong to speak of 'Root Canal Therapy' as a dead tooth; it is more correct to describe such a tooth as non-vital or, better, pulpless. Even though the central blood supply to the tooth has been

---

[152] Meinig, GE. Root Canal Coverup. *Price-Pottenger Nutrition Foundation Journal*, vol. 18, No. 3, pp.6, Nov. 1994.

lost, the tooth itself still retains its connection to the body via the periodontal membrane and the cementum."

This is like saying that even though the blood supply to your leg may be completely cut off, it would be wrong to suggest that the leg is dead, because it is still connected to your body by your hip joint! The Oxford dictionary defines 'non-vital' as 'fatal to life.' It defines 'dead' as 'no longer alive.'

The bacteria, yeasts and other organisms which enter the tooth do not die when the oxygen supply is reduced (which is what happens inside the root canal system). They undergo what is called a pleomorphic change and become 'anaerobic' bacteria. They literally change form and become bacteria that do not need oxygen to live. With the establishment of infection, the microbial flora changes from an initially predominant facultative gram positive flora, to a completely anaerobic gram negative bacteria when the canals have been infected for 3 months or more.[153]

> *"80% of patients' health problems can be partially traced to the mouth."*
>
> Dietrich Klinghardt MD, Ph.D. (www.neuraltherapy.com)

Other organisms such as yeasts, fungi and 'cell-wall-deficient forms' (Lida Mattman[154]) also inhabit this tissue. The dead teeth thus become a focus of infection which can cause numerous disease states throughout the body. Anaerobic bacteria produce incredibly potent neurologic and haemolytic toxins. A true 'toxin factory.'

Boyd Haley, Ph.D., a researcher at the University of Kentucky, has estimated that 75% of root-canalled teeth are infected. Another researcher, Hal Huggins, DDS,[155] has shown that the toxins liberated by infected root-canalled teeth are almost 1,000 times more toxic than botulism. Botulism, by the way, is the most toxic substance known.

In 1960, it was established by W. Meyer (Goettingen) that within devitalized teeth the dentinal canals and dental capillaries contain large microbial colonies. The toxins produced by these microbes in a tooth with a root filling can no longer be evacuated

---

153 Fabricius L, Dahlen G, Ohman AE, Moller AJR. Predominant indigenous oral bacteria isolated from infected root canals after varied times of closure. *Scand J Dent Res* 90: 134–144, 1982.
154 Mattman, LH. Cell Wall Deficient Forms: Stealth Pathogens. 3rd edition, USA: BioMed Publishing Group, 1997.
155 Huggins, HA and Levy, TE. Uninformed Consent: The hidden dangers in dental care. USA: Hampton Roads Publishing Co., 1999.

into the mouth, but must be drained away through the cross-connections and unsealed branches of the dental and capillary canals into the marrow of the jawbone. From there, they are conveyed to the tonsils, and thus the flow systems of the body. In fact, the conservative treatment may literally convert a tooth into a toxin producing 'factory' as described above.

With recent advances in molecular biological methods, the endodontic microflora is being continually reclassified. Molecular biological methods like PCR (Polymerase Chain Reaction) have enabled amplification of small amounts of nucleic acids and allowed for identification of bacteria that would be detectable by culturing techniques. A recent such study using PCR techniques revealed a number of bacterial species.[156]

---

156 George, M., Ivančaková, R. Root Canal Microflora, Acta Medica, (Hradec Králové) 50(1):7–15, 2007.

GRAM POSITIVE COCCI	GRAM NEGATIVE COCCI
Streptococcus anginosus	Capnocytophaga ochracea
S. gordonii	C. sputigena
S. oralis	C. curvus
S. mitis	
S. sanguinis	Veillonella parvula
Enterococcus faecalis	Campylobacter rectus
Peptostreptococcus micros	
Peptostreptococcus anaerobius	

GRAM POSITIVE RODS	GRAM NEGATIVE RODS
Actinomyces israelii	Fusobacterium nucleatum
A. naeslundii	Prevotella intermedia
Eubacterium alactolyticum	Prevotella melaninogenica
Eubacterium lentum	Prevotella denticola
Eubacterium timidum	Prevotella buccae
Eubacterium brachy	Prevotella oralis
Eubacterium nodatum	Prevotella loescheii
Propionibact. Propionicum	Porphyromonas gingivalis
P. granulosum	Bacteroides gracilis
Porphyromonas endodontalis	
Lactobacillus	

Table 1 – Bacteria Isolated from Root Canal of Teeth

Adapted from Sundqvist, 1992 a, b, 1994; Le Goff et al, 1997, R. M. Love, H. F. Jenkinson, 2002

What can be done?

So, what happens when we have a dead tooth in our mouths? Unfortunately, there are no good alternatives for this situation. The only treatment for dead tissue in the body is to remove it. It is impossible to sterilize the canals, but the drugs and antibiotics used do not penetrate the dentine tubules. Dr. Weston Price,[157,158] a famous dental researcher who wrote prolifically (two-volume work totalling 1,174

---

[157] Price, WA. Dental Infections: Oral and Systemic, being a contribution to the pathology of dental infections, focal infections and the degenerative diseases (Volume 1). USA: The Penton Publishing Company, 1923.

[158] Price, WA. Dental Infections and the Degenerative Diseases: Being a contribution to the pathology of functional and degenerative organ and tissue lesions (Volume 2). USA: The Penton Publishing Company, 1923.

pages), was even able to culture bacteria from teeth which had fuming formaldehyde poured over them. Even the recent dental literature reflects this:

"It is now known that complete sterilization of an infected root canal is very difficult to achieve and complete removal of all pulp tissue remnants frequently is not possible."[159]

Therefore, the treatment of choice is to extract a dead tooth rather than root-fill it. It is also important to remove any infected tissue from around the tooth. This usually requires a very easy surgical approach to access the end of the socket. Although this does not sound attractive, the results are generally positive and the actual surgery is usually very easy.

Dentists are usually taught to extract teeth with forceps and that any infected tissue left in the bony socket will be dealt with by the cells of the immune system. This does sometimes happen. Often, though, the bone will heal around the infected tissue, which remains indefinitely as an infected hole in the bone.

These areas are usually colonized by gram negative bacteria. They are called NICO Lesions (Neuralgia Inducing Cavitational Osteonecrosis). NICO lesions can act as foci of infection and also neural foci, just as the root treated teeth can. This is the main reason that a surgical approach is used for most extractions.

Dr. Bouquot[160] in 1992 reported 1,995 cases of neuralgia osteonecrosis (dead bone neuralgia) and relates these with facial neuralgia or trigeminal neuralgia. In 70% of these cases the facial neuralgia disappeared completely after the necrotic bone was surgically removed. NICO's are very difficult to spot on X-rays or MRI scans – one of the best ways of detecting a NICO is with Autonomic Response Testing (ART). If you touch the fingertip on the gum opposite the root of the extracted tooth while muscle testing, if there is a NICO the muscle will become weak.

Neural therapy using procaine can help to unblock the NICO and the muscle will test strong. The messages of the autonomic nervous system, travelling over the acupuncture meridians from that tooth area to the disabled or painful site have been blocked and neural therapy helps to repolarise the cell membranes and release the blockage.[161]

159 Phillip Delivanis Oral Surgery Vol 52 No 4, 1981.

160 Bouquot, JE. Brief review of NICO (Neuralgia-Inducing Cavitational Osteonecrosis). *Journal of Oral Surgery, Oral Medicine and Oral Pathology*, March 1992.

161 Meinig, GE. Root Canal Cover-Up. USA: Bion Publishing, 2000.

Dr Dietrich Klinghardt, in a study entitled, *The Tonsils and Their Role in Health and Chronic Illness,*[162] provides compelling literature and his own insights about how a root canal can damage overall health systemically. He mentions various ways:

1. By acting on the neural mechanism (by affecting the autonomic nervous system)

2. By having a toxic effect (release toxins altering the patient's biochemistry).

3. By having an allergic effect. If proteins are released from dying or dead teeth ('necrotoxins') the immune system may become sensitized and overreact. Once the patient is sensitized, there may be cross-reactivity with regular foods, amino acids and a whole host of chemicals and bio-chemicals. The patient's symptoms may be multiple chemical sensitivity or food allergies.

Dr Dietrich Klinghardt is a medical doctor, a neurologist and an expert in his field. He also cites many respectable researchers who have contributed to unravelling the mystery behind how root canals cause cancer, heart disease, allergies, multiple chemical sensitivities and any other known or unknown disease. It is crucial, therefore, that all dental foci are treated because they could be the causative factor of your severe chronic disease – from your weak immune system to your heart disease, to your cancer.

Recent research by Ralph Turk and Fritz Kronner in Germany has shown that even the act of drilling a tooth causes severe energy disturbance. Turk describes the modern dental turbine rotor as a sort of time bomb and that its damaging intensity has been completely missed by the clear majority of dentists. There are many likely reasons, not least being the fact that, despite water cooling, the temperature of the dentine rises by as much as 10 degrees after just a few seconds of drilling. *This is akin to cooking the tooth.*

This denaturation destroys the viability of the tooth and its ability to resist bacterial invasion. From over 6,000 cases studied, it was uniformly seen that, as soon as a tooth was visited by a high-speed drill, focal osteitis trouble began in connection with that tooth within 2 years.

It is possible to reduce the damage by taking sensible detoxification protocols before, during and after a dental programme. Such elementary measures would include

---

162 Available at http://www.neuraltherapy.com/a_tonsils.asp

vitamin C, charcoal (to absorb toxins), homeopathic support and immune drainage remedies, such as HEEL's lymphomyosot or Pascoe's Pascotox.[163]

Focal Infection Theory

A 'focus of infection' has been defined as *'a circumscribed area infected with microorganisms which may or may not give rise to clinical manifestations'*. A 'focal infection' has been defined as *'sepsis arising from a focus of infection that initiates a secondary infection in a nearby or distant tissue or organs.'*

Curtis, an eminent dentist, said many years ago that, *"...a focal infection is a localized or generalized infection caused by the dissemination of organisms or toxic products from a focus of infection. It probably would be better defined as a metastatic infection."*[164]

It has been known for over 150 years that focal infections in dead, root- canal treated teeth can in fact release organisms and their toxins into the body. These can then initiate disease states in other parts of the body. Stortebecker has even demonstrated that these organisms and their toxins can be transported directly back to the brain via the blood, and also by transport along the nerve fibres. Other researchers have demonstrated that parts of the brain can be directly infected by dead teeth.[165,166,167,168]

There is also research which demonstrates the presence of Tumour Necrotising Factor[169] at the end in the apical area of infected roots.[170,171,172,173] Tumour Necrosis Factor is capable of causing diseases and syndromes such as chronic wasting syndrome; anorexia and excessive weight loss; bone resorption through the activation of osteoclasts, as well as other inflammatory disease states.

---

163 Mumby, S. Virtual medicine: A new dimension in energy healing. Thorsons, London 1999.

164 Curtis, A.C.: Focal infection. American Textbook of Operative Dentistry.
7th ed. M.L. Ward, ed. Lea & Febiger, Philadelphia, 1840.

165 Black R., Laboratory model for Trigeminal Neuralgia. *Adv. Neuro.* 4:651-8, 1974.

166 Westrum LE., Canfield RC., Black R., Transganglionic degeneration in the spinal trigeminal nucleus following the removal of tooth pulps in adult cats. *Brain Res* 6:100:137-40, 1976.

167 Westrum LE., Canfield RC., Electron microscopy of degenerating axons and terminals in the spinal trigeminal nucleus after tooth pulp exterpation. *Am J Anat.* 149:591-6, 1977.

168 Gobel S., Bink J., Degenerative changes in primary trigeminal axons and in neurons in nucleus caudalis following tooth pulp extirpation in the cat., *Brain Res.* 132:347-54, 1977.

169 A member of a family of proteins, which induce necrosis (death) of tumour cells and possess a wide range of proinflammatory actions.

170 K.E Safvi *J. Endo.* vol 17 No 1, Jan 1991.

171 Bando Y, Henderson B, Meghji S, Poole S, Harris M. Immunocytochemical localization of inflammatory cytokines and vascular adhesion receptors in radicular cysts. *J Oral Pathol Med* 22(5):221-7, May 1993.

172 Wang CY, Stashenko P. Characterization of bone-resorbing activity in human periapical lesions. *J Endod* 19(3):107-11, March 1993.

173 Iwu C, MacFarlane TW, MacKenzie D, Stenhouse D. The microbiology of periapical granulomas. Oral Surg Oral Med Oral Pathol 69(4):502-5, April 1990.

Mechanisms of Focal Infection

The origin of many toxic or metastatic diseases may be traced to primary focal areas of infection. Two mechanisms can produce focal infection:[174]

1. An actual metastasis of organisms from a focus
2. The spread of endotoxins or toxic products from a remote focus to other tissues by the blood stream

Also in the same Journal of the American Dental Association we read:

"If the bacteria pass the barrier (of the abscess wall) a number of things may happen:

1. The bacteria may travel to another free surface where they begin to grow.

2. The bacteria can travel to distant parts of the body by way of the lymphatics or the blood. Some bacteria will be eradicated by the lymph nodes while others can greatly stress the lymph nodes causing lymphadonitis, which may convert to an abscess. If the bacteria get through the lymph nodes, they may:

(a) multiply in the blood, setting up an acute or chronic septicemia.

(b) be carried live to a suitable nidus where they infect the surrounding tissue.

(c) produce a slow but progressive atrophy with replacement fibrosis in various organs of the body.

3. The byproducts of bacteria such as endotoxins may reach remote parts of the body.

4. The bacteria at the focus may undergo autolysis or dissolution and again some of these endotoxins may cause allergic reactions in various tissues of the body."

The most dangerous of all odontogenous toxins are undoubtedly the thio-ethers, for instance dimethylsulfide. Thio-ethers are closely related, both in their structure and their effect, to mustard gas and other poison gases used in the First World War.

After root canal treatment when the pulp is removed, slowly over time the thio-ethers will be released into the circulation and paralyze the critical aerobic respiration of the cell.

---

174 Mechanism of Focal Infection J Am Dent Assoc Vol 42:619-633, June 1951.

The dental literature basically talks about the susceptible patient (regarding thio-ethers and other endotoxins) as being:[175]

- ❖ Those that are immune-compromised or have defective lymphatic drainage.
- ❖ Patients with heart disease, heart valve prosthesis and other chronic diseases.
- ❖ Patients that may be taking prolonged antibiotic, corticosteroid and immunosuppressive drugs.

Stortebecker had a disease model for multiple sclerosis, which is very persuasive. Through extensive research he was able to show that most plaques of nerve de-myelination (the unmistakable sign of MS) were located around blood vessels.[176] No-one else has noticed this important fact before.

He speculated that the back-pressure on veins had shunted toxic matter into the brain tissues, where foci of inflammation and myelin loss are instigated. What was particularly convincing was that MS cases with optic neuritis (leading to blindness) generally had bad teeth and inflammation plaques in the brain, whereas those who had leg weakness or paralysis, with de-myelination plaques in the spinal cord, had pelvic or other lower-body disease foci.

Even in the light of all this evidence, the dental profession generally still continue to suggest that focal theory is old fashioned and that root canal treated teeth do not act as foci of infection.[177,178] Yet one study cites at least 150 different species of bacteria at the end of the root of dead teeth stating: *"These infections are predominantly anaerobic."*[179] These bacteria can be extremely dangerous for people with defective heart valves, rheumatic fever and vascular diseases. The authors of this study add: *"Other forms of systemic diseases such as brain abscesses, haematological infection and implant infections have also been related to oral micro-organisms."*

Neural Focal Interference
So far, we have talked about root canal treatments and the microorganisms they contain causing various disease states in the body – this is one form of focus. There is another focus which was developed by two German doctors called the Heuneke brothers. What they found was that areas of dead tissue, scar tissue, foreign bodies,

175 Baumgartner, J. and Harrison, H. The incidence of bacteremias relate to endodontic procedures. *Nonsurgical endodontics J of Endodontics* Vol 3, No 5, May 1976.
176 Ibid.
177 Heimdahl A., Hall G, Hedberg M, Sandberg, H. Detection and Quantitation of Lysis-Filtration of bacteremia after different oral surgical procedures. *J Clin Microbiol* 28(1): 2205-9, 1990.
178 Debelian GJ., Olsen I., Tronstad L. Profiling of Propionibacterium Acnes recovered from root canal and blood during and after endodontic treatment. *Endod Dent Traumatol*, 8(6):248-54, 1992.
179 Debelian GJ., Olsen I., Tronstad L. Systemic diseases caused by oral microorganisms., *Endod Dent Traumatol*, 10(2):57-65 1994.

cystic tissue and infected tissue could interfere with the body's regulatory systems. They called these areas 'Foci of Neural Interference.'

Any chronic inflammation, any scar, any degenerative or other alteration can obviously satisfy this condition. The focus is embedded in the mesenchymal[180] base tissue and in that way has direct contact with the capillary system of the blood and lymphatic vessels and the neuro-vegetative nerve fibre. This produces the connection to the whole organism. Through any of these conduction systems, it will be able to cause distant actions in other organs. The focal nerve impulse will firstly be projected into the vegetative centres, where it can cause a vegetative dysregulation. On the other hand, focal toxins and bacteria will be infiltrated by the vessel systems where they can spread their infectious, toxic and allergenic properties *everywhere.*[181]

Dead and infected teeth fulfil all the criteria to become Primary Foci of Neural Interference. The imbalance in the regulatory system will then either create disease states in other parts of the body, which are remote from the original focus. These disease states will often coincide with areas of the body that are on the same acupuncture meridians as the primary focus. This has been verified by the work of Voll who was a German physician and electro-acupuncturist. For example, we often see disease states in the areas of the reproductive system, kidney and knees in relation to non-vital front teeth.

The mouth and teeth are a primary source of focal infection and neural interference fields. No other parts of the body have dead tissue routinely left in place. The only thing which seems to separate individual reactions is the state of that person's immune system, and genetic factors. Consequently, other factors which may reduce immune function will allow a greater reaction to the non-vital teeth (e.g. mercury from dental amalgam fillings will have a direct and deleterious effect on the immune system).

So, how can this be adressed?
The next obvious question is *'How do you fill the space?'* The solution depends on the location of the space and the condition of the adjacent teeth and or lack of teeth in the area. It will usually involve the creation of some sort of bridge or partial denture. Each person must be assessed individually.

---

180 The part of the embryonic mesoderm that consists of loosely packed, unspecialized cells that are set in a gelatinous ground substance, from which connective tissue, bone, cartilage, and the circulatory and lymphatic systems develop.
181 More Cures for Cancer Translation from the German by Dr. Josef Issels, Helfer Publishing E. -Schwabe, Bad Homburg FRG.

Some dentists prefer to recommend the fitting of titanium implants. I do not believe that this is a good solution as electric currents generated by these devices may also act as a neural interference field. Zirconium implants are the new ones being touted as 'safer,' but evidence has not yet been established that this is the case. There are of course very large profits to be made from each implant, which costs about $1,500 and more per tooth.

Very recently I was suffering from low back pain without understanding its cause. I had adjusted my spine using osteopathy and chiropractic manipulations by skilled practitioners a number of times, as well as my Primus Metatarsus Supinatus (PMS) using Prof. Rothbart's proprioreceptive insoles – but to no avail. I was taking glucosamine for over 6 months, along with other supplements.

There was a molar in the lower right quadrant of my mouth that was giving me pain. The X-ray showed that there was an infection in the bone that needed to be seen to immediately, and the only way of dealing with this was to have the tooth extracted. This took place under the supervision of a holistic (or biological) dentist who carefully injected Sanum isopathic remedies into the bone to help any anaerobic bacteria undergo pleomorphic changes into less pathogenic forms. I also used combinations of silver liquid protein 500ppm, grapefruit seed extract; echinacea and goldenseal, oregano oil and large doses of buffered vitamin C.

A little while after the extraction, my low back pain literally disappeared completely. I was absolutely convinced that it was the tooth extraction and clearing of the infection that was responsible for this dramatic turn in my health that was confirmed by Tom Warren when he wrote:

> *"I have been told about a woman who had a breast tumour. Oncologists (cancer specialists) do not like to operate if there are signs of other infection. Her physician asked the woman to have an abscessed tooth taken care of before surgery. Immediately after the dental appointment, while lidocaine was present in her system, the woman had a Thermography X-ray that revealed a thin white line extending from her tooth, down her neck, through the tumour in her breast and on down into her stomach. In light of the discovery, her physicians decided not to operate. Four months later the tumour disappeared. That was the first-time direct connection to disease following an acupuncture meridian was clinically observed and was an immeasurably important observation for western medicine. Every tooth has a separate acupuncture meridian running through major organs in the body."*

Teeth and Acupuncture Meridians

The acupuncture meridians are 12 in total and some of these pass through each tooth. Over the years there have been maps of teeth that have been modified and adapted by researchers familiar with testing the acupuncture meridians.

Below is a typical map of the teeth indicating the acupuncture meridians running through each tooth.

As an example, if we take the right upper (tooth 1) and lower (tooth 32) molars, the heart and small intestine meridian run through these two teeth. A focus in these teeth will likely lead to the following symptoms: Right shoulder, elbow, hand (ulnar), sacroiliac, foot, toes and middle ear; right heart, right duodenum, terminal ileum; CNS; anterior pituitary.

One thing I have alluded to above is the relationship between teeth and the acupuncture meridians, which are 'energy lines' that run through the body and 'energetically feed' organ systems. A tooth focus can directly block one of these meridians, causing energy blockages in various organ systems.

One example is of a 50-year old man who was athletic, conscious of his nutrition, affluent and generally enjoyed life to the full. On a routine medical examination for insurance purposes, he found that his PSA levels were high. Further examination of the prostate, including a biopsy, led to the diagnosis of stage II adenocarcinoma of the prostate. When he came to the Da Vinci Centre for the IDEL Diagnostic programme, one of the major issues that we discovered was an incisor on the right bottom quadrant (tooth 25) that is connected to the bladder and kidney meridian and runs through the prostate.

In fact, this tooth was capped after a riding accident four years previously, and the patient remembered quite specifically how a few months later he was getting prostate problems, including partial erectile failure and nocturnal micturition that he never suffered from before.

When an X-ray of this incisor was taken, it was clear that there was a large abscess at the root of the tooth. When the tooth was extracted a small sac of pus with a vile smell came out with it. If this tooth focus had not been identified and removed, then the chances are that this man would not be alive now, let alone completely cured and leading a full life again.

I have also seen several women with breast cancer who had tooth foci on the stomach meridian. This has been validated by other practitioners such as Dr. Thomas Rau from the Paracelsus Clinic in Switzerland,[182] who found that of 150 women with breast cancer, 98% had a disturbance on the stomach meridian – the breast belongs to the stomach meridian. Of these 150 women, there were only 3 patients who did not have a root canal in a tooth linked to the stomach meridian. These women were further compared with women in the same age range who did not have breast cancer – only 30% of these had root canals, which is a statistically significant difference.

Symptoms of Dead Teeth
The types of disease states which relate to dead teeth are so numerous that it is impossible in a chapter of this size to discuss them all. They range from head and neck pain all the way through to rheumatism and cancer. (183)

The most common symptom is in the form of head and neck pain. This may range from mild headaches to migraines to Trigeminal Neuralgia. Sinusitis is very often associated with non-vital and root canal treated teeth, especially if they are in the upper arch.

Dr. Weston Price found that most patients with non-vital teeth had some thyroid dysfunction. A number of other researchers and physicians are finding a relationship between cancer and non-vital teeth. Reduced immune function is common. Eye and ear problems are common with root treated teeth.

Rheumatic and arthritic changes are almost the norm amongst people with dead teeth in their mouths. Many heart problems[184,185] and nervous disorders are associated

182 Dr. Rau, Paracelsus Clinic, Switzerland – www.Paracelsus.ch
183 Genco R. Current View of Risk Factors for Periodontal Disease; *J. Periodontol* Oct 1996.
184 Beck J, Garcia R, Heiss G, Vokonas PS, Offenbacher S. Periodontal disease and cardiovascular disease. *J Periodontol* 67 (10 Suppl):1123-1137, Oct 1996.

with dead teeth. Multiple Sclerosis has also been linked to the toxins and organisms from dead teeth.[186,187]

The location of the tooth, the types of organisms inside it and the nature of the person's genetic makeup will determine the areas of disease found clinically. The one thing that is certain is that if you are sick you should look very carefully at all non-vital teeth, whether root treated or not.

At the Da Vinci Holistic Health Centre, all patients undergoing the IDEL Diagnostic Programme[188] will have their teeth checked using ART, Bioresonance testing, panoramic X-rays and other methods to determine whether there are tooth foci present.

Allergy to Dental Materials used to Restore Teeth

There are many types of dental materials that are used by dental professionals today ranging from gold alloys (containing palladium, silver, platinum and iridium), mercury fillings, acrylic denture material which contains methyl methacrylate, chrome cobalt partial denture framework, nickel based crowns and composite resin crowns containing polyurethane. It is possible that these dental materials can cause allergic responses resulting in intractable pain, chronic fatigue, food allergies, chronic sinusitis and headaches.

The dental liners or bases used under permanent restorative filling materials can also be the causative agent for an allergic response and body toxicity. A new toxicity disorder discovered by Dr. Omar M. Amin, Ph.D. (189) is Neurocutaneous syndrome (NCS).

The neurological aspects of NCS are characterized by pinprick and/or creeping, painful and irritating movement sensations – often interpreted as parasite movements – subcutaneously or in various body tissues or cavities including the head. In no case was the movement sensation related to parasites, which were always proved to be absent. Additional neurological symptoms include memory loss, brain

---

185 Herzberg MC, Meyer MW. Effects of oral flora on platelets: possible consequences in cardiovascular disease. *J Periodontol* 67 (10 Suppl):1138-1142, Oct 1996.
186 Stortebecker P. Chronic dental infections in the etiology of Glioblastomas. 8th int congress Neuropathy. Washington D.C. Sept 1978 *J Neuropth. Exp. Neurology* 37(s) 1978
187 Dental Caries as a cause of nervous disorders, 1981.
188 The IDEL Diagnostic Programme is a comprehensive diagnostic protocol involving many different testing protocols, including testing tooth foci with VEGA and ART – see
http://www.naturaltherapycenter.com/diagnosticstreatments/idel-diagnostic-programme/
189 For those interested in reading the full text of Dr. Amin's article, Toxicity from dental sealants causing neurocutaneous syndrome (NCS), a dermatological and neurological disorder, it is available on the following web site: www.holisticdental.org

fog and lack of concentration and control of voluntary movements, pain, depleted energy and a depressed immune system, all of which may invite various opportunistic infections. In many cases, lesions were associated with swellings in the arms and legs. Blood vessels may also become enlarged and elevated, the head may become hot and turn red and the gums and teeth may turn grey.

Electrogalvanism

It is well known and can easily be measured using a simple voltmeter and ammeter, that when two dissimilar metals are present in the mouth with the presence of saliva, an electric current will flow. Saliva acts as an electrolyte when it mixes with amalgam fillings, to create a measurable electric current of 900 millivolts (enough power to light a small torch bulb). This current overpowers the body's normal 450 millivolts, interferes with energy flow to the brain and is suspected to be a catalyst in many illnesses.

Other alloys, such as nickel in the metal base of bridges and under porcelain crowns, have been documented to lower the T-4 and T-8 lymphocyte levels.[190] In predisposed patients, exposure to nickel can be a contributory factor in the development of cancer of the lungs, nasal passages and larynx.

Any metal materials in the mouth such as gold crowns, chrome cobalt partial dentures, mercury fillings and titanium implants, will set the stage for galvanic currents.

In 1985, a research team (Knappworst, Gura, Fuhrmann and Enginalev) revealed that when mercury fillings were in close proximity to gold crowns, the mercury release was ten times greater when compared to mercury fillings alone.[191] Electrogalvanism is frequently the cause for the following symptoms:

- ❖ Lack of concentration and memory
- ❖ Insomnia
- ❖ Psychological problems
- ❖ Tinnitus
- ❖ Vertigo
- ❖ Epilepsy
- ❖ Hearing loss
- ❖ Eye problems

---

190 Eggleston, D. Effect of Dental Amalgam and Nickel Alloys on T-Lymphocytes: Preliminary Report, *J. Prosthetic Dent*, 51(5);617-623, 1984.
191 Stortebecker, P. Mercury Poisoning from Dental Amalgam - a Hazard to Human Brain. USA: Bio Probe.

❖ Mouth pain

Removing the mercury and other metals and replacing them with biocompatible, non-metal restorations will resolve the galvanic issue.

At the Da Vinci Natural Therapy Centre, all people undergoing a full diagnostic IDEL Diagnostic Programme will be asked to bring in a panoramic X-ray or Panorex. As you can see from the image below, the Panorex is a large, single x-ray film that shows the entire bony structure of the teeth and face. It takes a much wider area than any intra-oral film showing structures outside of their range including the sinuses, and the Temperomandibular Joints. It shows many pathological structures such as bony tumors, cysts, abscesses as well as the position of the wisdom teeth.

The teeth are then checked using Autonomic Response Testing (ART) to identify any tooth foci that will not be visible on the Panorex. These could be related to bacteria producing lethal toxins that block the acupuncture meridians. These foci can then be treated with low intensity laser therapy (LILT).

Panorex X-ray

We also get our patients to use the Soladey titanium oxide ionic toothbrush as it is extremely effective at killing bacteria and removing plaque that harbour them, all without toothpaste.

Soladey Toothbrush – No Toothpaste!
Dental plaque is a biofilm (usually colourless) that builds up on the teeth. If not removed regularly, it can lead to caries or periodontal problems such as gingivitis.

The microorganisms that form the biofilm are almost entirely bacteria, mainly Streptococcus mutans and anaerobes, including Fusobacterium and Actinobacteria.

Plaque can also make our teeth less attractive as they turn a brown colour and can cause bad breath.

Why do ordinary hand and electric toothbrushes often leave plaque on tooth surfaces no matter how carefully you brush or floss? Why do you have plaque/tartar when you visit the dentist for a check-up, even though you brush carefully? Because plaque attaches to teeth by an electrostatic bond, friction by itself is not enough to break this bond. This bond is due to plaque having a positive polarity and teeth having a negative   polarity.

Instead of using friction or sound (sonic) waves to try to "blast apart" this bond, there is now a patented IONIC technology that changes the polarity of the tooth surfaces from positive to negative.

This is the SOLADEY titanium oxide ionic brush. As you brush, plaque material is actively repelled by your teeth and drawn to the negatively charged bristles, even in hard-to-reach areas of your mouth. Unlike regular toothbrushes which require toothpaste - an abrasive compound - to help to remove plaque, the IONIC action works with or without toothpaste, making it gentler on the gums. It is probably the simplest but most advanced toothbrush in the world.

How does it work? There is a light-activated titanium rod (semiconductor) inside the handle. When exposed to any light source (a fluorescent bathroom light, a plain light bulb, or sunlight), the photo-sensitive titanium rod inside Soladey converts light into negatively-charged ions (electrons). The rod releases these ions, which blend with saliva to attract positive (hydrogen) ions from the acid in the dental plaque on your teeth.

In the presence of light, saturated low energy electrons in the wet semiconductor are transformed into high energy electrons resulting in a reduction reaction as shown below:

$$H+ + O_2 + e - = HO_2 \qquad 2H+ = + 2\,e - = H_2$$

$$2HO_2 = H_2O_2 \qquad H_2O_2 = 2HO$$

This reaction results in the reduction of H+ ions from the organic acid in the plaque causing its decomposition. The reaction influences plaque formation.[192,193] There is

---

192 Kusunoki, K., Oku, T., Koni, H., Nakaya, K, Mori, T, Hiratuka, V, Taguchi, M, Watanabe, Y and Miyake, T. A study on the effect of the solar energy conversion toothbrush on the control of dental plaque. *Journal of the Osaka Odontological Society* 49, 550-559, 1986.

also evidence that the toothbrush has a bactericidal effect against *Escherichia coli* and *Streptococcus mutans*.[194]

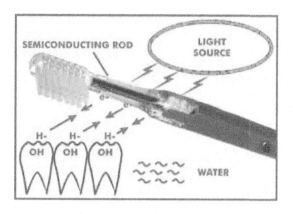

Soladey toothbrush with titanium semiconducting rod

A blind, two-way crossover clinical trial has shown that when the Soladey ionic brush was compared with an ordinary toothbrush with toothpaste as well as a placebo group, it was far superior at removing plaque in a shorter time period.[195]

193 Niwa, M and Fukuda, M. Clinical study on the control of dental plaque using solar energy conversion toothbrush equipped with a TiO2 semiconductor. *Odontology* 77, 598-606, 1989.
194 Moriaoka, T., Saito, T., Nara, K and Onoda, K. Antibacterial action of powdered semiconductor on a serotype g Streptococcus mutans. *Caries research* 22, 230-231, 1988.
195 Hoover, JN, Singer DL, Pahwa, P and Komiyama, K. Clinical evaluation of a light energy conversion toothbrush. *J Clin Periodontol* 19:434-436, 1992.

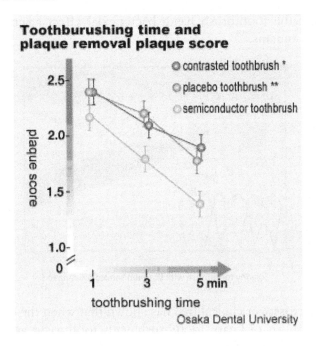

Plaque removal using Soladey brush

This brings us to the end of this chapter on the dangers of modern dentistry. The next chapter will examine the important topic of toxicity and how toxins is one of the most important underlying causes of many chronic diseases.

References

Boston University Medical Center. "Porphyromonas gingivalis accelerates inflammatory atherosclerosis in a mouse model." ScienceDaily. ScienceDaily, 4 January 2011.

Brown LJ, Oliver RC, Loe H (1989) Periodontal diseases in the US in 1981: prevalence, severity, extent, and role in tooth morality. Journal of Periodontology 60:363-370.

D'Aiuto F, Nibali L, Parkar M, Suvan J, Tonetti MS. Short-term effects of intensive periodontal therapy on serum inflammatory markers and cholesterol. J Dent Res.2005; 84:269-273.

D'Aiuto F, Parkar M, Andreou G, et al. Periodontitis and systemic inflammation: control of the local infection is associated with a reduction in serum inflammatory markers. J Dent Res.2004; 83:156-160.

Figueredo CM, Gustafsson A, Asman B, Bergstrom K. Expression of intracellular elastase activity in peripheral neutrophils from patients with adult periodontitis. J Clin Periodontol.2000; 27:572-577.

Fredriksson MI, Figueredo CM, Gustafsson A, Bergstrom KG, Asman BE. Effect of periodontitis and smoking on blood leukocytes and acute-phase proteins. J Periodontol.1999; 70:1355-1360.

Hua-Kung Wang, Yee-Chun Chen, Lee-Jene Teng, Chien-Ching Hung, Mei-Lin Chen, Shin-Hei Du, Hui-Ju Pan, Po-Ren Hsueh, and Shan-Chwen Chang. Brain Abscess Associated with Multidrug-Resistant Capnocytophaga ochracea Infection. Journal of Clinical Microbiology, Feb. 2007, p. 645–647 Vol. 45, No. 2.

Michael D. Williams, Caroline A. Kerber, and Helen F. Tergin. Unusual Presentation of Lemierre's Syndrome Due to Fusobacterium nucleatum Tergin. Journal of Clinical Microbiology, July 2003, p. 3445–3448 Vol. 41, No. 7.

Montebugnoli L, Servidio D, Miaton RA, Prati C, Tricoci P, Melloni C. Poor oral health is associated with coronary heart disease and elevated systemic inflammatory and haemostatic factors. J Clin Periodontol.2004;31:25-29.

Sanjeev Vasishtha, Henry D. Isenberg and Sunil K. Sood. Gemella morbillorum as a Cause of Septic Shock. Clinical Infectious Diseases. Vol. 22, No. 6 (Jun., 1996), pp. 1084-1086.

The World Oral Health Report 2003. Continuous improvement of oral health in the 21st century- the approach of the WHO Global Oral Health Programme

VIDEO TO WATCH

Mercury 101
https://iaomt.org/online-learning/mercury101/

Safe Removal of Amalgams
https://iaomt.org/online-learning/safe_removal/

Biologic Periodontics
https://iaomt.org/online-learning/biological_periodontics/

Hidden Pathogens
https://iaomt.org/online-learning/hidden_pathogens/

Chapter 8

Detoxification: The Health Secret of all Time

Earlier on, I talked about the importance of detoxification in regaining my own health – this was a critical step to my recovery and I have consequently learned that it should be the foundation of all healing protocols.

Because of my healing journey and new-found health, I have developed several detoxification protocols which I am now implementing with hundreds of my patients every year at the Da Vinci Holistic Health Centre in Cyprus (www.naturaltherapycenter.com).

I am certain that the topic of detoxification will one day become a true science; all the biochemical pathways mapped out showing how the body cleanses itself when the detox protocols mentioned here are used.

Do not underestimate the power of these simple protocols. As a clinician, I have seen miraculous changes in many chronically ill patients after detoxifying. In fact, there is an academically oriented clinical course entitled *"Detoxification and Toxicology"* that has been written for the Bachelor and Doctor of Science in Holistic Medicine.[196]

We will concentrate on talking about detoxification protocols, or different ways to detoxify, in this chapter.

Many diseases in our society are related to toxicity. Here are just some of the diseases that are linked to toxicity:
1. Parkinson's
2. Alzheimer's

---

[196] www.collegenaturalmedicine.com

3. Dementia
4. Heart disease
5. Chronic fatigue syndrome
6. Fibromyalgia syndrome
7. Cancers
8. Autoimmune diseases
9. Food allergies and intolerances
10. Arthritis
11. Digestive diseases like Crohn's disease, ulcers, colitis, and inflammatory bowel
12. Menstrual problems like heavy bleeding, cramps, PMS, menopausal symptoms, mood changes, and hot flashes

It might seem that everyone is toxic. This may be true to differing degrees.

What are Toxins?
A toxin is anything that is harmful or detrimental to the body.
Toxins can be internal (created by the biological processes of the body) or external (something that is introduced to the body, ingested, absorbed or inhaled).

The immune system, gastrointestinal (GI) system and skin are designed to protect you from toxins. However, you are exposed to toxic substances daily via what you apply to your skin, what you breathe and what you ingest.

Within your lifetime, you will consume up to 50 tonnes of food. Your GI system is responsible for breaking down these foods, digesting and absorbing components which are useful and eliminating the rest.

The liver works to remove toxins from the food you eat as well as toxins produced by your body. When the GI tract is not functioning well, the liver must do more work due to the additional burden placed upon it.

What Do Toxins Do to the Body?
When toxins build up, the ability for your body to remove them is quickly impaired. The body's self-regulation systems go out of balance, digestion becomes impaired and the liver and immune system become overwhelmed and cannot keep up.

The function of the large intestine slows down which in turn leads to congestion in the lymphatic system - which is designed to drain waste products from blood and tissues - thus forcing waste to re-circulate within the body.

When the liver is clogged, it allows toxins to travel into the body, instead of filtering them out. Toxins then get into the bloodstream and cause inflammation in other parts of the body. Thus, the body resorts to using the skin to purge the waste. Acne, rashes and eczema are signs that the body is trying to rid itself of toxins.

Toxins are also stored in body fat, causing weight gain and preventing the body from fully detoxifying itself.

How do you know that you are toxic?

Do you suffer from tiredness, lethargy, a 'heavy' feeling, digestive problems, bowel distension, headaches, muscle aches, poor concentration and memory, insomnia and many other symptoms too numerous to list? Well, all these symptoms can be related to toxins in your body that have accumulated over time.

Table 1 below shows some common signs and symptoms of toxicity:

Headaches	Backache	Runny nose	Fatigue
Joint pains	Itchy nose	Nervousness	Skin rashes
Cough	Frequent colds	Sleepiness	Hives
Wheezing	Irritated eyes	Insomnia	Nausea
Sore throat	Immune weakness	Dizziness	Indigestion
Tight or stiff neck	Environmental sensitivity	Mood changes	Anorexia
Angina Pectoris	Sinus congestion	Anxiety	Bad breath
Circulatory deficits	Fever	Depression	Constipation
High blood fats	Unexplained irritability	Chronic fatigue	Muscle twitching

Table 1. Signs and symptoms of toxicity

Signs and Symptoms of Toxicity

Life is toxic! There are toxins in the food you eat, the water you drink and the air you breathe. Even your own body produces toxins as a result of its many metabolic processes that keep you alive.

Signs that detoxification is needed if you have:

❖ Unexplained headaches or back pain
❖ Joint pain or arthritis
❖ Memory failure

313

❖ Depression or lack of energy
❖ Brittle nails and hair
❖ Abnormal body odour, coated tongue or bad breath
❖ Unexplained weight gain
❖ Psoriasis
❖ Frequent allergies
❖ A history of heavy alcohol use
❖ A history of natural and synthetic steroid hormone use
❖ An exposure to cleaning solvents, pesticides, diuretics and certain drugs.

Benefits of Detoxification

There are a number of benefits of detoxification such as:

❖ The digestive tract is cleansed of accumulated waste and fermenting bacteria.
❖ Liver, kidney and blood purification can take place, which is not possible during regular eating patterns.
❖ Mental clarity is enhanced as chemical and food additive overload is reduced.
❖ Reduced dependency on habit-forming substances such as sugar, caffeine, nicotine, alcohol and drugs.
❖ The stomach size is returned to normal as bad eating habits are stopped.
❖ The hormonal system is enhanced which is especially true for growth hormones.
❖ The immune system is stimulated.

It never ceases to amaze me that most symptoms, if not all, can disappear in less than 15 days! After detoxifying on an alkaline diet for 15 days, patients report high energy levels; clear and glowing skin with a brilliance that is obvious (I have said on many occasions that I should take before-detox and after-detox photos of patients - the change is striking!); weight loss of several pounds, which is an excellent motivating factor to continue with a detox programme; clear-headedness; higher thresholds for stress and tension; reduced cellulite; good body tone and a great feeling of being relaxed.

"How do you achieve this?" you may ask. Well, the secret lies in using a variety of detoxification protocols, which I will share with you below.
Detoxification has become a household word and a colloquialism that could mean anything from drinking a glass of carrot juice to entering a detoxification centre if you are an alcoholic or drug addict.

The term has now become a misnomer for many things that it is not. In the context that we are using the term, detoxification is the process of removing the toxins that have been accumulating in the body tissues and organs throughout a person's life.

These toxins will have been acting as metabolism blockers by literally poisoning the cells and not allowing them to function correctly.

You can have toxins stored in your body for years without experiencing any negative symptoms. It is only when the toxin levels become too high that you start to feel ill.

Sources of Toxins

So where do toxins come from? There are many sources, some of which I will mention here.

The three main sources are:

a) <u>Exogenous toxins</u>:

Exogenous toxins (Greek: 'from outside') are those that enter our bodies from the outside, i.e. food additives, pesticides, herbicides, fungi from food, industrial pollutants, viruses, bacteria, parasites and electromagnetic pollution such as X-rays, electromagnetic radiation and geopathic stress.

These external toxins may also come from other sources such as water, beverages, alcohol, medicines, accidents and injuries. Various industries have polluted our environment with an array of toxic heavy metals such as aluminium, antimony, arsenic, beryllium, bismuth, cadmium, lead, mercury, nickel, thallium and uranium.

Bisphenol A and Phthalates, commonly referred to as BPA, are toxic substances that exist in cheap plastic drinking bottles. While most bottles with BPA have been phased out, some still use them and should be avoided. A 2015 study confirmed that about 44% of canned food producers still use BPA-lined cans.

Amalgam teeth fillings contain 50% mercury, which is a potent neurotoxin. We will discuss this later when we talk about toxicity and heavy metals.

Processed foods contain artificial food additives, colours, flavours and preservatives.

Meat often contains hormones and antibiotics, which can cause hormonal disruption.

Caffeine and other stimulants, sedatives, alcohol, tobacco and illegal drugs, all must be filtered out of the body through the liver and kidneys.
Household chemicals are also guilty of introducing toxins into indoor living spaces. Common surface cleaners can emit dangerous fumes that may concentrate in small, enclosed areas. Even pet products may contain toxic elements that can harm both you and your pet.

In the past 100 years, around 75,000 new chemicals have been released into the environment. Chemicals that your body was never designed to cope with.

On top of all that, people are not getting the proper amount of sleep and exercise needed to stay healthy. Sleep and exercise play a critical role in relieving stress and eliminating harmful toxins.

b) Endogenous toxins:
Endogenous (Greek: 'from within') are toxins that are found or generated within the human body. This can occur when the body's normal metabolic mechanisms function inefficiently. For example, it typically takes several steps to convert the amino acid methionine into cysteine. If one step is sluggish, an intermediate called homocysteine accumulates in tissues. Accumulation of homocysteine can damage the vascular system and contribute to heart disease.[197]

Other toxins are associated with tuberculosis, syphilis or other diseases due to microbes; excess hormone secretions; constipation, producing toxins in the gut; pathogenic bacteria, causing food to putrefy and produce toxins in the gut;[198].

Hormones, such as oestrogen and androgen, get broken down and excreted in the liver after they are used. If the hormones are not properly taken care of by the liver, then hormonal imbalances and symptoms occur. Toxic build-up can occur when elimination mechanisms are inadequate due to poor nutrient intake or malabsorption of key detoxification nutrients.

Emotional stress is also a large contributor to toxins in the body. Research has shown that there is a connection between your emotions and well-being. When experiencing a traumatic or stressful event, it is common to react with anger, fear, grief, resentment etc. Repeated cycles of emotional stresses have a direct effect on the nervous and hormonal systems, which can indirectly affect our body's ability to detoxify.

Not dealing with your issues, and the emotions that get triggered by them, does not make the issue go away and only adds to the damaging effects on the body.

c) Autogenous toxins:

---

[197] Graham, I, Daly, L, Refsum H, et al. Plasma homocysteine as a risk factor for vascular disease. *JAMA*. 277;1775-1781, 1997.
[198] Donovan P. Bowel toxemia, permeability and disease: new information to support an old concept. In: Pizzorno JE, Murray MT. Textbook of Natural Medicine. St. Louis, MO: Elsevier Ltd; 1993.

Autogenous toxins (Greek: 'Born within') are generated within the body from miasmic influences, which are inherited tendencies that can pass through up to seven generations. Examples of these are psora, sycosis, tuberculosis, syphilinum and others. There is no detection of these pathogens with scientific testing, but their deep presence can affect the body's organs, primarily by inhibiting a good immune response and lowering its resistance.

Let's look at some specific sources of toxins that we encounter daily:
Cigarettes, alcohol, caffeine and drugs are all substances that the body cannot use for building and repair, so will add to the mounting waste. A lot of these toxic wastes are stored in the tissues and organs of the body.

Heavy metals such as mercury from fish and amalgam fillings; aluminium found in cheeses, baking powders, cake mixes, self-raising flour, cosmetics, toothpastes, antiperspirants and some drugs such as antacids. Cadmium is found in tea and coffee, as well as cigarette smoke. Lead is found in paints, fuels, rubber, plastics, inks, dyes, toys, building materials and hair restorers.

Arsenic is given to chickens as a growth promoter. Roxarsone - 4-hydroxy-3-nitrobenzenearsonic acid - is by far the most common arsenic-based additive used in chicken feed.[199] It is mixed in the diet of about 70% of the 9 billion broiler chickens produced annually in the U.S. In its original organic form, roxarsone is relatively benign. It is less toxic than the inorganic forms of arsenic-arsenite.

However, some of the 2.2 million lbs of roxarsone mixed in the nation's chicken feed each year converts into inorganic arsenic within the bird, and the rest is transformed into inorganic forms after the bird excretes it. Arsenic has been linked to bladder, lung, skin, kidney and colon cancer, while low-level exposures can lead to partial paralysis and diabetes.

Plastics containing Bisphenol A, the building block of polycarbonate plastics, which are everywhere: in pesticides as fungicides, antioxidants, flame retardants, rubber chemicals, a coating in metals, cans and food containers, refrigerator shelving, returnable containers for juice, milk and water, nail polish, compact discs, adhesives, microwave ovenware and eating utensils.

A diet that is high in animal fats will add to the waste. There are many different drugs and chemicals that are given to animals these days, ranging from antibiotics,

---

[199] Hileman, B. Arsenic in Chicken Production: A common feed additive adds arsenic to human food and endangers water supplies. *Chemical and Engineering News*. Volume 85, Number 15, pp. 34-35, April 9, 2007.

hormones, feed concentrates, etc. All these chemicals will accumulate in the fat cells of the animals that we then eat – so we slowly build up an accumulation of these chemicals over time.

Sluggish bowels can lead to a great deal of toxicity throughout the body.

Try to imagine a 10-metre tube running from mouth to anus packed with meat, sausage, fish, fruit salad, beef burgers, sugars, milk and other goodies – all fermenting and putrefying for days on end.

This fermentation produces highly toxic substances such as putrescine, neuracine and cadaverine. These are so poisonous that a small amount injected into a laboratory animal will kill it in minutes. All these toxic substances, apart from causing disease in the body, will also act as metabolism blockers, and will therefore have consequences on weight-loss too.

This process of 'self-poisoning' by these putrefying foods in the gut is called 'autointoxication.'

Refined foods such as white sugar, white flour, white rice, etc. are all deficient in nutrients, but calorie loaded. Apart from this, they also help to create a lot of sludge and debris in the body. If you remember from your childhood days, you probably used white flour and water to make a glue to make your kite, or to glue your coloured paper in your exercise book at school.

When eaten, white flour and its products become glue in the intestine and stick to the internal walls. When mixed with sticky sugar and fat, it becomes a rubber-like substance that blocks absorption of foods through the intestine, as well as being a constant source of toxins. If you don't believe me, read Dr. Jensen's book entitled, *Tissue cleansing through bowel management*[200]. There are also plenty of photos of what actually comes out of the intestine if you do a proper detox – disgusting!

Thousands of new, toxic chemical compounds are produced each year by the chemical industry, most of which are approved by various so-called 'Environmental Protection Agencies' (EPA's) without any serious toxicological studies. The cumulative number of toxic chemicals polluting our planet today exceeds 100,000.

Many claim that some of these chemicals, such as the flame retardants used in children's clothing, have potentially life-saving applications. But how many of these chemicals do we ingest or are absorbed by our bodies and those of our children?

---

[200] Jensen, B. Dr. Jensen's guide to better bowel care: A complete program for tissue cleansing through bowel management. USA: Avery Publishers, 1999.

And at what cost to our health? What is the capacity of the human body to eliminate them?

Has anyone conducted a general contracting cost-benefit analysis as to whether the benefits offered, for example, by fire hazard protection, truly outweigh the toxicity generated within us, our children and the environment? The answer is: *No.* There are no comprehensive, scientific answers, other than to confirm the obvious: toxicity levels in humans and animals across the globe are rising fast. Whether we realize it or not – *we are all toxic.*

In an article published in the October 2006 *National Geographic* entitled, *'The Pollution Within,'* journalist David Ewing Duncan had himself tested for 320 synthetic chemicals and certain heavy metals at a cost of $16,000, paid for by the magazine.

According to the article, Duncan was considered a healthy individual. Nevertheless, he had higher than average amounts of chemical toxins, such as flame-retardants (known as PDBE's), phthalates, Polychlorinated Biphenyls (PCBs), pesticides and dioxins, as well as heavy metals such as mercury.

Duncan's article alludes to some of the possible ways toxic chemicals may have accumulated in his body: some might have originated in childhood, while others may have been picked up in airplanes due to his extensive work-related travel. However, he and his doctors were merely speculating…

Duncan also describes his pre- and post-mercury toxicity results after a fresh fish dinner and breakfast. Duncan had fresh halibut for dinner and fresh swordfish for breakfast (cooked in his toxic non-stick pan), both of which were caught in the ocean just outside the Golden Gate Bridge in the San Francisco Bay area.

He tested himself for serum mercury before and after the meals, and found that his blood mercury levels had shot up from five micrograms per litre to over 12. The doctors conducting the tests advised him not to repeat that experiment ever again, yet I'm sure this dangerous diet is adhered to by thousands, unaware of the impact of toxicity on their health. After all, fish is promoted as a health food! Nevertheless, drawing conclusions on the experience of only one healthy adult is not robust, toxicological science. So, let us review the research.

New 21st Century Theory of Disease

Dr. Miller, of the Department of Family Practice, University of Texas Health Science Center at San Antonio, USA, believes that we are on the threshold of the new theory of disease that is triggered by toxic chemicals. She states in one of her papers[201]:

"In the late 1800's, physicians observed that certain illnesses spread from sick, feverish individuals to those contacting them, paving the way for the germ theory of disease. The germ theory served as a crude but elegant formulation that explained dozens of seemingly unrelated illnesses affecting literally every organ system."

She continues:

"Today we are witnessing another medical anomaly – the unique pattern of illness involving chemically exposed people who subsequently report multisystem symptoms and new-onset chemical and food intolerances. These intolerances may be the hallmark for a new disease process, just as fever is a hallmark for infection."

I strongly agree with Dr Miller and believe that many of the new diseases that we are seeing today such as Gulf War Syndrome,[202] Chronic Fatigue Syndrome, Myalgic Encephalomyelitis (ME), fibromyalgia, childhood diabetes, attention deficit hyperactivity disorder and others are all chemically related disorders.[203]

How exposed are you to these chemicals?

Check out below how prone you are to developing a chemically-triggered 21st century disease, by checking off the various categories. The more of these that apply to you, the higher your risk. Do you:

- ✓ Work with chemicals
- ✓ Use pesticides around the house and garden such as fly spray, weed killer or flea powder
- ✓ Use non-environmentally friendly cosmetics, toiletries and household cleaners
- ✓ You are responsible for disposal of chemicals used in medicines such as mercury preservatives in vaccines and flea shampoo
- ✓ Eat nonorganic fruit, vegetables and meat products
- ✓ Eat contaminated seafood, usually containing mercury

---

[201] Miller C. Are We on the Threshold of a New Theory of Disease? Toxicant-induced Loss of Tolerance and its Relationship to Addiction and Abdiction. *Tox. Ind. Health*. 15:284-294, 1999.

[202] Miller, C. and Prihoda, TA Controlled Comparison of Symptoms and Chemical Intolerances Reported by Gulf War Veterans, Implant Recipients and Persons with Multiple Chemical Sensitivity. *Tox. Ind. Health* 15:386-397, 1999.

[203] Miller, C. Prihoda, T. The Environmental Exposure and Sensitivity Inventory (EESI): A Standardized approach for measuring Chemical Intolerances for Research and Clinical Applications. *Tox. Ind. Health* 15:370-385, 1999.

✓ Eat too many processed foods, full of preservatives, colourings, flavourings and other additives
✓ Drink unfiltered tap water containing aluminium and fluoride
✓ Consume soft drinks from aluminium cans
✓ Have mercury amalgam fillings in your mouth
✓ Live in a major city with all the air pollution.

These chemicals are accumulative, so do not think that a little exposure will do you no harm – it simply takes longer to reach critical levels in the body before symptoms appear.

Signs and Symptoms of Chemical Poisoning

In clinical practice, I am often very vigilant in trying to detect symptoms that are related to chemical sensitivity and other toxicity issues. If the patient suddenly develops the following symptoms, then chemical exposure should be suspected:

✓ Dark blue, black or pink circles under the eyes
✓ Wrinkles or abnormally puffy bags under the eyes, as well as wrinkles on hands and knuckles
✓ Bright red cheeks, nose tips or ear lobes
✓ Unstable legs
✓ A spaced-out look and feeling
✓ Itchy nose
✓ Licking lips frequently
✓ Fuzzy thinking, confusion; difficulty in concentrating, thinking clearly or remembering
✓ Joint or arthritic pains
✓ Runny nose or nasal congestion causing sinusitis and blocked nose
✓ Extreme fatigue, even when rising in the morning
✓ Headaches

One study that tried to assess exposure to Bisphenol A (BPA) and 4-tertiary-octylphenol (tOP) in the American population found 92.6% and 57.4% of the persons, respectively had these chemicals in their urine.[204] These are industrial chemicals used in the manufacture of polycarbonate plastics and epoxy resins (BPA) and non-ionic surfactants (tOP). These products are in widespread use in the United States and the rest of the world.

Ways to Address Toxicity: The good, the bad and the ugly

---

[204] Calafat AM, Ye X, Wong LY, Reidy JA, Needham LL. Exposure of the U.S. Population to Bisphenol A and 4-*tertiary*-Octylphenol: 2003-2004. *Environ Health Perspect* Jan;116(1):39-44, 2008.

Let's start with the ugly first: the typical misguided response to the toxicity onslaught is to visit the average doctor, who will note a few toxicity-induced symptoms, and come up with a superficial diagnosis.

At first, a diagnosis appears simple: flu, sinusitis, eczema, tonsillitis, or otitis. Over time, diagnoses get complicated: asthma, arthritis, sacroiliatis, heart disease, renal disease, liver disease, cancer or any of the currently labelled chronic degenerative diseases which can strike.
This ugly, symptom-based approach amounts to a classically wrong diagnosis.

The main causative factor, TOXICITY, remains undetected. Hardly anyone is searching for it, let alone finding it! Tragically, the ugly approach has become the norm, instead of the exception. Depending on the wrong diagnosis, which is typically a mere description of the symptom, the typical physician will prescribe chemical drugs to ingest, or refer you to other specialists who may contemplate removal of body parts (pardon the cynicism here, but this is the truth, as I experienced it from allopathic doctors – hopefully there will always be the exception among such practitioners).

With the ugly approach, the worse the disease, the worse the treatment gets. Cancer, the dreaded disease, is the perfect example.

The reasoning goes: many toxins are proven carcinogens, so they could well be the cause of a person's cancer, right? Wrong! The ugly approach sees the world differently. Even at this advanced stage of body toxicity, when the body's immunity and vitality has been seriously compromised by carcinogens, the default medical intervention is to load the body with even more toxins: potent chemotherapeutic agents that are super-toxic, or cancer-causing radiation treatments to remove the original cancer.

You also need additional drugs (Erythropoietin Stimulating Agents) to counter the decrease in red blood cell production caused by chemotherapy, which add their own serious side-effects. By then, the tumour is reduced, the cancer has metastasized and the patient is either dead or bankrupt – or likely both. 'Common sense' at its best!

What we should be doing, medics and patients alike, is exactly the opposite. Should we not be addressing the cause of the problem - the toxins - instead of chasing and suppressing the symptoms? We should be reducing the toxic load, not increasing it.

We should be improving the tissue integrity, not cutting it apart. It seems evident to me that the common-sense approach would dictate addressing the safe removal of the toxins. Assuming our interest lies in achieving real, long-term relief for the patient.

Indeed, between the ugly and the good approach, there is also a bad way to address toxicity-caused illnesses.

If you try to release toxins from the body too fast, or too clumsily, the body may be tipped over the edge. This is an issue that many well-meaning practitioners underestimate – either because of inadequate technical know-how, insufficient experience or poor judgment – with disastrous results vis-à-vis the recovery prospects of their patients.

Unfortunately, there are plenty of bad ways out there to deal with toxicity-induced diseases. Therefore, sound and continuous research by the patient and practitioners to minimize such a risk is integral.

Meanwhile, a growing group of medical practitioners have 'jumped on the bandwagon' so to speak, using their medical licenses to chelate people with various heavy metals – using more drugs such as EDTA, DMSA, DMPS and the like. This can often lead to disastrous consequences as these drugs mobilize metals quicker than the body can eliminate them, while stripping the body of the good minerals.

In other words, the typical MD's knowledge of toxicology needs improvement, to say the least. There are natural, gentler ways of detoxifying the body of heavy metals and other xenobiotics.

I hope that this book, based on extensive research, will provide food-for-thought to the many out there that are lost and confused about these complex issues.

Let's move now to the main detoxification treatments and protocols that I use at the Da Vinci Centre, which effectively deal with the toxicity within my patients' bodies and are instrumental to the recovery of many diseases, including chronic degenerative disorders.

The Da Vinci Centre Detoxification Diet – clean, clean, clean!

The 15-day Alkaline Detoxification Diet (15-DADD)

Most of the patients that come to me for a wide variety of health problems will be placed on the Da Vinci Centre's 15-day Alkaline Detoxification Diet (15-DADD). This is a diet that I have put together through clinical experience, as well as studying the work of other practitioners[205,206,207,208] who are very well versed in the field of detoxification.

Most of my patients can safely follow this 15-day detoxification programme, except for a few who have other diseases such as diabetes, cancer, heart conditions, low blood pressure and some neurological diseases. There are modified protocols for all the aforementioned, but these should be supervised by a qualified health practitioner.

These more complex patients need more thought and each detoxification regime can be tailored to suit each patient. Therefore, I take a careful history from each one, as well as examining all their clinical findings. These include blood tests, blood pressure, conducting an Iridology examination (looking at the iris, the coloured part of the eye, using an iris microscope which gives me further health information), as well as other diagnostic instruments that I have at my disposal such as Live Blood Analysis, VEGA testing, Biological Terrain Analysis, heavy metal testing, Autonomic Response Testing, Thermography and more[209].

Generally, most patients will be able to tell me what their problem is and its severity, as they have usually received a medical diagnosis before arriving on my doorstep.

Given that all is OK to begin the 15-day detox diet, I suggest that they eat only fresh fruit, salads, freshly squeezed juices, steamed vegetables and vegetable soups for 15 consecutive days. This means that they ONLY eat these foods for the duration, most of which will be rich in the live enzymes, which are the tools required to flush out the toxins from the body. You must be patient and put your mind to it.

I cannot emphasize just how important the detoxification diet is to your success!

---

[205] Ballie-Hamilton, P. The Detox diet. UK: Penguin, 2002.

[206] Scrivner, J. Detox Yourself. UK: Judy Piatkus (Publishers) Ltd., 1998.

[207] Wade, C. Inner Cleansing: How to Free Yourself from the Joint-Muscle-Artery-Circulation Sludge. New York: Parker Publishing Co., 1992.

[208] Cabot, S. Juice Fasting Detoxification. USA: The Sprout House, 1992.

[209] www.naturaltherapycenter.com

What will I be eating during the 15-DADD?

I strongly suggest that you try to eat as many raw fruits and vegetables as possible, including at least 1-3 fruit and vegetable juices daily. Carrot juice has a strong effect on the digestive system, provides energy, serves as an important source of minerals, promotes normal elimination, has diuretic properties and helps to build healthy tissue, skin and teeth. So, I recommend as many carrot juices as they can handle, mixed with beetroot juice (about 1/3rd of a glass), which are powerful cleansing agents of the body. Beets are said to really cleanse the blood and kidneys. In nature, homogenous colours do not occur by accident – it is no coincidence that the red beetroot affects the blood!

I also encourage the use of a little 'green juice' mixed with each carrot juice. This can be anything from fresh parsley, lettuce, kale, collard greens, Swiss chard, alfalfa, cabbage, spinach, turnip greens, watercress, celery, cucumber, green pepper, scallions, coriander, or any other green vegetable in season. You can place a couple of inches of the green juice in the glass, and top up with carrot juice. All green vegetables contain chlorophyll, which is very oxygenating for the body. It is also an effective antiseptic, cell stimulator, red blood builder and rejuvenator – therefore helping to remove toxic sludge faster. Greens are also super-rich in live enzymes.

I also suggest that each meal should begin with raw fruit or vegetables, seasoned with a little lemon, ginger, garlic, coconut or desired herbs. This way, they are available for digesting the fat, protein, and carbohydrates from the meal that follows. The enzymes in vegetables control or restrict the amount of waste deposited on your adipocytes. Remember to chew all foods thoroughly.

These are the foods that I allow during the detoxification phase – no other family of foods is allowed. You may eat as many of the following foods as you wish, but it is best to eat only when you feel hungry. Wash all fruit and vegetables in a bowl of water with 4-5 tablespoons of grape vinegar added (not apple cider vinegar), to help wash away any pesticide/herbicide residues. Rinse afterwards with clean water. Here are the foods that you can eat in plenty – in fact, the more you eat and drink, the quicker you detoxify:

• **SALADS** – use any type of fresh vegetables you like, in any combination. Use organic vegetables when available, and include bean sprouts when in season. Salad dressings should be kept simple – a little virgin olive oil with fresh lemon or lime juice, or cider vinegar. Add plenty of fresh onion and garlic – these are very detoxifying!

- **STEAMED VEGETABLES** – eat any variety you like, including broccoli, cauliflower, potatoes, beetroot, carrots, etc. Steam as opposed to boil, and eat with a little herbal salt, lemon and a little virgin olive oil, with plenty of garlic. You may also have jacket potatoes with a little olive oil, garlic and parsley dressing.

- **STIR-FRIED VEGETABLES** – this is a quick, easy way of cooking vegetables healthily. Use no more than four cups of chopped, hard or medium-hard vegetables or eight to twelve cups chopped leafy greens in a 14-inch wok to avoid crowding the pan. It's important that the vegetables are very dry, otherwise, the vegetables will steam and braise in the pan and lose their crisp texture. Giving the vegetables a whirl in a salad spinner is the easiest solution, but you can also pat them thoroughly with kitchen towels.

- **VEGETABLE SOUPS** – again quick and easy to make, and very nutritious, providing all the vegetables that our bodies require. It is easy to digest and is generally low in calories. Studies have shown that we tend to eat 20% less calories overall when we eat soups before a main meal. You can make nutritious leak and broccoli soups, as well as tomato and clear soups with various vegetables, adding onion and garlic for their detoxification benefits too.

● **VEGETABLE/FRUIT JUICES** – drink a minimum of 1-3 per day, and try to include one cocktail comprising one-third of a glass of raw, green juice (spinach, parsley, cabbage and any other green vegetables), topped up with carrot juice. There is no limit to the amount of fresh vegetable and fruit juices that you may drink in a day.

● **FRESH FRUIT** – choose the fruit of your choice (preferably organic) and eat as much as you like, whenever you like. You could begin the day with 2-3 pieces of fruit, which are gentle on the digestive system. Make a tasty fruit salad and eat it in the morning as this helps to detoxify. Fruit is rich in antioxidant phytonutrients which are beneficial to the body in many ways; protecting us from chronic diseases.

● **HERBAL TEAS** – choose any of your choice. Chamomile is a good relaxant; aniseed and mint is good for the digestive system; Kombucha; dandelion tea or 'coffee' (which is excellent for purifying the blood and detoxifying and stimulating liver function); Sage tea, (which is a blood cleanser); or Nettle tea, (which is excellent for driving away excess fluid out of the tissues and is a wonderful cleanser for all the detoxification organs). Drink as many as you like, with a little honey on the tip of a teaspoon if you like, but plain is best.

You will also need to drink at least 8-10 glasses per day of still mineral water to flush out the toxins – this is VERY IMPORTANT, so please take note!

When the 15 days are over, you should carry on eating the above for a couple more days while gently adding a little protein such as fresh steamed or grilled fish, organic chicken, pulses, a soft-boiled organic egg or a little cheese. Go gently on the protein for a couple of days before you begin eating normally again so that you do not overload your digestive system.

Lots of Food and Calories
This may appear to be an awful lot of calories, since there are no restrictions on the amount of such foods consumed over the 15-day period. The purpose of this diet, however, is to DETOXIFY – to remove the toxins from the fat cells and tissues as well as the organs, so that the body can return to its optimum level of functionality. I have yet to see anyone going through the 15-DADD put on any weight, so don't worry about counting calories – most people lose one or more kilos (2-4 lbs) over the 15-day period.

I had one gentleman weighing 150 kg (nearly 24 stone) who lost 10 kg (22 lbs) in 15 days, but I believe that most of this was accumulated fluid due to a drinking problem. On a biochemical and microbiological level, there is much going on during the detoxification.

The pH or acidity/alkalinity of the body is being adjusted back to normal, and any nasty pathogens in the body are encouraged to reverse their course. This is based on the work of Enderlein, Neissens and Beauchamp who were proponents of pleomorphism as opposed to monomorphism.
With our bad eating, smoking and drinking habits, body chemistry is unbalanced in most people. This unbalanced body chemistry will be another metabolism blocker that will not allow the body to digest, assimilate, eliminate or get rid of fatty deposits optimally.

Detoxification Symptoms:"The healing crisis"

When the body detoxifies, it goes through various biochemical and physiological changes.[210] Generally, on the first day of fasting the blood sugar level is likely to drop below 65-70 mg/dl. The liver immediately compensates by converting glycogen to glucose and releasing it in the blood. After a few hours, the basal metabolic rate is likely to fall to conserve energy. This means that the heart, pulse and blood pressure will drop. More glycogen may be used from muscles, causing some weakness.

As the body requires more energy, some fat and fatty acids are broken down to release glycerol from the glyceride molecules and are converted to glucose. You may notice the skin becoming quite oily as these fatty acids and glycerol increase in the blood. The skin is one of the largest detoxification organs, so you may get some skin problems such as pimples, acnes or a pussy boil – this is all part of the body trying to cleanse. The complexion may become pallid for a day or two as the wastes accumulate in the blood.

The incomplete oxidation of fats may result in the formation of Ketones resulting in ketoacidosis. Combined with high levels of urea, resulting from protein metabolism, this state can cause several symptoms which may suppress appetite; they affect the satiety centre in the hypothalamus.

Generally, this takes a few days to happen and you may notice your appetite dwindling. You may get pains in different joints, or organs such as the lungs. There may be a considerable amount of yellow mucus released from the throat and expelled. The sinuses may also begin clearing with more mucus secreted.

Given that the body is releasing these toxins quickly during the first few days of the detoxification process, it should not surprise you to experience some changes in your body that may cause certain symptoms. Initially, for the first 2-3 days these symptoms can be a little unpleasant, SO BE WARNED!

A fair number of people will have headaches, nervousness, diarrhoea, upset stomach, energy loss, furry tongue, halitosis (bad breath), as well as acne or other skin rashes, a general feeling of malaise, frequent urination due to the toxins irritating the bladder and some of their existing symptoms may be exacerbated. When the toxic residues enter the blood, they affect mind and body functions.

These may be unpleasant symptoms for the first couple of days, but they are a NORMAL part of the detoxification process, and in natural medicine we call this the HEALING CRISIS. All these symptoms indicate that the DETOX IS WORKING!

---

210 Salloum, TK. Fasting Signs and Symptoms: A Clinical Guide. USA: Buckeye Naturopathic Press, 1992.

This is a temporary and transient crisis, it will pass – so hang on in there and don't worry that there is something wrong with you.

There was always something wrong with you, and now you are doing something about it – you are reversing this toxic process that your body has adapted to.

If you are a coffee drinker, then the symptoms will be more pronounced, as your body will be in a state of withdrawal. Yes, coffee is a drug and when you come off it you go into withdrawal, meaning that your body will start asking for a dose of what it is addicted to. When it doesn't get it, then it screams for it louder and louder, usually in the form of headaches, migraines, muscle pains, general weakness and lack of concentration.

Enduring a cleansing crisis is the hardest part of the healing process. To stop feeling bad, most people want to eat, but do not eat during a cleansing crisis! The body is overloaded with the work of removing toxins. Digestion makes matters worse. Drinking one or two glasses of sodium bicarbonate (baking soda) – one teaspoon in each glass drunk twice daily - will help to neutralize the ketoacidosis.

Helter-skelter rides are common – the 'downward slope' is when the body is vigorously cleansing and the blood gets swamped with toxins causing you to feel down, moody, depressed and achy, like having a bad cold. You feel weak and lethargic. The mind rationalizes: 'I feel horrible: this can't be working.' You can maintain a normal routine of work on a dip but it requires willpower and determination. It also helps to know that the longer the down period, the greater the fasting high.

Phases of Detoxification

There is a lot going on in the body during the detoxification process – most of the work is happening in the largest detoxification organ of the body – the liver. The detoxification phases in the liver are composed of two phases, known as Phase I and Phase II. These phases chemically biotransform toxins into progressively more water-soluble substances through a series of chemical reactions so that they can be excreted from the body.

Phase I: Detoxification

This phase of detoxification usually involves oxidation, reduction, or hydrolysis. A family of enzymes commonly referred to as cytochrome P450 mixed-function oxidases perform the most important processes – detoxifying xenobiotics and endogenous substances.[211]

---

211 Grant DM. Detoxification pathways of the liver. *J Inher Metab Dis*. 14;421-430, 1991.

At least 50 enzymes in 10 families governed by 35 different genes allow Phase I to take place. Many forms of cytochrome P-450 enzymes are involved in Phase I reactions. The highest concentration of cytochrome P-450 occurs in the liver, which is the most active site of metabolism. The lungs and the kidneys are secondary organs of biotransformation, with about one-third of the liver's detoxification capacity. Cytochrome P-450 has also been found in the intestines, adrenal cortex, testes, spleen, heart, muscles, brain, and skin.

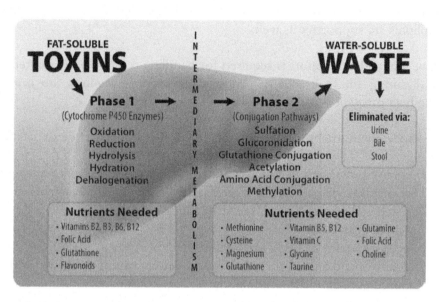

Our understanding of these detoxification pathways over the last couple of decades has helped clinicians understand how they can help patients overcome toxic effects.[212] Sluggish, imbalanced, or impaired detoxification systems can result in the accumulation and deposition of metabolic toxins, increased free radical production and its ensuing pathology, impaired oxidative phosphorylation, and reduced energy.

Nutrients Required for Detoxification Phase
The action of detoxification enzymes in both Phase I and Phase II detoxification pathways depends on the presence of various nutrients.[213,214] For example, alcohol dehydrogenase, an enzyme that converts alcohols (such as ethanol) to aldehydes in an oxidation reaction, depends on an adequate supply of zinc to function properly.

---

212 Davies MH, Gough A, Sorhi RS, Hassel A, Warning R, Emery P. Sulphoxidation and sulphation capacity in patients with primary biliary cirrhosis. *J Hepatol.* 22(5):551-560, May 1995.
213 Anderson KE, Kappas A. Dietary regulation of cytochrome P-450. *Annu Rev Nutr.* 11:141-167, 1991.
214 Bland JS, Bralley JA. Nutritoinal upregulation of hepatic detoxification enzymes. *J Appl Nutr.* 44(3&4):2-15, 1992.

In the next metabolic step, the enzyme aldehyde oxidase changes the aldehyde into an acid that can be excreted in the urine. Aldehyde oxidase depends on an adequate supply of molybdenum and iron. Other minerals that are required by enzymes include manganese, magnesium, sulfur, selenium, and copper.

Other supporting nutrients involved in cytochrome P-450 enzymes include vitamins B2, B3, B6, B12 and folic acid. The tripeptide glutathione and the branched-chain amino acids leucine, glycine, isoleucine, and valine are also required. Flavonoids and phospholipids are supportive as well.

Protective antioxidant support is required for handling reactive oxygen intermediates produced during Phase I activity. Antioxidant support requires the carotenoids, including beta-carotene, vitamin C and E and coenzyme Q10.

To summarize, the nutrients required during Phase I and Phase II detoxification are:

- ❖ B-complex vitamins: necessary co-factors used in Phase 1 detoxification
- ❖ Digestive enzymes: may be necessary to ensure that protein is adequately digested and glycine is readily available
- ❖ Essential fatty acids
- ❖ N-acetyl cysteine (NAC): an immediate precursor to glutathione, a potent antioxidant and among the most import detoxification nutrients for the liver
- ❖ Reduced glutathione
- ❖ Selenium, zinc, magnesium and manganese; possibly iron and copper if used with caution
- ❖ Taurine
- ❖ Vitamins C and E and beta carotene
- ❖ Inositol & Methionine: lipotropic agents (help with the breakdown of fat in metabolism) that work to transport fat out of the liver
- ❖ High ORAC vegetable extract blend with polyphenols (a phytonutrient)

Most of these are available in one high-potency multivitamin/mineral formula that we use called HMD MULTIS. The fatty acids can be obtained from KRILL OIL. All supplements mentioned here are obtainable from www.worldwidehealthcenter.net.

In addition, liver herbs can be used to aid detoxification (traditionally known as 'blood cleansing' herbs):

- ❖ Dandelion root, beet leaf & Yellow Dock: cholagogue (stimulates liver secretions and bile flow)
- ❖ Artichoke leaf: promotes regeneration of the liver and promotes blood flow in that organ; stimulates bile flow

❖ Silymarin (bioflavonoid found in Milk Thistle): according to research, this herbal extract stabilizes the membranes of liver cells, preventing the entry of virus toxins and other toxic compounds including drugs and supports the protection of the liver and promotes its regeneration

❖ Turmeric: a cholagogue like dandelion.

❖ Caraway, dill seeds, sassafras tea

Most of these can be found in the herbal formula that we use called HEPATO PLUS.

Here is a more detailed diagram showing these important nutrients:

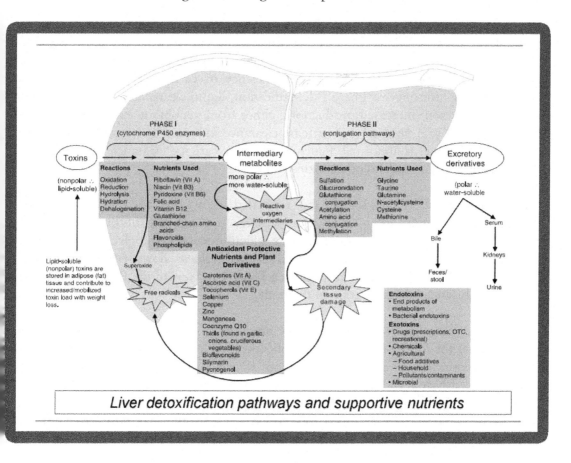

Liver detoxification pathways and supportive nutrients

Usually, the enzymatic reactions in Phase I decrease chemical toxicity. However, toxic or reactive chemicals can form during Phase I that are more toxic than the original compound. This is known as bioactivation. When Phase II detoxification proceeds normally, these chemicals are then rendered harmless and excreted. However, if there is an imbalance in the active levels of Phase I and II

333

detoxifications, these toxins will remain in the body. Imbalance between Phase I and Phase II is associated with increased symptoms of nervous, immune, and endocrine system toxicity.

Toxic chemicals produced during Phase I include teratogens (causing fetus malformation), mutagens (causing cell mutation), and carcinogens (causing cancer). For example, benzo[a]pyrene, a chemical found in coal tar and cigarette smoke, is biologically inert until it is converted by the mixed-function amine oxidase system into a metabolite that can then initiate cancer causing activity. During Phase I, many compounds also form dangerous reactive free radicals - chemicals with an unpaired electron that can cause tissue damage. A buildup of free radicals can increase the risk of cancer.

The level of functioning of Phase I can be measured with a simple caffeine metabolism test. A known quantity of caffeine is ingested, and saliva samples are taken twice at specified intervals. The efficiency of caffeine clearance is directly related to the efficiency of Phase I detoxification. Rapid clearance of caffeine shows enzyme induction (increased production), either from xenobiotic exposure or toxins within the body. A slow rate of caffeine clearance indicates that cytochrome P-450 activity in the liver is abnormal. Patients with slow caffeine clearance have difficulty eliminating xenobiotics and other toxins.

The function of Phase II can be evaluated through the ingestion of both acetaminophen and aspirin. This test measures the recovery of the products of glutathione conjugation, sulfur conjugation, glucuronidation, and glycine conjugation (acylation) in the urine. Comparison to normal values allows evaluation of the efficiency of Phase II. A high ratio between Phase I and any of the Phase II pathways implies imbalanced detoxification in the body.

The detoxification process requires large amounts of caloric energy, which comes mainly from the food we eat. If we do not eat enough protein, the body breaks down vital tissue protein to produce the energy it needs. This decreases the available amounts of Phase I and Phase II enzymes, amino acids, and peptides, because the body breaks down protein to amino acids and peptides. The greater the toxic burden of the body, the higher the need for protein, carbohydrate, fat, and micronutrient intake.

Supplements that Help the Detoxification Pathways
Some of the nutrients required for the proper functioning of the detoxification pathways have already been mentioned above. To reiterate, it is strongly advised that you drink at least 10 glasses of mineral or reverse osmosis water daily, so that you can

flush out the toxins quicker. All supplements mentioned here are obtainable from www.worldwidehealthcenter.net

We have already mentioned taking a multivitamin formula to help optimize your levels of vitamins and minerals, which are crucial raw materials for many of the detoxification pathways of the body. Choose one that has high levels of vitamins and minerals, not just the RDA levels – at the Da Vinci Center we use a high-potency formula called HMD MULTIS.

In addition, taking a couple of grams of vitamin C three times daily during the detoxification process will also help. Vitamin C will help to absorb certain toxins, as well as helping the immune system cope with a heavy burden of toxins that it needs to get rid of. I usually recommend a Calcium/Magnesium Ascorbate in powder form, which is an alkaline form of vitamin C, and is much gentler on the stomach and gut than plain ascorbic acid.

At the Da Vinci Center we use one in capsule form called VITAMIN C (Mixed Blend). Take 2 caps x 3 times daily, or you can open these up and place them in some juice or water.

Other supplements that we recommend include the following:
HEPATO PLUS - this is a herbal combination, specifically designed to provide extra support to the detoxification organs and systems of the body – particularly during periods of over-indulgence in food, alcohol or smoking.

Beneficial for...
- Liver cleansing
- A sluggish liver and gallbladder
- Body cleansing and detoxification
- Blood purifying support
- High energy levels
- Cholesterol levels
- Body odour
- Digestive health
- Indigestion
- Relieving symptoms of occasional over-indulgence in food and drink
- A colon cleansing program
- Those with a poor diet
- Those with a high toxic load

You can take one capsule x 3 times daily. Each capsule contains:
- ❖ Artichoke extract (40:1), 2.5% cynarin (equivalent to 4800mg of fresh artichoke)
- ❖ Parsley powder
- ❖ Beetroot extract (5:1) (equivalent to 400mg of fresh beetroot powder)

❖ Turmeric powder (95% Curcumin)
❖ Burdock root extract (5:1) (equivalent to 200mg of fresh burdock root)
❖ Fennel seed extract (4:1) (equivalent to 120mg of fresh fennel seed powder)
❖ Dandelion root extract (4:1) (equivalent to 100mg of fresh dandelion root powder)
❖ Liquorice root extract (5:1) (equivalent to 100mg of fresh liquorice)
❖ N-acetyl L-cysteine
❖ Alpha lipoic acid
❖ Garlic (black aged garlic) extract (100:1) (equivalent to 500mg of fresh garlic powder)
❖ Ginger root powder
❖ Cayenne (Capicum Frutescens) extract (8:1) (equivalent to 30mg of fresh cayenne powder)

Another herbal formula called COLFORM. This is a fast-acting, herbal colon cleanser and bowel support formula with 10 active herbal ingredients, including glucomannan.

COLFORM is a well-known herbal colon cleanser and bowel support combination, based on a formula by American master herbalist, Dr. John R. Christopher.

Beneficial for...

• Constipation
• Sluggish bowels
• Haemorrhoids
• Clearing bowel 'pockets'
• Diverticula
• Internal cleansing and detoxification
• Stool softening
• Prior to, following or between colonic hydrotherapy treatments

You should take one capsule x 3 times daily. Each capsule contains:

❖ Rhubarb powder
❖ Barberry powder
❖ Burdock root powder
❖ Cayenne powder
❖ Ginger root powder
❖ Rhubarb root extract (30:1)
❖ Fennel seed powder
❖ Aloe vera extract (200:1)

❖ Clove bud powder
❖ Dandelion root extract (4:1)

Another herbal remedy called <u>CONSTFORM</u>, based on one of Dr. John R. Christopher's formulas, is good to add when there has been a history of constipation.

It is a fast-acting colon cleanser, designed for the chronically constipated in need of strong treatment for a blocked bowel.

Beneficial for...

- Chronic constipation
- Internal cleansing
- Lower bowel function
- Bowel regularity
- Laxative abuse
- Use by colonic hydrotherapists before, during and after treatments

You can take one capsule x 3 times daily. Each capsule contains:

❖ Rhubarb powder
❖ Barberry powder
❖ Glucomannan 90%
❖ Alfalfa powder
❖ Cayenne powder
❖ Garlic powder
❖ Aloe vera extract (200:1)
❖ Dandelion root extract (4:1)
❖ Ginger root extract (20:1)
❖ Nettle leaf extract (4:1)

Another herbal formula that I recommend to my patients during the 15-day detox is called <u>PARAFORM PLUS ONE</u>. This one is designed to eliminate parasites from the intestine; we pick these up from food and water all the time, so a couple of times per year it is good to detox from these too.

The ingredients have been hand-picked for their anti-parasitic, anti-bacterial, anti-microbial, anti-fungal and anti-viral activities.

Beneficial for...

- Internal parasites, flukes and worms
- Candida albicans overgrowth
- Irritable Bowel Syndrome (IBS)
- Diarrhoea
- Constipation
- Fungal infections
- Mouth sores and herpes
- Certain skin conditions, such as acne and eczema
- Colon cleansing
- Travel abroad to locations where food hygiene and/or water quality may be less then ideal

Each capsule contains:

- ❖ Magnesium caprylate – **175mg**
- ❖ Cinnamon powder – **100mg**
- ❖ Cloves powder – **100mg**
- ❖ Shiitake mushroom powder – **100mg**
- ❖ Garlic powder extract (10000mg/g) – **75mg**
- ❖ Glucomannan (95%) – **50mg**
- ❖ Pumpkin seed P E 4:1 (40%) (equivalent to 200 mg pumpkin seed powder) – **50mg**
- ❖ Chicory root P.E 4:1 (equivalent to 120mg chicory root powder) – **30mg**
- ❖ Grapefruit seed P.E 5:1 (equivalent to 100mg grapefruit seed powder) – **20mg**
- ❖ Cayenne extract 7:1 (equivalent to 100mg cayenne powder) – **14.3mg**
- ❖ Fenugreek seed P.E 4:1 (equivalent to 48mg fenugreek seed powder) – **12mg**
- ❖ Olive leaf extract 15:1, 6% Oleurpein (equivalent to 50mg olive leaf powder) – **3.35mg**

Yet another supplement that I recommend during the detox that gives the body a good energy boost is called SUPER GREENS PLUS. This is a 100% organic (Soil Association registered) superfoods powder, that can be used as a plant protein powder, light meal shake or daily nutrient booster. In fact, it is one of the most nutrient-dense organic superfood combinations per serving you will find.

It provides a broad range of vitamins, minerals, antioxidants and powerful phyto-nutrients through its multiple organic superfood, superfruit and herbal ingredients.

High in vegetable-source proteins, this full-spectrum blend also contains over 20 natural enzymes and 70 beneficial nutrients.

A great all-round supplement to support energy levels, cleanse, detox, and alkalise the body – daily organic nourishment made easy!
For every 300 g of powder, it contains:

*Activated Pre-Sprouted Barley
*Apple
*Linseed / Flaxseed
*Wheatgrass
*Quinoa
*Barley Grass
*Alfalfa
*Kelp (Ascophyllum)
*Spirulina
*Acai Berry
*Carrot
*Turmeric
*Bilberry Fruit
*Spinach Leaf
*Lemon Peel

Stay with the detoxification process, and allow yourself time to rest, particularly during the first few days. It is best starting on a Friday, given that you will have the weekend at home to get organized and rest when you need to.

I do not recommend vigorous exercise during this initial period, but a 20-30-minute walk with a friend or loved one in an open-air park is fine. You need to conserve your energy levels for the detoxification process. Under normal circumstances, the body uses 80% of its energy for detoxification, which is a substantial amount, and this will increase during the 15 days of this intensive detox programme.

The Good News!
The good news is that after the initial healing crisis you WILL FEEL A LOT BETTER. This is literally a guarantee that I can give you personally, as I have witnessed it hundreds of times with my patients, as well as myself.

I personally detoxify twice a year for 15 days, and another 7 days in the summer when fruit and juices are plentiful here in Cyprus.

I KNOW how it feels when your body begins to get rid of the toxins and you are over the healing crisis – a clarity of mind that is crystal clear, increased concentration, increased energy levels, better sleep, calmer, more reflective state of being, increased awareness of your environment, better digestion, your constipation improves, body pains dwindle or melt away, arthritis improves, chests and throats clear, skin colour and tone greatly improves and I have had many clients who cut down or actually stopped smoking, as the body rebels harder during a detox programme.

These are all benefits that you will experience, so STICK WITH THE PROGRAMME and achieve OPTIMUM HEALTH. Once you experience this state of optimum health you will wonder what the hell you were doing when you had moderate health, just like most people walking the planet today.

The Alkaline Detox Diet is one of the most positive steps you can take and should be treated and enjoyed that way – treat yourself for 15 days, eat as much as you like, whenever you like, of the foods that you are allowed during the detox.

Before Starting the Detox Programme
There are a few indications which would exclude some people from starting the detox programme and you should not do so if any of the following apply:

❖ You are pregnant – the toxins released during the detoxification process can harm the embryo because the embryo's capacity to detoxify is limited due to its poor organ functionality at such early stages of development.

❖ You are breastfeeding – toxins released into the mother's blood will travel to the milk, so the baby will get a dose of toxic milk that will not help them in any way. Wait until after the baby is weaned off the breast and meanwhile you could start eating healthily.

❖ You are presently being treated for an illness or condition such as diabetes or heart problems without medical supervision. It is important for your doctor or health practitioner to know what you are doing. With diabetics, for example, it is possible that you might go into a hypoglycemic episode where your blood sugar levels fall below normal, due to the increased insulin production by the pancreas.

I have seen this several times – as the pancreas begins to clear of toxic overloads, it begins to function better, so it can begin to produce MORE insulin than before, resulting in a sudden decrease of blood sugar levels. This is fine if a health practitioner is aware of what is going on, and can adjust the dosage of drugs to suit.

❖ You are recovering from a serious illness without expert medical supervision – if you are recovering from cancer, any type of operation, an accident or other serious disease, then you should be extremely careful of detoxifying by

340

yourself. The toxins released in the body could upset the healing process and period of convalescence. Seek guidance from an experienced health practitioner who has experience in detoxifying. It is pointless asking a doctor who has no idea of detoxifying, as you are more than likely going to get a negative report, just from pure ignorance. Seek the help of an experienced person in these matters, and take note that not many medical doctors are knowledgeable of the detoxification process, nor have experience in these matters. Only very few do, so do not take it for granted that all are knowledgeable because they are doctors.

❖ You are taking any prescribed or non-prescribed medication – again, the toxins mixed with the drugs could exacerbate further the healing crisis and cause more symptoms than are necessary.

❖ You are not ready at this moment in time to begin – the detox programme does require a little discipline and organization so would not be suited to a person who is travelling continuously, or eating out continuously with business associates, or who is under a lot of stress from marital or domestic problems. We need to prepare ourselves psychologically and emotionally before we begin. If you feel that this is not the right time for you, then postpone it for another time when you are ready.

Preparing for the Detox

Preparing for the detox is not difficult, nor is it costly, but should be done some time BEFORE you decide to begin. There are several things that you need to gather before you start. A checklist of essentials is outlined below:

❖ A large stock of fresh vegetables and fruit in season – kept in the fridge for freshness. If you have access to ORGANIC FRUIT and VEGETABLES, then this should be your obvious first choice. Organic produce is free from the pesticides and chemical fertilizers that are harmful to the body, but are also richer in nutrients due to the organic fertilizers that are used. One famous doctor, Dr. Gerson, said, *"The soil is our second metabolism."* What he meant by this profound statement was that the nutrient quantity and quality of the soil is going to determine the quality of our bodily functioning. Organic produce has been 'fed' the right ingredients of minerals, trace elements and vitamins that our bodies require to function optimally. I sincerely wish I had a steady supply of organic produce at my disposal here in Cyprus where I work and live, but unfortunately, we are not that health conscious as a nation to begin organic farming yet.

❖ A good thermos flask – you can use this for transporting freshly squeezed fruit or vegetable juices to and from work. It is important to remember, however, that the live enzymes and vital energy in freshly squeezed juices have a life-span of ONLY THREE HOURS. So, it is crucial that you drink the juice within these 3 hours, and try to keep the juice as cool as possible – heat can destroy these very vulnerable enzymes. You may also use the flask to transport herbal teas, either hot or cold (with ice cubes) if you wish.

❖ A good quality juicer – there are many different types of juicers on the market, and it is a true science to choose the right one. Most of the juicers on the market for domestic use are centrifugal juicers. If you are buying one, try to find the best that money will buy as this is going to be a sound health investment that will see you through many years of life. There are cheaper ones at half the price that will probably only last a year or less, so choose carefully. You could pick up a good one for less than $100, but if you can pay to buy the Rolls Royce of juicers, go for something like a Champion juicer (about $300), which will extract 25% more nutrients from vegetables and juices than the centrifugal juicer. The Champion juicer is a masticating juicer – it grinds the fruit or vegetable into a paste before spinning at high speed, to squeeze the juice through a screen set into the juicer bottom. The ultimate in juicers is the Health Stream Press which can extract up to 50% more juice than a centrifugal juicer, but can cost from $500 to over $2,000 for the automated press.

❖ A steamer – metal (stainless steel) or bamboo – the type you place over or in the pan of hot water to steam vegetables. Steaming is far more preferable to boiling because when you boil vegetables in water they lose minerals such as potassium, which is crucial to health. Steaming vegetables decreases the losses of these important minerals.

❖ Extra virgin olive oil – this is extracted using a cold press method from whole, ripe, undamaged olives. It is made without heat and is unrefined, as compared with olive oil that is not virgin or extra virgin. It still contains many of the natural factors unique to olives, which are normally lost through degumming, refining, bleaching and deodorizing. Virgin olive oils do not suffer nutrient losses and molecular changes that negatively affect human health. Choose this oil over ones that do not have the word 'virgin' or 'extra virgin' on the label.

❖ Fresh garlic – have plenty of fresh garlic at hand - it would be wise to eat one clove a day as this contains more than 200 chemical compounds, most of them having therapeutic qualities. Eating fresh parsley and lemon juice, or sucking on a whole clove can help to neutralize garlic odour on the breath. Garlic can inhibit and kill bacteria, fungi and parasites; lower blood pressure, blood cholesterol and blood sugar; prevent blood clotting; protect the liver and contains anti-tumour properties. It can also boost the immune system to fight off potential disease and maintain health.

Regarding detoxification, which particularly interests us here, garlic can stimulate the lymphatic system, which expedites the removal of waste from the body. It can nourish most of the organs such as the heart, stomach, circulation and lungs, as well as protect the cells from damage by nasty free radicals (molecules that harm the body). The sulphur elements in garlic also help to stimulate certain enzyme systems that are beneficial for detoxifying, such as the liver's glutathione pathways, which help to remove toxins from the body; there are going to be plenty of these passing through the liver in the next 15 days.

So, now you understand why garlic is so important. It is one of the true wonders of nature, and I cannot understand why people dismiss it because of its odour, yet we accept so many other disgusting smells such as smokers smelling like ashtrays!

❖ A brush made of natural fibre – this is going to be used for SKIN BRUSHING (see details below).

❖ Water – you will need a large supply of either mineral or distilled water throughout the detoxification process. I suggest that you drink at least 10 glasses daily – this may mean having a glass next to you at home and the workplace and keeping it topped up. You will be surprised how many glasses you can drink in a day if you do this systematically. It really is a matter of habit, but what I have found is that if you don't have the water to hand, you will not remember to drink it. Water is crucial to detoxification. It is part of the flushing process, which gets the toxins that are released by the cells out of the body. After a lot of research regarding water filters, I have personally settled for the reverse osmosis unit with a vortex energizer – there are many companies now that can fit the unit under your sink and add a separate small tap specifically for the drinking water. This is connected to your tap water, but the reverse osmosis filter will eliminate literally everything from chlorine, fluoride, heavy metals, pesticide residues as well as micro-organisms – it is squeaky clean water that you can drink and cook with.

❖ Fresh lemons or cider vinegar – what you use is really a matter of taste, but both are excellent and healthy condiments. Cider vinegar made from apples is very rich in potassium, a mineral that is required by all cells during metabolism. In his book, *'Cider Vinegar'*, Cyril Scott talks about how cider vinegar can help overweight people, citing several case histories. He recommends two teaspoons of cider vinegar in a tumbler of water, to be taken on rising in the morning. Exactly how it works is an enigma, but even if it does not work for weight loss, it will certainly help to alkalize the blood and help clean it.

❖ Herbal teas – there are several herbal teas that you could drink every day throughout the detox programme. Green tea is excellent. Apart from being rich in vitamin A, E, C, calcium and iron, it contains healthy phytonutrients called Epigallocatechin Gallate (EGCG), which inhibit the growth of cancer and lowers cholesterol levels. Dandelion 'coffee' is also excellent, as this herb purifies the blood, detoxifies and stimulates the function of the liver. It's also a natural diuretic. It's good to drink teas that help to drain the detoxification organs and get rid of the toxins. Another good one is stinging nettle tea, which helps to drive excess fluid out of the tissues and helps with metabolism by increasing the elimination through the kidneys. Other goodies are chamomile, peppermint, rosehip, blackcurrant, elder flower, strawberry and Melissa. Most of these can be found in good health food shops – either in tea bags, or loose.

The Theory of Autointoxication

The compelling suspicion that a stagnant bowel filled with putrefying matter can leak out and become a source of infection for the rest of the body was first suggested by the ancient Egyptians. In the 19th century, this became known as 'The theory of autointoxication – self poisoning from one's own retained wastes.' This idea has been enthusiastically embraced by every subsequent generation. One of the main causes is constipation.

Constipation

Constipation has done more to provide the health profession with an obvious solution to un-diagnosable ailments than any other simple complaint. It is defined as 'The difficult or infrequent passage of faeces' and it is associated with the presence of dry, hardened stools.

Constipation is a national pastime and slow bowels are more common today than years previous. For one thing, people not only ate better 100 years ago, they were more active and got out doors more.

When the bowels slow down, toxins are not eliminated but are reabsorbed and carried back to the liver for recycling and elimination. Reabsorbed bile salts have been linked to increased cholesterol levels. Therefore, high cholesterol is a major precursor of constipation. Also, when the bowels get slow and toxin levels increase, the pathogenic microorganisms grow to out-number the normal flora, causing dysbiosis.

Although friendly bowel flora such as Acidophilus (small intestine) and Bifidobacteria (colon) are needed to correct this, it is the clogged bowels that are the major problem. When the bowels move again, everything else will fall into order.

Our endocrine glands (which control metabolism), are also involved since it is our thyroid that controls metabolism and metabolism affects how our bowels function. In this way, constipation can be seen as a symptom of hypothyroidism. Low body temperatures (a symptom of hypothyroidism) are very common today –although they are not 'normal' – as many authors have reported.

Intestinal toxaemia (a form of blood poisoning), is caused by the absorption of bacteria and their toxins through the intestinal wall. The large intestine (colon) is the most prolific source of bacterial contamination in the entire body. Thirty-six toxic substances have been isolated from the human colon, including such compounds as indole, skatole, phenol and cresol.

When these kinds of toxins are passing through the intestinal wall, they can enter the lymphatic or portal system and be directly transported to the liver. Temporary increases in the toxic load of the liver occur during periods of stagnation in the colon. Any prolongation of this state will impede the detoxification and bacteria-killing function of the liver. The importance of this function cannot be overlooked when one realizes that blood from the intestinal tract enters the liver before it is delivered to the tissues of the body.

An overburdened liver, which cannot handle the toxic load from the intestine, transfers the task of detoxification onto another organ - the kidney. Unfortunately, the kidney is not able to reduce the amount and kind of toxins that enter the liver, nor can it detoxify them as efficiently as the liver. The toxins that the kidneys do not remove from the blood increase circulating body-toxin levels.

The Oxford Dictionary defines constipation as, *'Irregular and difficult defecation.'* The question is, *'What is a regular bowel movement when there is no norm?'* Regularity becomes a meaningless expression when some people have a bowel movement regularly every Sunday morning, while others regularly empty their bowels after every meal.

Defecation is a reflex action, stimulated by distension of the rectum with faeces. It is under voluntary control in adults and normally takes place only when time and circumstances are suitable. The presence of food in the stomach stimulates a reflex action called peristalsis, which moves food residue into and along the colon. Mass peristalsis gives us the feeling that we need to empty our bowels. This reflex action usually occurs after the first meal of the day but can also be stimulated by only drinking some liquid on rising.

If the call to defecate is persistently neglected, the reflex mechanism becomes less sensitive and constipation can result. This is likely to happen when there are time constraints causing hurry and stress (stress ceases peristaltic action in the colon).

Some healthy people don't defecate every day and do not have any discomfort. Many others open their bowels every day with excruciating agony – passing dark, rock hard, compacted stools. Both cases would be considered constipated.

Ideally, one should defecate as many times as we have a proper meal, usually 3 times per day. Although the main rule is that we should have a bowel movement at least once a day. The stool should be fibrous, light in colour, float in the water, break up easily and cause no pain or discomfort to pass – in fact no toilet paper should be needed. Pain or discomfort whilst passing hard or dry stool at less than daily intervals can be considered as constipation. Many people have suffered heart attacks as a result of vigorous efforts to have a bowel movement as continuous efforts to evacuate material from the rectum increases the heart rate, blood pressure and respiration.

Referred to essentially as a Western disease, constipation is virtually unheard of among third world people adhering to traditional fibre-rich diets. Constipation is implicated in many Western diseases such as diverticulosis, obesity, varicose veins, cancer of the colon and rectum, appendicitis and haemorrhoids. These are all very rare in undeveloped countries.

Whatever the causes of constipation, it is important that you should try to use some gentle herbal formulas and supplements in order to help the transit time of the gut.

At the Da Vinci Center, I use the following formulations to help my patients. They can all be combined if required and the dosages can vary depending on the condition and the patient:

1. CONSTFORM
2. COLFORM
3. OXYGUT

Nature Needs Some Help and Urgently

* In the U.S., approximately 80 million people suffer from bowel problems.
* 100-120,000 a year lose their lives – usually from bowel cancer.

❖ Colon cancer is the second leading killer in the Western World.
❖ Behind these statistics are also those saved by colostomies (surgical removal of the large intestine), which in the US only approximately 250.000 people a year receive.
❖ In UK and the rest of Europe, the numbers are more or less the same.

Bowel experts all over the world now agree that poor bowel management is the root of most health problems. The faulty Western commercialized diet is the focal point of the problem. A diet high in meat, white sugar, white flour, fat, and low in dietary fibre and water is believed to be connected with constipation.

The root of the problem is clearly indicated by laxative sales, estimated at *600–800 million dollars a year.*

Laxatives aggravate the problem of constipation by interfering with the colon's ability to eliminate normally on its own. The chemicals within laxatives irritate and stimulate the colon to abnormally contract, to expel the irritating substances. In addition, the oral route of administration is the least optimal method for evacuation of the colon because crucial digestive processes occurring in the stomach and small intestine are interfered with. Most laxatives and purgatives precipitate dehydration.

Hippocrates took the view of not disturbing and messing up the entire peptic system with harsh laxatives, as the problem lies at the extreme end of this same system. Standard enemas, even highly recommended as first aid, only cleanse the rectum and last portion of the colon, missing out most of the large intestine.

Colon Hydrotherapy is an extended and more complete form of an enema. This method extends beyond the rectum to cleanse the entire colon and offers greater therapeutic benefits. It addresses the cause or source of the constipation problem. Other methods treat only the symptoms and provide temporary relief of the problem.

Why constipated? The biggest reasons? Dietary (lack of natural dietary fibre and consumption of devitalized foods, especially white sugar, white flour and all their by-products); neglecting the urge to eliminate; dehydration (too little water); stress; too little exercise (sitting for long hours); abuse of stimulants and drugs; irregular hours (work – rest, wake – asleep) and pathological conditions.

The most common signs and symptoms due to an impacted, constipated colon are:
❖ Infrequent or difficult bowel movements; hard compacted stools and low stool weight
❖ Tiredness, fatigue, lethargy, lack of energy, poor concentration and irritability

- ❖ Bloating and flatulence
- ❖ Headaches, mental depression or dullness
- ❖ Irritable Bowel Syndrome, diverticulosis, colitis, leaky gut, cancer of the bowel, Crohn's Disease, appendicitis, hiatus hernia
- ❖ Malabsorption, bad breath and a coated tongue
- ❖ Haemorrhoids, varicose veins, obesity and cellulite

Colon Hydrotherapy

Colon Hydrotherapy is one of the most powerful and effective ways of cleansing and detoxifying our entire system. The mucous membrane of the large intestine is the first and most important defence system against toxic substances (followed by the liver, the lymph system, lungs and the skin), thus a very important part of the body's immune system.

As I outlined above, nearly all doctors and practitioners of natural medicine take the view that most disease originates in an unhealthy colon.

Exogenous toxins such as poor nutrition, sterilized and denatured foods, environmental toxins and poisons, abuse of medicines and narcotics as well endogenous toxins from emotional conflicts and stress, clog detoxifying channels on an on-going basis.

Having three bowel movements a day does not negate the fact that after years of dietary indiscretion, a gradual build-up of mucus and undigested foods begin to form in the lining of the colon.

Dehydration and stagnation occur. Our bodies are being poisoned by these toxic substances which can cause inflammation, damage the intestinal wall and cells, and intoxicate the nerves and glands. These toxins can also be absorbed through the walls of the colon into the blood and lymph; ultimately to into the cells and tissues. The resulting toxaemia can become a chronic condition, but for most of us it creates erratic conditions in the body that we call *disease*.

Heavy Metal Detoxification

We will discuss this in a separate chapter on toxicity, but we can briefly mention that heavy metals such as arsenic, aluminum, antimony, cadmium, lead, mercury and uranium are insidious in today's world. There is probably not a person on this planet that does not have some of these in their system, leading to heavy metal toxicity, which is the cause of many illnesses.

The early signs of heavy metal poisoning are vague or often attributed to other diseases. These include headaches, fatigue, muscle pain, indigestion, tremors, constipation, anemia, indigestion and tremors. Mild toxicity symptoms include impaired memory and distorted thinking ability. Severe toxicity can lead to death.

Hair mineral analysis is a convenient but often unreliable screening test. The most accurate measurement is by blood analysis of actual toxin levels within the red blood cells. Many toxic metals tend to accumulate inside the cell, where most of the damage is done.

One of the safest and most effective ways to remove heavy metal toxicity is to use a natural heavy metal chelating therapy named 'The HMD Ultimate Detox Protocol'[215]. The main formulation that mobilizes the metals is called HMD™ – you will need to take 50 drops, three times a day shortly before meals, in some water or juice.

In addition, there are two other drainage remedies that can be taken along with the HMD™, and are part of the HMD Ultimate Detox:

Chlorella (500mg) for absorbing the stray heavy metals that may get reabsorbed from the gut. Recommended adult dosage: 2 tabs three times per day.

'Organic Lavage' combines several organic herbs that help to clean the blood and help the kidneys, liver and lymphatic system to open up and drain the toxins out of the body. Recommended adult dosage: 25 drops x 3 daily for 3-6 months, along with the HMD™ and chlorella.

Killing Uninvited Guests

Schmidt and Roberts in their 1989 *'Foundations of parasitology* [216] book noted that 25%–30% of people living in the south-eastern US (mainly children) were infected with whip worm (the trichuris species)[217].

Meanwhile, the Centers of Disease Control also stress that parasitic infections affect persons living in developed countries, including America. Zoonotic diseases, i.e. those transmitted from animals, are often caused by parasites, and infected people can even experience symptoms so severe they become life-threatening.

Food can become contaminated if livestock (i.e. cows and pigs), are infected with parasites such as cryptosporidium and trichinella. People can acquire trichinellosis by

---

[215] www.worldwidehealthcenter.net
[216] Schmidt, GD and Roberts, LS., Foundations of Parasitology (4th ed). USA: Times Mirror/Mosby College Publishers, 1989.
[217] For a brief history of human parasitology, visit the site: http://cmr.asm.org/cgi/content/full/15/4/595. Further information can also be found at: http://www.alternative-doctor.com/allergies/parasites.htm

ingesting trichinella-infected, undercooked meats. Cryptosporidiosis can be passed to humans if orchards or water sources near cow pastures become contaminated by infected bovine faeces; or if tainted fruit is consumed without being washed adequately beforehand.

In addition, pets too can act as parasite hosts and pass them on to humans. Young animals, such as puppies and kittens, are more likely to be infected with Ascaris and hookworms. According to official CDC data:

"Trichomonas is the most common parasitic infection in the USA, accounting for an estimated 7.4 million cases per year. Giardia and cryptosporidium are estimated to cause two million and 300,000 infections respectively in the US annually. Cryptosporidiosis is the most frequent cause of recreational water-related disease outbreaks in the US, causing multiple outbreaks each year. There are an estimated 1.5 million new toxoplasma infections and 400 to 4,000 cases of congenital toxoplasmosis in the US each year; 1.26 million persons in this country [US] have ocular involvement due to toxoplasmosis; and toxoplasmosis is the third leading cause of deaths due to food-borne illnesses (375+ deaths).[218] "

In the EU, the European Food Safety Authority (EFSA) was set up in January 2002 following a series of food crises, which have hardly subsided since then; mad cow/sheep/goat disease, foot-and-mouth disease, bird flu and so on. In its latest report, the EFSA says the most commonly reported zoonotic infections in humans in the EU are, by far:

"... those caused by bacterial zoonotic agents that can be shed by asymptomatic farm animals: the 2004 data indicates salmonellosis (192,703 reported cases) and campylobacterosis (183.961) – followed by yersiniosis (10,381), human listeriosis (1,267), parasitic zoonoses is 2,349 (trichinellosis, toxoplasmosis and echinococcosis put together). Compared to the main bacterial food-borne infections mentioned above (395,455 put together), reported human cases of 'classic' zoonoses are relatively low: brucellosis (1,337), tuberculosis due to M. bovis (86) and rabies (two imported)."

But perhaps even harder to accept is that the parasites within you are infected by their own parasites in turn – parasites within parasites! The story is endless. For an enlightening exposition on the nature of symbiotic, as well as parasitic endobiotic relationships (microorganisms living within other organisms), Dr. Peter Schneider's

---

[218] The CDC's A-Z index listing of Parasitic diseases can be accessed at:
http://www.cdc.gov/ncidod/dpd/parasites/index.htm

article, *'Prof. Enderlein's research in today's view. Can his research results be confirmed with modern techniques?'*[219] is enlightening.

Parasites are everywhere. In their most pathogenic states cause havoc in body, mind and spirit. Doctors respond with a range of treatments intended to suppress the symptoms, while failing to attack their source – the parasites themselves.

So, what can we do about these parasites we carry? Dr. Hulda Clark, Ph.D., N.D., a naturopathic physician, has brought the issue of parasitically-caused diseases and other types of toxicity back into the spotlight in recent years, dealing with this subject at length in her book, *'The cure for all diseases.'*[220] Clark describes various methodologies and procedures to cleanse the body from these nasty creatures. This is not the only herbal parasite cleanse that is used at the Da Vinci Centre. Sometimes other therapies are combined using Sanum remedies, homeopathics, other herbal formulas and bioresonance therapy.

At the Da Vinci Holistic Health Center, we use Bioresonance diagnostics to identify the specific parasites in question and can therefore design bespoke anti-parasite programmes. However, generally we use the PARAFORM PLUS ONE (one capsule x 3 times daily, away from food) mentioned above, along with a PARAFORM TINCTURE (2 teaspoons in the morning, in a little water away from food). Both of these can be taken together.

The Liver and Gallbladder Flush
The liver is the gateway to the body and in this 'chemical age' its detoxification systems are easily overloaded. Thousands of chemicals are added to food and over 700 have been identified in drinking water.

Plants are sprayed with toxic chemicals, animals are injected with potent hormones and antibiotics, and a significant amount of our food is genetically engineered, processed, refined, frozen or cooked. All this can lead to destruction of delicate vitamins and minerals, which are needed for the detoxification pathways in the liver. The liver must try to cope with every toxic chemical in our environment, as well as damaged fats that are present in processed and fried foods.

This is why it is crucially important to cleanse your liver, much like you clean your house, bedroom, car and external self. Cleansing at least once per year is a good

---

[219] Schneider, P. Prof. Enderlein's Research in Today's View: Can his research results be confirmed with modern techniques? First published in the German language in the *SANUM-Post magazine* (56/2001) Semmelweis-Institut, Germany, 2001.
[220] Clark, HR. The Cure for All Diseases. San Diego, CA: New Century Press, 1995.

thing. When the liver gets overloaded it cannot metabolize fats and cholesterol easily, and this is when your cholesterol level start increasing and gall stones form.

As well as this, the liver itself becomes 'fatty.' Fatty livers are usually found in about 50% of people over the age of 50 – this is often seen by radiologists over time when examining patients routinely. Any imbalances in the liver will have a direct effect on the gallbladder, since it's the liver that produces the bile and gallstones.

Let's look at the gallbladder and how this organ can be easily cleansed, with amazing health benefits.

The gallbladder is a pear-shaped organ that stores about 50ml of bile until the body needs it for digestion. Bile is a bitter, yellow/green alkaline fluid secreted by hepatoacytes (special cells) in the liver. The human liver can produce close to one litre of bile per day. The bile stored in the gallbladder is between 5-10 times more concentrated and potent that the bile secreted directly by the liver. This bile is discharged into the duodenum (the first part of the small intestine) mainly for the emulsification (breakdown) of fats during digestion. This is why people who have had their gallbladder removed are likely to have a tough time digesting fatty foods.

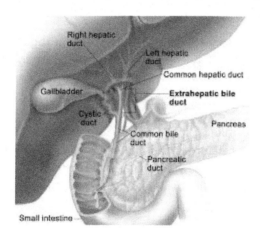

Gallstones
If the tubing of the gallbladder is filled with gallstones, then this can cause a number of health problems including allergies or hives. However, some people have no symptoms. These stones cannot be seen by ultrasound scan or X-rays as they are not actually in the gallbladder, but in the ducts. They may also not be calcified stones. There are many types of gallstones, most of which have cholesterol crystals in them. They can be black, red, white, green or tan coloured.

As the stones grow and become more numerous, the back-pressure on the liver causes it to make less bile. This is also thought to slow the flow of lymphatic fluid. Imagine if your garden hose had small stones in it; the result would be that much less water would flow. When there are gallstones present, much less cholesterol leaves the body, resulting in elevated cholesterol levels.

Moreover, gallstones are porous so can pick up all the bacteria, cysts, viruses and parasites that are passing through the liver. These masses or 'nests' of infectious material hang around the liver and supply the blood flowing through it with lots of fresh bugs daily. This is one way that parasites are circulated and reproduce. These parasites and infectious nests must be removed, and the simplest way of doing that is to remove the gallstones.

The Pathogenesis of Gallstones

The stones consist mainly of cholesterol, bilirubin and calcium salts, with smaller amounts of protein and other materials. In Western countries, essentially all gallstones, whether cholesterol or pigmented, arise in the gallbladder. In Asia, a significant fraction of pigmented stones originate in the bile ducts. In Western countries cholesterol is the principal constituent of more than three quarters of gallstones.

In the simplest sense, cholesterol gallstones form when the cholesterol concentration in bile exceeds the ability of bile to hold cholesterol in solution. Non-cholesterol stones are categorized as black or brown pigment stones, consisting of calcium salts of bilirubin.

Most of the stones are made of cholesterol (75-80%), with bilirubin stones being rarer and consisting of calcium bilirubinate, with large amounts of mucoprotein. Brown pigment stones are usually the hardest and smallest of the stones and these are usually made of calcium salts of unconjugated bilirubin, with variable amounts of protein and cholesterol.

Gallstones Effect Many Millions of People

It is estimated that 20% of the world's population will develop gallstones in the gall bladder at some stage in their lives. This figure does not take account the numerous stones that accumulate in the liver and its ducts.

In the United States, over 10% of the total population has gallstones. Each year 1,000,000 new patients are diagnosed. Performance of 500,000 cholecystectomies (gallbladder removal) leads to an annual expense of more than $5 billion in direct costs.

Gallstone prevalence varies with age, sex and ethnic group. Ultrasound surveys show a female:male ratio of 2:1 in the younger population and an increasing prevalence in both sexes with age. After the age of 60, 10-15% of men and 20-40% of women will have gallstones. Childbearing, oestrogen-replacement therapy and oral contraceptives increase the risk of developing gallstones.

Ultrasound scan of gallstones

How do we remove gallstones without resorting to surgery?
Cleansing the liver of gallstones dramatically improves digestion, which is the basis of your whole health. You can expect your allergies to disappear, too, with each cleanse you do! Incredibly, it also eliminates shoulder, upper arm, and upper back pain. You'll also have more energy and an increased sense of well-being.

I have personally witnessed the removal of gallstones from hundreds of patients. Some of them with gallbladder symptoms expelled many stones that did not even appear on an ultrasound, probably because they were trapped in the liver and gallbladder ducts and were not sitting in the gallbladder where the radiologists usually look.

Most, however, did not have any symptoms at all, yet would flush out literally hundreds of stones – no exaggeration! One woman in her 50's had three scans and the radiologists found nothing. She had pains in the gall-bladder region for 20 years. When she did the gall bladder flush she removed 280 stones the first time around, and about 200 the second time! Here's her first flush with the gallstones – the coins are there to indicate size ratios and are Cypriot.

Gallbladder stones flushed naturally

About a week before I did my first gall bladder flush (on myself), I went to see a friend who is an ultrasound specialist. He checked my gall bladder and found it as clean as a whistle. When I flushed a week later I removed 5 LARGE stones (about the size of a walnut), and about 150 smaller stones, including gravel – here is a photo of some of them:

My stones on the first gallbladder flush

It is believed by many naturopathic doctors that EVERYONE has gallstones, even children, with all the junk food that they eat these days (some less than others), and I have validated this many times in clinical practice.

The cleanse that I recommend below takes place within a period of less than 14 hours and can be done at home over the weekend. It is a harmless, pain-free and natural way of removing stones, without requiring invasive procedures such as surgery, laser, etc. Now *that* is a statement that will not be believed by the majority of general surgeons performing their gallbladder removals!

I had a personal experience of a 78-year old nun from a local convent here in Cyprus who was under my care for various health problems, including gallstones. She collected her stones in a jam- jar after her flush and took them to the surgeon at the local hospital here in Larnaca. His first reaction was, *But that's impossible; you can only remove gallstones surgically or with a laser!'* The nun looked at him in amazement and said, *But Doctor, do you think I am lying to you?'* whilst holding her rosary beads. The surgeon adamantly persisted his point of view. The nun said, *'OK Doctor, you scanned me about 3 weeks ago, and you found stones and said that I require an operation. Is it possible that these stones disappeared by themselves?'* He replied, *'No, this is not possible, once they are in the gallbladder they will stay there until they are removed, and yours were quite large, too.'* The nun wisely replied, *'OK Doctor, if this is the case, then why don't you scan me again and let's see if they are in the gallbladder or in the jam jar?'* So off they went to the ultrasound room, where he performed another scan. They emerged 30 minutes later after a thorough examination.

There were absolutely NO STONES in the gallbladder at all and now the surgeon looked really surprised. After a short silence, he perked up and said, *'I cannot see any stones now so this may have been a wrong diagnosis, but you certainly have quite a lot of sludge, so the operation should proceed.'* The nun was flabbergasted and did not know what to say, but before leaving, they agreed to have the stones analyzed in the hospital lab – the results came back: 'GALLBLADDER STONES!'

The moral of this interesting story is: do not try to persuade your doctors and surgeons. There is a mindset akin to brainwashing where it is difficult for them to accept new concepts and treatments, particularly when they are based on the principles of Nature, who they are not too friendly with! Just keep the information to yourself. It is your health that you are trying to optimize, so why go through all the hassle of creating enemies with your doctor? Who you may need on other occasions.

Remember that many years ago, people and scientists were convinced that the world was flat, and it's ironic that there are still these believers in the 21st Century!

Preparations for the Gallbladder Flush
OK, enough of the stories, let's proceed with the details of the gallbladder flush, beginning with the ingredients that you should first collect:

Apple juice (which is high in Malic acid and pectin); it acts as a solvent in the bile to weaken adhesions between solid globules, while softening the stones. This is crucial to the success of the procedure as it enables them to pass HARMLESSLY through the gall ducts.

The apple juice should be coarse, unfiltered and free of additives and preservatives – you will need to drink close to ONE LITRE (3-4 GLASSES) DAILY FOR 14 DAYS PRIOR TO THE FLUSH. In the worst-case scenario, if you cannot find fresh apples to juice, then you can use packaged apple juice, which should still contain these ingredients, but see if you can pick up some organic ones. An alternative to apple juice, which is just as effective, is taking Malic Acid in capsule form (magnesium malate). You will need to take one capsule, three times daily for 14 days before attempting the flush).

Four tablespoons of **Epsom salts** (magnesium sulphate). This allows magnesium to be absorbed into the bloodstream, therefore relaxing smooth muscles that surround the gallbladder ducts. This enables larger stones that may otherwise create spasms to pass through a relaxed bile duct. This is a very crucial part of the therapy and you CANNOT do the flush without taking these salts, which are freely available in most pharmacies. Ask for the B.P. variety for internal use, not those used for soaking in the bath – you will require about 70 grams per flush.

Half a cup of **Extra Virgin Olive Oil**, which stimulates the gall bladder and bile duct to contract powerfully, thus expelling the stones into the duodenum or small intestine. Once you drink the cup of olive oil and citrus fruits it enters the gut and the gallbladder which, detecting huge quantities of fat or oil, begins to go into spasm, expelling all the waste rubbish that has been stored for years.

At least a couple of large **grapefruits** (oranges will do if there are no grapefruits) mixed together with the juice of two fresh **lemons or limes**. The more acidic the juice, the faster the transit of the olive oil through the stomach and into the duodenum, which helps prevent or minimize nausea.

I have supervised hundreds of such cleanses using exactly this protocol that I am recommending here, without one patient suffering any harm whatsoever. But please follow the instructions carefully, and it must be said that you have ultimate responsibility, given that none of you are actual patients of mine.

On the day of the gallbladder flush there are some rules to follow:
1. Take no medications, vitamins or pills that you can do without on the day of the flush. They could prevent success.

2. Eat a NO-FAT breakfast and lunch such as cooked cereal with fruit, fruit juice, brown bread with a little honey (no butter, milk or margarine), baked potato or other vegetables with salt only.

3. 2:00 PM – Do NOT drink or eat anything after 2:00 PM – only mineral water is fine, non-fizzy.

4. 6:00 PM – Drink one serving (3/4 cup) of ice cold Epsom salts. Mix one tablespoon Epsom salts into 3/4 cup cold water and stir well. You may add 1/8 teaspoon of vitamin C powder to improve the taste. You may drink a little water afterwards, or rinse your mouth out. Epsom salts can also be mixed in with apple juice to make it taste nicer, or a few drops of lemon or lime can be added; or a little orange juice.

5. 8:00 PM – Repeat the Epsom salt drink as above.

6. 9:45 PM – Pour 1/2 mug (a large 10 oz. mug) of olive oil and squeeze 1/2 cup of orange or grapefruit juice into this, with the juice of two whole fresh lemons. Shake or stir hard until the oil and fruit juice mix thoroughly. Visit the bathroom now, shower, brush your teeth, go to the toilet etc. so that you are ready to lie down as soon as you have taken the olive oil mixture.

7. 10:00 PM – Drink the olive oil and juice you have mixed. Drinking through a plastic straw helps it go down easier. Drink it standing up, not sitting or lying. You may use a little honey between sips to help it down. Try to drink it as quickly as you can, within 5 minutes.

TIPS: If you find it difficult drinking the olive oil mixture by itself, it is possible to mix it with prune juice or grape juice with a tablespoon of honey and put it in a blender for a minute or so.

If you can obtain ozonated olive oil – maybe your naturopath has an ozonator and can make some ozonated olive oil for you – it may be better to use this as it will kill off any bacteria, parasites or other micro-organisms that may be lingering in the bile when it enters the intestine.

LIE DOWN IMMEDIATELY, ON YOUR RIGHT SIDE! You may fail to get stones out if you don't. The sooner you lie down, the more stones you will get out. Try to keep perfectly still for 20 minutes as the more you move the less stones your gallbladder will expel. You may feel a train of stones travelling along the bile ducts like marbles. There is no pain because the bile duct valves are open, thanks to the Epsom salts. GO TO SLEEP.

NEXT MORNING – upon awakening take another dose of Epsom salts. Drink 3/4 cup of the mixture. You may go back to bed. Don't drink this before 6:00 a.m.

2 HOURS LATER – take your 4th and last dose of Epsom salts. Drink 3/4 cup. You may again go back to bed and rest if you wish. Between the first and this dosage of Epsom salts, expect to frequent the toilet more often with diarrhea.

AFTER 2 MORE HOURS – you may begin to eat. Start with fruit juice or a carrot juice. Half an hour later eat some fruit. One hour later you may eat regular food but keep it light – salads, steamed vegetables, fruit, juices, etc. It's probably a good idea to drink some prune juice too as this will help to clear the gut.

BY SUPPER you should feel well. There are occasions when you may feel a little unwell for a couple of days, particularly if you have not done a liver flush before the gallbladder flush. Parasites in the liver can also cause symptoms to linger. Other times this may be due to stones and debris remaining in the colon and causing irritation and inflammation. Colon hydrotherapy or a good, deep enema can help this problem.

IN THE MORNING expect diarrhea. Try to catch the gallstones in a sieve placed on the toilet pan so that you can see them. If any of you have a digital camera, please take photos and send me a copy for my clinical archives – admin@docgeorge.com.

Most of the stones will be SOFT and green, breaking easily, or even dissolving. All these green stones are as soft as putty thanks to the malic acid in the apple juice, and are mostly made of cholesterol. Some stones may be dark, near black in colour because of the bilirubin they contain. Other stones may be small and hard, made of calcium and oxalates (see image below). You may see all these types in one flush, but most of them will be the soft green ones made of cholesterol, as about 80% of the stones in the gallbladder are made of these.

A few days after the flush (maybe 10-15 days) stones from the rear of the liver will have travelled 'forward' towards the main bile ducts leaving the liver, and fill the gall bladder again! This is why it is sometimes necessary to do up to 6 cleanses (perhaps one each month) in order to get rid of all the stones. If a cleanse produces no more stones, your liver can be considered to be in excellent condition!

Small hard stones on the right of image

Helpful Tips

On rare occasions, some people may feel nauseous. This is related to the toxic bile leaving the gallbladder, causing discomfort and the feeling of wanting to vomit. There are a few things that may help in such cases:

- ❖ Taking one hydrochloric acid tablet at bedtime will help reduce any nausea during the night – these are sold in health food stores.
- ❖ If you have a tendency to get nauseated from the oil, take 2 tablespoons of Aloe Vera juice after your doses of oil and citrus juice.
- ❖ Placing a hot water bottle over the liver area (under the right ribcage) during the night also helps relieve nausea.

Many people complete this procedure with minimal discomfort, and nearly everyone feels much better after completing it. Flushing the liver and gall bladder in the manner described (if the gall bladder is present) stimulates and cleanses these organs like no other process does.

Oftentimes, people suffering for years from gallstones, lack of appetite, biliousness, backaches, nausea, and a host of other complaints, will find gallstone-type objects in the stool the day following the flush. These objects are light to dark green in colour, very irregular in shape, gelatinous in texture, and of sizes varying from 'grape seed' size to 'cherry' size. If there seems to be a large number of these objects in the stool, the flush should be repeated in 2-4 weeks.

In the next chapter we will look at how energy medicine and bioresonance therapy can help balance our bodies energetically and help in alleviating symptoms of many diseases.

361

Chapter 9

Curing with Energetic Medicine and Bioresonance

Everything is vibration
The human body is a symphony of sounds. Every chakra, organ, bone, tissue and cell has its own resonant frequency; its own sound. Together, they create a unified or composite frequency with its own sound, like the instruments of an orchestra coming together. Ideally, the individual sounds and frequencies comprise a harmonious whole. That is, when the body is functioning as it should. However, when an organ is out of time or out of tune with the rest, then the entire body is affected. This disharmony leads to states of disease and disintegration.

Every living and none living thing has its own resonant frequency – everything is vibration. Every organ of the body has its own individual resonant frequency, much like the note of a tuning fork. All bacteria, viruses, parasites and fungi also have their own frequencies.

It's interesting that the latest quantum physics theory, born only a decade or so ago, arrives at a similar conclusion. It's called String Theory and it basically suggests that the physical universe is built out of sound vibrations, kind of as if everything is the result of some huge cosmic guitar being played somewhere. It's a mind-blowing concept that is held by some of the sharpest minds in the physics community, including Steven Hawking.

In essence, everything in the world is made up of energy. We are all constantly vibrating masses of microscopic particles that are always in motion. Every object, person and organ has a healthy vibration rate called resonance. If that vibration is out of resonance, disease results.

Every organ, every bone, every tissue, every system, all are in a state of vibration. Now, when we are in a state of health, the body puts out an overall harmonic of health. However, when a frequency that is counter to our health sets itself up in some portion of the body, it creates a disharmony that we call *dis-ease*.

When an organ such as the liver gets sick, the frequency usually drops. The lungs resonate at a frequency of 72 cycles per second, also known as Hertz. If the lungs develop an infection, then the frequency will change, usually dropping a few Hertz.

At the University of California, Los Angeles, nanotechnologist Jim Gimzewski is pioneering a new science he calls sonocytology - the study of cell sounds. His first experiments began with yeast cells, using a nanotechnology tool called an atomic force microscope to detect sound-generating vibrations and then using a computer to enhance the volume. The yeast cells were heard to produce harmonics of around 1,000 Hz.

In musical terms, they were "singing" in the range of C-sharp to D above middle C. Killing the yeast cells with alcohol made the pitch rise dramatically, as if the cells were screaming. Cellular harmonics were also affected by temperature, speeding them up or slowing them down. Genetic mutations were found to make a slightly different sound than normal cells. Dead cells emitted a low rumbling like radio static.

Distinguishing between the sound signatures of healthy and diseased cells may be a part of the medicine of the future.

Healing Frequencies

The healing nature of the frequency spectrum lies in the ability of a living organism to absorb a very precise range of frequencies that can physically create a healing effect on certain organs and organic systems.

In many cases the healing effect of frequencies is achieved by the ability of the frequency to create a very accurate effect on specific bacteria and viruses by sending highly matched Healing Frequencies capable of neutralizing their chemical structure.

"Put a cat and a bunch of broken bones in the same room" some veterinary schools joke, *"and the bones will heal."* Only two years ago, scientists discovered that vibrations between 20-140 Hz are anabolic for bone growth and will also help to heal fractures, mend torn muscles and ligaments, reduce swelling, and relieve pain. Fauna have found that a cat's purr not only matches this vibration, but its dominant frequencies are 25 and 50 Hz - the optimum frequencies for bone growth and fracture healing. All cats, including larger ones such as pumas, ocelots and lions, have further sets of strong harmonics at the exact Hertz that generate muscle strength, increase joint mobility and provide therapeutic pain relief.

Richard Gerber, M.D. states in his book, *Vibrational Medicine:*

> *"When viral and chemical environmental stressors are introduced into the human biological system, the place where they will cause the most damage will be partially determined by the weakest link in the physiologic/subtle energy chain.*
>
> *From an energetic standpoint, the human body, when weakened or shifted from equilibrium, oscillates at a different and less harmonious frequency than when healthy. This abnormal frequency reflects a general state of cellular energetic imbalance within the physical body.*
>
> *When a weakened individual is unable to shift their energetic mode to the needed frequency a certain amount of subtle energetic help may be needed. When supplied with a dose of the needed energetic frequency, it allows the cellular bioenergetic systems to resonate in the proper vibrational mode, thereby throwing off the toxicities of the illness."*

Bioresonance

Each body has its own unique frequency. When the interaction of these frequencies is balanced, you feel peaceful and at perfect harmony with yourself as well as towards other people. When they are off balance, it can have significant negative effects.

An unbalanced body is unable to fulfil its energy contribution to the system. This can have negative psychological and physical consequences on an individual. Anger, depression, constipation, lack of concentration, and sexual dysfunctions are just a few examples of symptoms due to unbalanced internal frequencies.

If we can produce the same frequency as a healthy lung using a frequency generator, then we can help the lung to recuperate its normal functioning. The body heals and rebalances itself when it is connected to healthy frequencies. This is the principle of BIORESONANCE.

If we take a crystal wine glass as another example, this also has its own resonant frequency of around 500 Hertz. If we can produce a sound at the same frequency and stand the glass in front of a speaker, then the glass will absorb this frequency and break. This is the phenomenon of RESONANCE.

In the same way, microbes also have their own resonant frequencies – if we can match these frequencies then the microbes will absorb this energy and burst.

There have been many researchers that have worked on energy medicine and Bioresonance this century, such as Dr. Rife, Dr. Voll, Dr. Schimmel, Dr. Morell and others. In addition, unknown to the West, the Russians have worked in the background and made ground-breaking discoveries in this field.

The Russians conducted extensive studies on over 25,000 people. They established an accurate system of analysing and reinforcing energetic health of the organs and their connection to specific areas on the skin (dermal-visceral zones). The Russian space program uses this technology because it enables convenient and non-invasive monitoring and enhancing of the health of their cosmonauts.

Over the last 17 years, Russian scientists, spearheaded by Dr. Konoblov, a medical doctor and Ph.D. physicist, have developed small, portable devices that are innovative and cutting-edge, at only a fraction of the cost of previous generation machines.

These devices produce weak electromagnetic fields at varying frequencies that can penetrate the body's cells and bring them back to optimal balance and health.

Deta Elis Bioresonance Devices
The Russian company initially called DETA ELIS and now DEHOLDINGS, has developed a number of therapeutic devices. One of these is called the DEVITA AP (Fig. 1) and is designed to resonate with different microorganisms to destroy them. It is no bigger than a mobile phone and can comfortably be carried in one's pocket, or placed under the pillow and ran at night while sleeping.

The other device (Fig 1) is called the DEVITA RITM and is designed to resonate at the same frequencies as normal organ systems, hence helping to upregulate these organs, bringing them back to normal functioning.

Both these devices can be programmed using the DEINFO USB (Fig 1) which contains more than 3,000 programmes for eradicating many microorganisms including parasites, protozoa, bacteria, fungi and viruses, as well as many other programmes for all the organ systems of the body.

Fig 1. The DEVITA AP and RITM portable Bioresonance devices
www.deta-elis-uk.com

The Hippocratic Oath states, *"Do no harm"* when treating people. These gentle devices achieve exactly this – they can heal without being invasive and causing side-effects. The devices can be used with children and pets, and can therefore act as your "family doctor".

The devices have undergone clinical trials with many thousands of patients suffering many different health problems, as well as being certified by the Ministry of Health of the Russian Republic. These devices have also been patented in 73 different countries, and have won many certificates and awards.

They are presently manufactured in Germany and have a CE as an electromagnetic wellness device.

I strongly believe that bioenergetic and informational medicine is going to be the medicine of the future. These discoveries on energetics are now gradually percolating into the consciousness of medical practitioners. Researchers, healthcare professionals and the public are realizing that these energetic healing modalities are here to stay.

In clinical practice, I have used various energetic diagnostic and healing modalities that have completely cured difficult chronic diseases, where more orthodox approaches could not help. Other users of the Deta Elis devices are getting good results in different diseases, so this is encouraging.

Having said this, however, these devices are not a cure-all for all diseases – nothing is! We can use and respect the technology knowing that it will do us no harm with the potential to heal on levels that other remedies and drugs cannot.

A Little History

In 1923, George's Lakhovsky[221], a Russian engineer working in France, built a simple apparatus capable of registering microvoltage measurements from human cells, plants and microbes. In his studies of normal and diseased cells, Lakhosvky found that there were marked differences in their oscillation patterns.

Each group of cells emitted frequencies specific to its organ or tissue of origin. Cancerous cells emitted a different, abnormal pattern. Lakhovsky also discovered that harmful factors such as faulty nutrition, environmental pollutants such as toxic chemicals or heavy metals, bacteria or viruses weaken and distort cellular electro-magnetic fields prior to the onset of illness and death.

A little later, Professor Harold Saxton Burr[222], of Yale Medical School, carried out his own investigation of human-energy related phenomenon. His systematic measurements of the electromagnetic fields emitted by different bodily tissues and organs confirmed Lakhovsky's findings concerning the difference in the electrical emissions of healthy and diseased organs and tissues. He called these the 'L-fields' with 'L' representing "Life." Thanks to the controlling L-fields, new molecules and cells in the body are constantly being rebuilt, arranging themselves in the same pattern as the old ones.

With the advancement of scientific research technology, the number of discoveries regarding the human energy field grew. In 1967, the magnetic field around the human heart was observed and recorded using a sophisticated Superconducting Quantum Interference Device (SQUID) at the Massachusetts Institute of Technology in Cambridge, Massachusetts by Zimmermann and his colleagues.[223,224]

Professor Tiller[225] believes that the magnetic elements in living cells are repositories for voluminous amounts of information, the pathological content of which contributes to the development and sustainment of chronic diseases. All of the major assaults that the body is not able to overcome (toxins, infectious agents and physical or emotional traumas) become imprinted onto these cellular recordings in a CD-like fashion and then continuously feed back into the body's chemistry, negatively altering it.

---

[221] Lakhovsky, G. The Waves Which Cure (Gauthier-Villars and Co), 1929.

[222] Burr, H.S. Bluprint for Immortality, Neville Spearman Publishers, 1972.

[223] Zimmermann, J.E. Josephson effect devices and low frequency filed sensing. *Cryogenics* 12:19-31, 1972.

[224] Zimmermann, J.E., Thiene P, Harding J T. Design and operation of stable rf-biased superconducting point-contact quantum devices, and a note on the properties of perfectly clean metal contacts. *Journal of Applied Physics.* 41:1572-1580, 1970.

[225] Tiller, W. Energy Fields and the Human Body. Frontiers of Consciousness, edited by J. White. New York, Avon Books, 1974.

German physicist Professor Herbert Frohlick[226] of the University of Liverpool, a world-renowned authority on human energy research, summarized his fifty years of research in the field by concluding that every structure in the body, including the entire chemistry of the body down to the chromosomes, is energy-operated and driven by electromagnetic fields that are created by flows of charged ions. He received the Max Planck Medal, the highest award for physics in Germany.

How does the body work energetically?

When students of medicine and biology study the cell, the diagrams that they study are very simplistic in the sense that they only look at the structural components; the different organelles contained inside the cell and their function. However, to be able to understand the energetic systems of the body, we need to understand the basic anatomy of the body's Living Matrix.

It is the living matrix or extracellular matrix (ECM) that communicates with each cell of the body forming a complex web of interconnectedness. Figure 2 is a summary of these interconnections – notice how the tissues surrounding the digestive tract, nerves, bones, blood vessels, muscles and underlying the skin contain a sparse but active number of generative cells that form and continuously modify the extracellular matrix and play an important role in injury repair and defense against disease.

These cells are part of a structural, energetic and informational continuum. This fibre system is now recognized by many scientists as an important communication system that affects all metabolic systems as well. It is part of a semiconducting, oscillatory continuum that allows all parts of the biological organism to communicate with each other. One research scientist, Adey, in 1993 referred to this as *"whispering between cells."*[227]

---

[226] Hyland, GJ and Rowlands, P (ed). *Herbert Frohlich FRS: A Physicist Ahead of his Time.* (2nd edition), UK: University of Liverpool, 2008.
[227] Adey, WR. Whispering between cells: electromagnetic fields and regulatory mechanisms in tissue. *Frontier Perspectives.* 3:21-25, 1993.

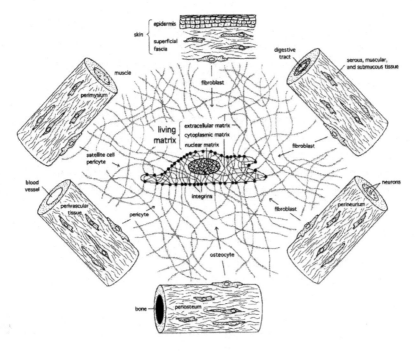

Fig. 2 The Living Matrix

In trying to understand the energy dynamics of the living matrix, the field of physics plays an important role. In the structure of the living matrix there is a degree of coherent crystallinity – this is like an ordered crystal matrix that is very important to the structure-energy-communication model of living tissue.

Interestingly, many of the key molecules that make up the living matrix such as collagen, elastin, keratin, DNA, actin and myosin are all helical, much like a helical spring. If we can understand how the helical spring can convert energy from one form to another, then we will better understand how the living matrix can respond to different energies.

This system is comprised of two main structures: the visible and invisible connective tissue that extends from the molecular level of our body throughout our energy field and the element of water.

It was back in 1941 that Albert Szent-Györgyi,[228] who had received the Nobel Prize in 1937 for the synthesis of Vitamin C, gave the Korányi Memorial Lecture in Budapest, Hungary. He said:

---

[228] Szent-Györgyi, A. The Study of Energy Levels in Biochemistry) *Nature* 148:157-159, 1941.

"If a great number of atoms are arranged with regularity in close proximity, as for instance, in a crystal lattice, the electrons cease to belong to one or two atoms only, and belong to the whole system…A great number of molecules may join to form energy continua, along which energy, excited electrons may travel a certain distance."

What this means is that free electrons can move around the body quickly and transfer energy and information wherever they wish. This is clarified further by Dr. Donald Coffey and an eminent group at Johns Hopkins School of Medicine.[229] They were studying the nuclear matrix and its interconnections with both DNA and with molecules that extend across the nuclear envelope and connect to the cytoskeleton.[230]

In 1991, the same group produced an inspiring report on the way signals propagate through this matrix, which they termed a tissue tensegrity matrix system.[231] The tensegrity aspect had evolved from the work of Buckminster, Fuller and others.[232] Tensegrity is defined as a continuous tensional network (called tendons) supported by a discontinuous set of compressive elements (called struts).
The 1991 report by Pienta and Coffey gave precise language and experimental validation to the transfer of energy and information through the living matrix:

"Cells and intracellular elements are capable of vibrating in a dynamic manner with complex harmonics, the frequency of which can now be measured and analysed in a quantitative manner...a tissue-tensegrity matrix system…is poised to couple the biological oscillations of the cell from the peripheral membrane to the DNA."

The helical molecules in living systems are piezoelectric semiconductors which have the ability of emitting and absorbing and converting light energy into vibrations that can travel through the living matrix. Due to the transverse Hall effect, these helical molecules can also respond to magnetic and biomagnetic fields.

Whenever a therapist applies any type of stimulus to the living matrix, whether it is by touch on the skin, inserting an acupuncture needle, using a pulsing

---

229 Presented by James L. Oschman, Ph.D.in a lecture entitled "The development of the living matrix concept and its significance for health and healing in a speech commemorating the London premier of The Living Matrix: a new film on the science of healing and the Science of Healing Conference at Kings College, London on March 13, 2009.
230 Berezney, R., Coffey, D.S. Isolation and characterization of a framework structure from rat liver nuclei. *Journal of Cell Biology* 73:616-637, 1977.
231 Pienta K.J., Coffey D.S. Cellular harmonic information transfer through a tissue tensegrity-matrix system. *Medical Hypotheses* 34:88-95, 1991.
232 Tensegrity is a naturally occurring construct first recognized and developed by sculptor Ken Snelson and visionary R. Buckminster Fuller. For a detailed discussion, go to Dr. Stephen M. Levin's web site, http://www.biotensegrity.com

electromagnetic field such as the PAPIMI that we will discuss below, the vibratory energy from these stimuli will be converted by the helical molecules of the living matrix into signals that will travel throughout the living matrix.

Informational Medicine

There are also many phenomenon in healing that are not governed by quantity, space and time. These phenomenon and related treatment modalities are outside modern-day medicine since they are not covered and explained by modern-day physics. These can be placed into the category of 'Informational Medicine' and would include homeopathy, psychology, emotional freedom technique, distant healing, prayer healing, radionics, Hellinger Family Constellations and more. Of these, homeopathy was the first systemically developed form of informational medicine in recent history.

Informational medicine consists of words, signs, symbols, rituals and pictures – the use of information in all its forms. Even though this has not been recognised formally by modern medicine, it no doubt exists and is a powerful healing modality that goes beyond the placebo effect.

There are many informational modalities that are often misunderstood as being energetic. Since these modalities do not use substance or energy to diagnose or heal, there is no way that atomic physicists using quantum mechanics can measure the energy, as it does not exist as an energy system but an information system.

Alongside the levels of matter and energy, information forms a third level of existence that is guided by its own laws which differ in many aspects from those of matter and energy. They can, however, co-exist. Matter and energy can be transformed into each other, as can information be transformed into energy or vice versa. Information can also be *transported* via energy.

However, a new aspect that is unknown in modern physics, maybe except for Global Scaling[233], is that information can be transmitted *without* energy. This is possible because pure information is not ruled by time and space. It may be difficult to conceive, but our world is holographic in its structure, which means that every part contains all other parts. This implies that any part can affect every other part and can be a measure of every other part.

---

[233] The Theory of Global Scaling assumes that matter resonates harmonically at its lowest level of energy. This lowest level global scaling theory is not merely designated the "physical vacuum"; however, the frequency spectrum of the natural oscillations of the vacuum comprises many orders of magnitude and is fractally developed, like a melody. This "melody of creation" is, according to the theory, the cause of the logarithmic-hyperbolic, scale invariant, fractal distribution of frequencies of most varied measure – from the elementary particles to the galaxies.

To illustrate this, let's look at an example. It is well known that silver particles in a beaker of water will kill bacteria. What is not so well known is that if the colloidal silver was placed in a nearby gas discharge tube, the electromagnetic emissions from this will also kill the bacteria. If one also closely simulated the silver spectrum using light energy, the electromagnetic radiation from this light source would also kill the bacteria.

We can clearly see that it is not the physical contact of the silver ions with the bacteria that are killing them, but the specific information pattern inherent in the silver atom that is responsible. So, manipulating the information aspect of the silver can alter the information aspect of the bacteria in such a way as to 'kill' the bacteria.

The diagnostic methods described in this book use the human energy field to derive health-related information. For instance, thermography records the thermal properties of the human energy field. The VEGA EXPERT measures electrical energy flow in specific energy channels of the body, known as meridians which are all connected to the Living Matrix. This will be registered after stimulation with a different energy field (a food item, a medical drug, a toxin, a mineral or a vitamin supplement).

Autonomic Response Testing (ART) is a way of measuring energy changes in the autonomic nervous system, which is connected to the Living Matrix - using this method it is possible to understand what stresses the body on an energetic level.

Some people gifted by birth, such as mystics and healers, have been speaking and writing about the energetic nature of the human being and the interconnections with the sea of energy around us for thousands of years. Barbara Ann Brennan, a healer as well as a physicist, bridged her natural gift with the science of physics in her book entitled, *Hands of Light: A guide to Healing through the Human Energy Field.*[234]

Many writers have contributed to this body of knowledge as well, some naturally gifted, others less so. Many were ordinary scientists, relying on indirect observation using special instruments or biochemical tests to infer on the impact of energetic treatments.

Vibrational Medicine by Dr. Richard Gerber[235], and *Energy Medicine: The Scientific Basis*[236] by James Oschman provide excellent overviews of the scientific basis of energy medicine. The fact remains that many energetic therapeutic interventions work, some

---

[234] Brennan, BA. Hands of Light: A guide to Healing through the Human Energy Field. USA: Bantam Books, 1987.
235. Gerber, R. Vibrational Medicine (3rd edition). USA: Bear and Company, 2001.
236. Oschman, J.L. Energy Medicine: The Scientific Basis. UK: Harcourt Publishers, 2000.

of them with exceptional results. The practitioners who employ them do not wait for the blessing of conventional medicine, with all its vices, to be ready to explain the why and the how.

Visual Medicine: Seeing the effects of energy on water

Masaru Emoto[237] is a Japanese author known for his controversial claim that if human speech or thoughts are directed at water droplets before they are frozen, images of the resulting water crystals either take on a beautiful geometric pattern or a disorganized, ugly one, depending upon whether the words or thoughts were positive or negative.

Emoto claims this can be achieved through prayer, music or by attaching written words to a container of water. Dr. Emoto is at the forefront of the study of water. By using high-speed photography under high-power microscopy to photograph water freezing quickly, he has shown that thoughts and feelings affect physical reality. By producing different focused intentions through written and spoken words and music and literally presenting it to the same water samples, the water appears to "change its expression".

Fig 3. Crystalline patterns of water

He found that water from clear springs and water that has been exposed to loving words shows brilliant, complex, and colorful snowflake patterns (Fig 3). In contrast, polluted water, or water exposed to negative thoughts, forms incomplete, asymmetrical patterns with dull colors.

---

[237] Emoto, M. *The Journal of Alternative and Complementary Medicine*. February 2004, 10(1): 19-21.

The implications of this research create a new awareness of how we can positively impact the earth and our personal health. The success of his books[238] outside Japan has been remarkable. Dr. Emoto has been called to lecture around the world as a result and has conducted live experiments both in Japan and Europe as well as in the US to show how indeed our thoughts, attitudes, and emotions as humans deeply impact the environment.

The Human Bioenergetic System

Humans consist of more than physical nerves, muscles and bones. We are part of a larger dynamic, multidimensional system of energy and light; we are simply much more than the physical body. Our physiological systems comprising of organs and tissues are not only supported by oxygen, glucose and other nutrients, but also by higher vibrational energies which provide life to the physical body.

These higher energies are regulated by the chakra-nadi system and the physical-etheric interface, which include the acupuncture meridian system. The etheric energies provide ways of organizing cellular structure and function.

The fine network of nadis distributes high-frequency energies coming in through the chakras to all the body's organs and tissues. This high-frequency energy helps to provide balance and order at the molecular level of expression. It's like a higher dimensional homeostatic system. When energetic disturbances occur at these higher frequency levels, these will manifest in the physical body as symptoms and disease.

---

[238] Emoto, M. *Messages from Water, Vol. 1,* Hado Publishing, 1991; Emoto, M. *Messages from Water, Vol. 2,* Sunmark Pub, 2001; Emoto, M. *The Hidden Messages in Water*, Beyond Words Publishing, 2004.

If we could widen our perspective and see humans in their multidimensional anatomy, consisting of higher vibrational bodies, chakras, nadis, and meridians (Fig 4), then it would be possible to explain much of what allopathic medicine cannot explain about disease processes. Humans are not closed, physiological boxes but open energy systems in a dynamic equilibrium with a multidimensional electromagnetic environment.

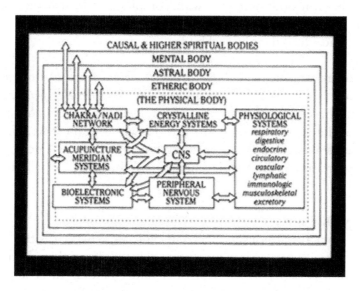

Fig 4. Human Multi-dimensional Bioenergetic System

The real future of Holistic Medicine will depend on the integration of vibrational medical therapies and clinical practice alongside all the other healing modalities. The holistic physician will need to integrate the physical, emotional, mental and spiritual elements of life in order to truly cure the patient on all these levels. The ultimate approach to healing will be to remove the subtle-energy imbalances that led to the manifestation of illness in the first place.

Even though allopathic physicians have acknowledged for some time that stress contributes to diseases such as stomach ulcers, ulcerative colitis, psoriasis, asthma and more, there have been very few attempts to address the underlying pathogenesis of these diseases, other than using anxiolytic drugs such as valium and the like. These drugs may help in the short-term with acutely stressful situations, but only tend to suppress the symptoms and overlook the primary, underlying causes. It is much more constructive for the holistic physician to integrate and rebalance the elements of the mind and body with the element of spirit.

For many years, physicians have looked at and treated the physical body as a separate entity to the mind and the spirit. There has begun a paradigm shift away from this dualistic thinking of old into a new model that accepts the health effects of the mind on the physical body.

Still, it is early days, and the majority of medical doctors are still only trying to direct therapeutic strategies toward particular organ systems instead of treating the whole person. Humans are greater than the sum of their physical organs and physiological systems. The physical body interacts with complex subtle structures and networks that help the life-force and energies of consciousness to maintain a homeostasis required for the health of the physical body.

Many practitioners will say, "*Well that's all well and good, but how can we measure these 'subtle energies' and help get a better understanding of how they adversely affect our patients?*" This is an excellent. There are many different technologies and techniques that have been developed over the years for doing just this. However, it must be said that all these technologies are still in the process of development and there is not one system that can purport to measure the subtle energies of the body on all their levels and correlate them with the physical body yet.

Subtle Energy Diagnosis
Personally, as a practicing holistic medicine clinician, I have had the opportunity of using many of these 'subtle energy measuring devices'. Even though these are not yet fully developed, it is better to get a broader understanding of at least some of the subtle energies that have been responsible for their health problems, as opposed to ignoring these completely.

Let's look at some of these modalities that I mainly use in the Da Vinci Holistic Health Centre and am very familiar with. This is by no means a comprehensive list of all the measuring devices – it would take another book much thicker than this one to list them all. We will examine the Vegetative Reflex Test (VRT) using the VEGA and the DETA PROFESSIONAL devices; Bioresonance therapy using the BICOM and PROFESSIONAL; as well as Rife frequency generators.

The Vegetative Reflex Test using Bioresonance Devices
One system, which is beginning to grow in popularity among doctors and dentists, are devices known as VRT Bioresonance devices. There are a number of them now on the market, but I personally use the VEGA EXPERT VRT device (Fig 5), and the Deta Elis PROFESSIONAL (www.deta-elis-uk.com) device (Fig 6).

Fig 5. The VEGA VRT device

Fig 6. Deta Elis PROFESSIONAL device

Both the VEGA and PROFESSIONAL[239] Vegetative Reflex Test (VRT) represent an advanced development of the "Electroacupuncture according to Voll" (EAV)[240] concept. It features a combination of electronic measurements of skin resistance on specific energy meridian points (acupoints) that disclose vital health information through vegetative (autonomic) reflexes and resonances.

These devices can highlight the underlying causes of illnesses by using homeopathic bionosodes. This is usually a small portion of diseased tissue from a diseased organ that is ground up and made into a homeopathic remedy. When a particular bionosode is placed on the honeycomb or resonator plate of these devices, it induces a resonance reaction in the acupoint, which infers a relationship between the diseased organ being tested and the related organ of the patient.

If the patient does not have a diseased liver, for example, then they will not resonate with a bionosode of a diseased liver placed on the honeycomb of the device. Even

---

[240] Voll, R. The phenomenon of medicine testing in electro-acupuncture according to Voll. *American Journal of Acupuncture* 8:97-104, 1980.

bacteria, viruses, fungi, stealth organisms and more can be tested for resonance with the patient and be identified much quicker than any other type of biological testing.

The Vegetative Reflex Test (VRT) can help the clinician in the following ways:

❖ Discovery of pathophysiologic processes that escape the standard clinical examination.
❖ Determination of the existence of focal infections.
❖ Determination of sub-clinical infections and energetic functional conditions in different quadrants of the body, as well as different organs.
❖ Show the condition of the immune system and of the immune- related tissues (spleen, thymus and lymph nodes).
❖ Determination of emotional stress and disturbances.
❖ Identification of the pathogenesis of disease (the root causes and where they began from with their interrelationships).
❖ Testing for allergies from environmental factors as well as food intolerances.

Personally, as a clinician, I have found VRT testing very useful in the following cases and circumstances:

❖ When all conventional diagnostic tests (physical and biochemical) reveal no clues to the cause of a patient's complaints, the disorders are most likely functional in nature rather than morphological. The VEGA reveals about 80% of the otherwise un-diagnosable cases of migraines, backaches, chronic fatigue syndrome, systemic Candidiasis, bowel distention, IBS, Crohn's disease, sleep disturbance and more.
❖ When conventional examination cannot fully or correctly explain the patient's complaints, the VEGA is highly indicative. It is superbly suited for the diagnosis of functional ailments (about 70% of all patients) and of clinically obscure, sub-clinical disorders. These make up about 20% of all indications.

There are about 40% of patients who have many symptoms but conventional laboratory tests yield negative results. These patients are often referred to psychologists or psychiatrists resulting in needless suffering and are a waste of time and money.

These Bioresonance devices are capable of going beyond the diagnosis of energetic imbalance levels in particular systems. It is frequently capable of finding the actual causes of the energetic dysfunction, as well as potential cures for the disorders.

380

Bioresonance Therapy

New methods are evolving all the time which move us closer to the goal of individualized treatment. One such method, BIORESONANCE, also known as BRT (Bioresonance therapy), can be used to treat a wide range of disorders. BRT has been tested and approved throughout Europe and Canada, and it is in use in 85 countries worldwide. In Germany, where it was developed by Regumed,[241] BRT has been in use for over 25 years.

Bio-resonance promises not only to address the unique needs of each patient, but also, as it becomes more widespread, to provide an answer to the nagging question: *"Why do some individuals do well with one type of medication, while others improve only slightly or not at all?"*

At the Da Vinci Natural Health Centre we use a couple of Bioresonance devices: the BICOM, a German-made device (Fig 7) and the DETA PROFESSIONAL made by Deta Elis, a Russian company (Fig 8). The patient's body signals are conducted from the right hand into the input of the device using a brass electrode. These devices can filter out the disharmonious frequencies and invert them. These inverted therapeutic oscillations are now given back to the patient via the left hand using another electrode.

Fig 7. BICOM Bioresonance Device

---

[241] http://www.regumed.de

Fig 8. DETA PROFESSIONAL

Central to its application is the idea that all life is made of energy. Although humans tend to think of themselves as relatively solid creatures, we are just a mass of compressed energy. We emit our own electromagnetic fields and, as with all things, we each have our own unique "vibration," or oscillation. This oscillation can easily be measured with electronic equipment. When we are healthy, our bodies produce a smooth, regular oscillation. When the body is under stress, the pattern becomes jagged and irregular.

The treatment of pathological oscillations involves returning them back to the body in a modified form - in this case, as a mirror image. This action is based on the principle well-known in physics, that oscillations are influenced by their exact mirror image. Returning the oscillation to the patient in this modified form can diminish, or even eliminate, the pathological oscillations of the allergen or toxin, allowing the body's own healthy oscillations to become dominant. If the practitioner decides that medicine would also be useful in treatment, the oscillation of that specific medicine could also be returned to the patient.

Fig 9 Returning Oscillations of Bioresonance Therapy

These returning oscillations (Fig 9) help to balance the patient electromagnetically, and are again fed into the Bioresonance device for further analysis. The process is repeated constantly in fractions of a second. The pathological signals in the body are consequently reduced and finally extinguished and the physiological endogenous regulatory forces can regulate the biological process unhindered.

There has been a lot of recent media coverage on exposure to electromagnetic fields causing illness by altering the body's own electric "chemistry". However, practitioners of bio-resonance believe that the reverse is also true; healthy electrical signals transmitted into the body, in this case via hand-held electrodes, can re-harmonize it. Similar to homoeopathy and acupuncture, bio-resonance aims to relieve the body of stress factors and improve its regulatory systems.

There is considerable ongoing research in the field of Bioresonance, specifically using the BICOM device. One such study was conducted by Machowinski at the Naturopathy Outpatients Clinic of the Carsten's Foundation, University of Heidelberg, under the direction of Dr. Gerhard.

It was a prospective, randomized controlled study with 28 patients suffering with chronic hepatocellular damage, as reflected by elevated laboratory values of hepatic enzymes such as GOT, GPT and gamma-GT. There were 14 patients in the treatment group using the BICOM and 14 in the control group not receiving any treatment.

On completion of the study, the hepatic values of the BICOM-treated group were within normal limits, while the values of the control group were still within the pathological range with no change (Table 1). The following table shows the percentage decrease in the values:

Hepatic values	Decrease towards normal of excess values (BICOM treatment)	Decrease towards normal of excess values (Control group)
GOT	42 %	4 %
GPT	50 %	5 %
Gamma-GT	38 %	7 %

Table 1. Results of BICOM and control group

In the treatment group, the geometric mean values for the degree of improvement were 45% for GOT values (5% for control group), 55% for GPT activity (control group displayed a slight deterioration) and 45% for gamma-GT activity (slight deterioration in the control group).

It is clear from the experimental evidence presented that treating minor hepatocellular damage with BICOM therapy in the frequency range between 10 Hz and 150 kHz can bring about reconstitution of damaged hepatic cells.

Dr. Rife Technology
Another famous technology that uses the principle of energy medicine is the frequency generator invented by one of the most incredible geniuses of our time, Dr. Royal Raymond Rife, who back in the 1930's had cured 16 terminally-ill cancer patients with this electronic resonance device. This was an incredible feat, not only then, but also by today's standards. He had invented a Universal microscope[242] (Fig 10) with nearly 6,000 parts that could magnify up to 17,000x without killing the specimen. This is how he identified the cancer virus.[243]

---

242 Siedel, RE., Winter, EM. The New Microscopes, Annual Report, Smithsonian Institute, USA, pp. 193-220, 1944.
243 Annual Report of the Board of Regents of The Smithsonian Institution, 1944, The Rife's Microscope, The Smithsonian Report, 1944.

Fig 10 Universal Microscope

Royal R. Rife, born in 1888 (Fig 11), discovered that when a cell was exposed to some form of energy to which it is resonant, this energy would be absorbed by the resonant structure. Should the resonant energy be greater than the cell can effectively dissipate, Dr. Rife found that this cell would fail structurally, often resulting in cell death.

A simple way to understand resonance is to think of an opera singer who can break a wine glass with her voice. The wine glass resonates at a certain frequency. If the opera singer can match that natural frequency with her voice, then the glass will absorb this resonant energy and smash.

Fig 11. Dr Rife with his Universal Microscope

This simple principle can be applied to living organisms too, such as bacteria and viruses. This is what Dr. Rife managed to do. He discovered a resonant frequency that he called the mortal oscillatory rate (MOR) for over 55 major bacterial diseases. He also found the MOR for cancer after arduous years of experimentation using the sophisticated Universal microscope that enabled him to see micro-organisms live, without killing them by staining. Using this equipment, he isolated the cancer virus that he called the "BX" virus.

In time, Rife was able to prove that the cancer micro-organism has 4 forms:[244]

1. BX (carcinoma)
2. BY (sarcoma - larger than the BX virus)
3. Monococcoid form in the monocytes of the blood of over 90% of cancer patients.
4. Crytomyces pleomorpha fungi

Rife wrote in his 1953 book:

> *"Any of these forms can be changed back to the 'BX' within a period of 36 hours and will produce in the experimental animal a typical tumour with all the pathology of true neoplastic tissue, from which we can again recover the 'BX' micro-organism. This complete procedure has been duplicated over 300 times with identical and positive results."*

---

244 Rife, RR. History of the development of a successful treatment for cancer and other virus, bacteria and fungi. Rife Virus Microscope Institute, San Diego, USA, 1953.

There is no doubt that Rife was a perfectionist to the greatest degree.

What did Rife mean when he said that the other forms could be changed back to the 'BX' form? If we take what Pasteur has taught the world as the absolute truth, then no micro-organisms can change back to other types. Pasteur taught bacteriology based on Monomorphism; there is basically one micro-organism that causes each of the different diseases.

So, for every disease, there is a different bug. However, this is not what Dr. Rife and other researchers such as Beauchamp, Gaessens and Prof. Enderlein saw in their microscopes.[245] Using a darkfield condenser with an iris objective, they could see different forms changing in front of their own eyes. This went directly against Pasteur's theory of Monomorphism, to one of Pleomorphism.

It seems rather remote that all these researchers had reported seeing the same phenomenon of pleomorphism using their microscopes. It is also interesting that monomorphism - one bug for each disease - is still the paradigm that is taught in all medical schools around the world.

By using Live Blood Analysis, it is possible to show that the more toxic the internal milieu of the body, the more these micro-organisms change forms to more and more virulent and pathological types which causes degenerative diseases. The ultimate stage would be the 'BX' virus that Rife had not only isolated, but found in over 90% of cancer patients.

As Rife declared in 1953:

> *"These successful tests were conducted over 400 times with experimental animals before any attempt was made to use this frequency on human cases suffering from carcinoma and sarcoma."*

In 1934, Dr. Rife opened a clinic, which successfully cured 16 of 16 cases within 120 days. Working with some of the most respected researchers in America, along with leading doctors from Southern California, he electronically destroyed the cancer virus in patients, allowing their own immune systems to restore health.

A Special Research Committee of the University of Southern California oversaw the laboratory research and the experimental treatments until the end of the 1930s. Follow-up clinics conducted in 1935, 1936 and 1937 by the head of the U.S.C.

---

245 Poehlman, Karl H. Synthesis of the Work of Enderlein, Bechamps and other Pleomorphic Researchers. Explore Vol. 8, No. 2, 1997.

Medical Committee verified the results of the 1934 clinic. In his 1953 book, Dr. Rife wrote about the cancer clinics on December 3rd 1953:

> *"The first clinical work on cancer was completed under the supervision of Milbank Johnson, M.D. which was set up under a Special Medical Research Committee of the University of Southern California. 16 cases were treated at the clinic for many types of malignancy. After 3 months, 14 of these so-called hopeless cases were signed off as clinically cured by the staff of five medical doctors and Dr. Alvin G. Ford, M.D. Pathologist for the group.*
> *The treatments consisted of 3 minutes' duration using the frequency instrument, which was set on the mortal oscillatory rate for 'BX' or cancer (at 3 day intervals). It was found that the elapsed time between treatments attains better results than the cases treated daily. This gives the lymphatic system an opportunity to absorb and cast off the toxic condition that is produced by the devitalized dead particles of the 'BX' virus. No rise of body temperature was perceptible in any of these cases above normal during or after the frequency instrument treatment. No special diets were used in any of this clinical work, but we sincerely believe that a proper diet compiled for the individual would be of benefit."*

Independent physicians utilizing the equipment successfully treated as many as 40 people per day during these years. In addition to curing cancer and other deadly diseases, degenerative conditions such as cataracts were reversed. Rife had been able to determine the precise electrical frequency that destroyed individual micro-organisms responsible for cancer, herpes, tuberculosis, and other illnesses. His work was described in Science magazine, medical journals, and later the Smithsonian Institution's annual report.[246]

Unfortunately, Rife's scientific theories and method of treatment conflicted with orthodox views. His work was stopped and both the research and the treatments were forced underground. The AMA took him and his associates to court. This trial would start Rife on a long road of deterioration, alcoholism and depression, as the deaths from cancer mounted year after year. While the court case was taking place (and afterwards), the AMA visited all the doctors involved. Those who didn't stop using the Frequency Instrument would lose their medical license.

One of his main co-supporters, Milbank Johnson died under mysterious circumstances (possibly poisoned), and records of Rife's work were destroyed. No medical journal was ever permitted to print Rife's work, except one by the Franklin Institute that slipped by the censors. In 1946, Rife's problems forced him to sell off his laboratory piece by piece.

Doctors secretly continued curing cancer patients for 22 years after the original

---

246 Lynes, B. 1992. The Cancer Cure that Worked. Marcus Books, Ontario, Canada.

success of the 1934 clinic, but always with opposition from medical and governmental authorities.

However, from 1950 to the mid-1980s, a number of research scientists, working independently, have slowly been verifying the scientific principles upon which Rife's clinical cures of the 1930s were based. A body of recognized scientific evidence now overwhelmingly supports the original cancer theories articulated and demonstrated by Rife 50 years ago. This includes modern AIDS researchers.

In the next chapter we will look at emotional, psychological and spiritual factors can play a significant role in the cause and maintenance of chronic diseases.

Chapter 10

Emotional, Psychological & Spiritual Roots of Disease

Emotional pain often exacts a greater toll on the quality of your life than physical pain. The stress and negative emotions associated with any trying event can even lead to physical pain and disease.

In fact, emotional stress is linked to health problems including chronic inflammation, lowered immune function, increased blood pressure, gut and stomach problems, altered brain chemistry, increased tumour growth and more.

Of course, emotional pain can be so severe that it interferes with your ability to enjoy life and, in extreme cases, may even make you question whether your life is worth living.

Whether it's a simple spat with your spouse or long-held resentment toward a family member or friend, unresolved conflict can go deeper than you may realize - it may be affecting your physical health.

The good news: Studies have found that the act of forgiveness can reap huge rewards for your health, lowering the risk of heart attack; improving cholesterol levels and sleep; reducing pain, blood pressure, and levels of anxiety, depression and stress. And research points to an increase in the forgiveness-health connection as you age.

"There is an enormous physical burden to being hurt and disappointed," says Karen Swartz, M.D., director of the Mood Disorders Adult Consultation Clinic at The Johns Hopkins Hospital. Chronic anger puts you into a fight-or-flight mode, which results in numerous changes in heart rate, blood pressure and immune response. Those changes, then, increase the risk of depression, heart disease and diabetes, among

other conditions. Forgiveness, however, calms stress levels, leading to improved health.

Psychological Inflammation and Physical Illness

A study published in the Proceedings of the National Academy of Sciences suggests that psychological stress directly interferes with your body's ability to regulate inflammation, which leads to the progression of disease.

Stress wreaks havoc on the mind and body. Until now, it has not been clear exactly how stress influences disease and health. Now researchers have found that chronic psychological stress is associated with the body losing its ability to regulate the inflammatory response. The research shows for the first time that the effects of psychological stress on the body's ability to regulate inflammation can promote the development and progression of disease.

"Inflammation is partly regulated by the hormone cortisol and when cortisol is not allowed to serve this function, inflammation can get out of control," said Sheldon Cohen, a Professor of Psychology at Carnegie Mellon University, which sponsored the research.

Cohen states that psychological stress causes immune cells to become insensitive to cortisol's regulatory effect. In turn, runaway inflammation promotes the development and progression of many diseases.

Cohen's earlier work showed that people suffering from psychological stress are more susceptible to developing common colds, and used the common cold as the model for testing his theory. He showed the common cold to be a side effect of the inflammatory process that is triggered by the body's attempts to fight infection.

In other words, if your life causes you emotional stress that weighs on you daily, then you are on the path toward chronic inflammation and physical disease.

Stress and the Gastrointestinal Tract

Let us now move on from this important spiritual component of our lives, the power of prayer, back to the biological mechanisms of how stress can affect the GI tract specifically.

The stress response causes several detrimental events in your gut, including:

❖ Decreased nutrient absorption

❖ Decreased oxygenation to your gut

❖ As much as four times less blood flow to your digestive system, which leads to decreased metabolism

❖ Decreased enzymatic production by as much as 20,000 times.

It is interesting to note that we have the same type of tissue in our gut, as we do in our brain. During foetal development, one part turns into your central nervous system while the other develops into the nervous system of your gut.

These two systems are connected via the Vagus nerve - the tenth cranial nerve that runs from your brain stem down to your abdomen.

This "brain-gut axis" is what connects your two brains together, and explains why you get butterflies in your stomach when you're nervous, for example.

Likewise, stress results in alterations of your brain-gut connection, which can contribute to, or directly cause, numerous gastrointestinal disorders, including:

❖ Inflammatory bowel disease (IBD)

❖ Irritable bowel syndrome (IBS)

❖ Peptic ulcer

❖ Gastroesophageal reflux disease (GERD)

❖ Food antigen-related adverse responses (food allergies)

❖ Other functional gastrointestinal diseases

Harvard Reviews How Stress Can Cause Stomach Disorders

The wise Father of Medicine, Hippocrates, once said 2,500 years ago, *"All diseases begin in the gut."* It's also widely known that stress is a trigger that causes multiple chronic disease processes to occur.

These two health dogmas are intricately intertwined, as stress is detrimental to your gut health, and together stress and a damaged gut can contribute to multiple inflammatory diseases and conditions, such as:

❖ Crohn's disease

❖ Ulcerative colitis

❖ Multiple sclerosis

❖ Type 1 diabetes

❖ Rheumatoid arthritis

❖ Osteoarthritis

❖ Lupus

❖ Chronic skin conditions

❖ Kidney problems

❖ Urinary conditions

❖ Allergic and atopic conditions

❖ Degenerative conditions

❖ Chronic fatigue syndrome

❖ Fibromyalgia

❖ Myalgic encephalomyelitis (ME)

❖ Inflammatory bowel diseases

To put it simply, chronic stress (and other negative emotions like anger, anxiety and sadness) can trigger symptoms and full-blown disease in your gut. As Harvard researchers explain:

> *"Psychology combines with physical factors to cause pain and other bowel symptoms. Psychosocial factors influence the actual physiology of the gut, as well as symptoms. In other words, stress (or depression or other psychological factors) can affect movement and contractions of the GI tract, cause inflammation, or make you more susceptible to infection."*

In addition, research suggests that some people with functional GI disorders perceive pain more acutely than other people do because their brains do not properly regulate pain signals from the GI tract. Stress can make the existing pain seem even worse. Interestingly, the connection works both ways, meaning that while stress can cause gut problems, gut problems can also wreak havoc on your emotions. The Harvard researchers continue:

> *"This connection goes both ways. A troubled intestine can send signals to the brain, just as a troubled brain can send signals to the gut. Therefore, a person's stomach or intestinal distress can be the cause or the product of anxiety, stress, or depression. That's because the brain and the gastrointestinal (GI) system are intimately connected — so intimately that they should be viewed as one system."*

Imbalances in Your Gut Can Make You Depressed, Anxious and More

Research using a probiotic containing the friendly bacteria Bifidobacterium longum NCC3001 has been shown to normalize anxiety-like behaviour in mice with infectious colitis.

Research published in 2011 also demonstrated that probiotics have a direct effect on brain chemistry under normal conditions - in such a way that can impact your feelings of anxiety or depression.

In addition, other research found that the probiotic Lactobacillus Rhamnosus had a marked effect on brain chemicals that lowered the stress-induced hormone corticosterone, resulting in reduced anxiety and depression-related behavior.

The authors concluded:

> *"Together, these findings highlight the important role of bacteria in the bidirectional communication of the gut-brain axis and suggest that certain organisms may prove to be useful therapeutic adjuncts in stress-related disorders such as anxiety and depression."*

Interestingly, neurotransmitters like serotonin are also found in your gut. In fact, the greatest concentration of serotonin, which is involved in mood control, depression and suppressing aggression, is found within your intestines, not your brain!

Psychic Masochism

There are probably a number of people that you have encountered who simply don't "let go." Why do we remain in these detrimental psychological states of conflict, anxiety, anger and frustration, even when we know they are not helping anyone and causing us to become ill?

A psychiatrist from the days of Freud by the name of Edmund Bergler answered that very question. So far, the mental health community has shunned Bergler's ugly truth. Here it is in layman terms:

We *like* misery.

Unconsciously, misery and unhappiness are so familiar and self-justifying that we cling to them, regardless of the consequences.

So, we end up subconsciously doing things that give us more of what we hate. When a chance for true happiness and fulfilment appears, we turn away. Bergler called it **psychic masochism,** or the tendency to take unconscious pleasure in *displeasure.* The result is self-sabotage, which may be the one universal mental health concern. In general, we gravitate toward the negative, refusing to let go of the negativity as if our very lives depended on it.

Learn how self-sabotage develops and what to do about it by watching this free video. It's a real eye opener.

We Live in an Insensitive World

We have all watched on television as a family comes out of the courthouse with a guilty verdict for the killer, and unbelievably, they state that they have forgiven the killer! Some would find this concept bizarre. Those who think about it a bit more, however, may realize that harbouring a grudge, anger and hurt against someone who has harmed you only causes damage to you!

In real life, it's not killers that we deal with on a day to day basis, it's the people we have everyday dealings with. The most important are our friends and loved ones.

It is a fact that we live in a world where many people are insensitive to others feelings and needs – it is quite an egocentric world, and selfish behaviour from others is likely to hurt us in many ways.

Common offences include betrayals of trust, rejection, lies and insults.

Whether you've been cut off in traffic, slighted by your mother-in-law, betrayed by a spouse, or badmouthed by a co-worker, most of us are faced with a variety of situations that can cause us a lot of stress and inflammation that leads to disease.

We have no control over these wrongs committed by others – we can encounter insensitive or angry people at any time of our lives.

What Happens When You are Hurt

Once hurt, people can rehearse painful memories and harbour grudges. This can perpetuate negative emotions and the physiological responses to these emotions.

When people hold a grudge, they stay in the victim role and perpetuate the negative emotions. Some people hold onto this for reasons of 'saving face' or to give themselves some sense of control. This is because a lack of control causes stress. However, nursing a grudge is a commitment to staying angry and this keeps all the negative health effects going.

Revenge is Disease

Society's main metaphor for revenge is disease. By default, we tend to think of revenge as a sickness that invades a vulnerable host (perhaps one whose resistance to the infection has been weakened by a poor psychological constitution or a bad childhood), consumes the host (morally, physically, and psychologically), and then has destructive effects on the avenger and the object of his or her vengeance.

Sometimes this disease spreads from one avenger-host to another until the outbreak reaches epidemic proportions. When you hear reporters describe "outbreaks of violence" that are fuelled by the lust for vengeance, that's the disease metaphor at work.

This disease model of revenge received modern psychology's seal of approval in 1948, when an influential psychoanalyst named Karen Horney described how the desire for revenge could absorb people for a moment in time, or for lifetime — becoming, effectively, a chronic illness:

> *"This drive can be the governing passion of a lifetime to which everything is subordinated, including self-interest. All intelligence, all energies, then, are dedicated to the one goal of vindictive triumph."*

Horney went on to argue that people prevented from exercising their vengeful impulses may exhibit symptoms such as headaches, stomach aches, fatigue, and insomnia. In short, the desire for revenge produces such a powerful psychological toxin that it literally makes you sick.

So, what do we do in these circumstances where others have hurt and upset us? One of the most powerful healing tools that we all internally possess is to forgive these people, and move on. The alternative would be to harbour these feelings and allow them to ruminate inside us, causing inflammation and disease.

One of the definitions of forgiveness involves letting go of the negative feelings you have and adopting a merciful attitude or good will towards the offender.

What is Forgiveness?

Generally, forgiveness is a decision to let go of resentment and thoughts of revenge. The act that hurt or offended you might always remain a part of your life, but forgiveness can lessen its grip on you and help you focus on other, more positive parts of your life. Forgiveness can even lead to feelings of understanding, empathy and compassion for the one who hurt you.

Forgiveness doesn't mean that you deny the other person's responsibility for hurting you, and it doesn't minimize or justify the wrong. You can forgive the person without excusing the act. Forgiveness brings a kind of peace that helps you go on with life.

What are the Benefits of Forgiving Someone?

Letting go of grudges and bitterness can make way for happiness, health and peace. Forgiveness can lead to:

- ❖ Healthier relationships
- ❖ Greater spiritual and psychological well-being
- ❖ Less anxiety, stress and hostility
- ❖ Lower blood pressure
- ❖ Fewer symptoms of depression
- ❖ Stronger immune system
- ❖ Improved heart health
- ❖ Higher self-esteem

Why is it So Easy to Hold a Grudge?

When you're hurt by someone you love and trust, you might become angry, sad or confused. If you dwell on hurtful events or situations, grudges filled with resentment, vengeance and hostility can take root. If you allow negative feelings to crowd out positive feelings, you might find yourself swallowed up by your own bitterness or sense of injustice.

What Are the Effects of Being Unforgiving?

If you're unforgiving, you will:

- ❖ Bring anger and bitterness into every relationship and new experience
- ❖ Become so wrapped up in the wrong that you can't enjoy the present
- ❖ Become depressed or anxious
- ❖ Feel that your life lacks meaning or purpose, or that you're at odds with your spiritual beliefs
- ❖ Lose valuable and enriching connectedness with others

398

How Do I Reach a State of Forgiveness?

Forgiveness is a commitment to a process of change. To begin, you should:

❖ Consider the value of forgiveness and its importance in your life at a given time
❖ Reflect on the facts of the situation, how you've reacted, and how this combination has affected your life, health and well-being
❖ Actively choose to forgive the person who's offended you, when you're ready
❖ Move away from your role as victim and release the control and power that the offending person and situation have had in your life

The Challenges of Forgiveness

Forgiveness can be a challenge for several reasons. Sometimes forgiveness can be confused with condoning what someone has done to us: "That's OK. Why not do it again?" The distinction between accepting someone's bad behaviour as "okay" and accepting that it happened and you must let go of anger to move forward, can be difficult because these two are easily confused.

Forgiveness can also be difficult when the person who wronged us doesn't seem to deserve our forgiveness. It feels like we are letting them "off the hook" when *they* are the one who wronged *us*. It's hard to remember that forgiveness benefits the forgiver more than the one who is forgiven.

Ultimately, forgiveness is especially challenging because it's hard to let go of what's happened. It can be difficult to accept some things in life, and forgiving someone who has committed unacceptable behaviour can be difficult when we are having trouble letting go of anger about the events and accepting what happened to us.

Can You Learn to Be More Forgiving?

Forgiveness is not just about saying the words. "It is an active process in which you make a conscious decision to let go of negative feelings whether the person deserves it or not," Swartz says. As you release the anger, resentment and hostility, you begin to feel empathy, compassion and sometimes even affection for the person who wronged you.

Studies have found that some people are just naturally more forgiving. Consequently, they tend to be more satisfied with their lives and have less depression, anxiety, stress, anger and hostility. People who hang on to grudges, however, are more likely to experience severe depression and post-traumatic stress disorder, as well as other health conditions.

But that doesn't mean that they can't train themselves to act in healthier ways. In fact, 62% of American adults say they need more forgiveness in their personal lives, according to a survey by the non-profit Fetzer Institute.

Making Forgiveness Part of Your Life

Forgiveness is a choice. You are choosing to offer compassion and empathy to the person who wronged you. The following steps can help you develop a more forgiving attitude - and benefit from better emotional and physical health:

Reflect and remember - that includes the events themselves, and also how you reacted, how you felt, and how the anger and hurt have affected you since.

Empathize with the other person - for instance, if your spouse grew up in an alcoholic family, then anger when you have too many glasses of wine might be more understandable, says Swartz.

Forgive deeply - simply forgiving someone because you think you have no other alternative, or because you think your religion requires it, may be enough to bring some healing. But one study found that people whose forgiveness came from understanding that no one is perfect could resume a normal relationship with that person, even if that person never apologized. Those who only forgave in an effort to salvage the relationship wound up with a worse relationship.

Let go of expectations - an apology may not change your relationship with the other person or elicit an apology from them. If you don't expect either, you won't be disappointed.

Decide to forgive - once you make that choice, seal it with an action. If you don't feel you can talk to the person who wronged you, write about your forgiveness in a journal or even talk about it to someone else in your life whom you trust.

Forgive yourself - the act of forgiving includes forgiving yourself. For instance, if your spouse had an affair, recognize that the affair is not a reflection of your worth, says Swartz.

Forgiveness and Health

Lack of forgiveness has been implicated in the following health problems:

1. Stressing the hormonal system that reacts to stress – the part that involves the production of stress hormones such as cortisol and adrenaline. This will also negatively affect other hormones too, as well as the autonomic nervous system

which regulates many bodily functions. These reactions place the body under considerable stress.

2. Mental illness; anxiety, depression

3. Heart disease, heart attack, hypertension, premature death

4. Immune suppression. Studies have shown effects on levels of immune protective cells and anti-cancer cells (Natural Killer cells)

5. Gastrointestinal problems

6. Effects on the reproductive system

7. Anything that follows from increased stress responses would also theoretically occur e.g. irritable bowel syndrome, Crohn's disease, ulcerative colitis, pain, muscle tension, fatigue, infectious illnesses and more.

Empathy

Being able to develop feelings of empathy can help move the person towards forgiveness. Empathy is placing yourself in the perpetrators shoes so that you have some sort of understanding of "where they were coming from".

This may help you understand why they did the offending behaviour. Empathy has been found to reduce stress responses in the body as well as cardiac risk.

Please note that forgiveness still allows you to hold the offender responsible for the offence and does not involve denying it happened, nor ignoring, minimizing, tolerating, condoning, excusing or forgetting the offence.

Now, it's not that easy to just decide to forgive. There is usually a process that most people can go through naturally. Some people are more predisposed to forgive – it's in their nature. Some have more difficulty, or there are circumstances that make it difficult.

It's possible to cultivate a more forgiving attitude by developing empathy and understanding that we are all human and not perfect. If you have been hurt and are finding it difficult to move forward to feeling better about it, you may benefit by seeing someone for psychological help.

In the end, its only you that suffers. So, go ahead and forgive, but not necessarily forget for the sake of your health and relationships.

When we do not forgive, we hold on to bad experiences, to the pain, to the trauma. This can cause fear, depression, frustration, anxiety, self-hatred, and loneliness. It's self-destructive. A writer said that non-forgiveness results in emotional, physical and spiritual bondages. He said that 90 percent of all health, marital, family and financial problems come from non-forgiveness.

According to Dr. Steven Standiford, chief of surgery at the Cancer Treatment Centers of America, refusing to forgive makes people sick and keeps them that way. Forgiveness therapy is thus now being used to help patients with cancer and other chronic illnesses.

Of all cancer patients, 61% have forgiveness issues, Dr. Michael Barry, author of *The Forgiveness Project*, said, *"Chronic anxiety and anger produce excess adrenaline and cortisol in the body which depletes the production of natural killer cells or antibodies which are the body's foot soldiers in the fight against cancer, most people do not realize what a burden anger and hatred are until they let them go."*

Spirituality and Well-being

As the director of Duke University's Center for Spirituality, Theology, and Health, Dr. Harold Koenig has been studying the connection between spirituality and well-being since 1985. Koenig's latest project is a $1.5 million study comparing the outcomes of secular and spirituality-based therapies.

How did you come to study the connection between spirituality and health?

"I became interested in the topic as a medical resident. When I asked people with illness how they were coping, they would often talk about their religious faith. I was very moved by their responses and began to look for ways to study it. Many other researchers are exploring this intersection. There's been a tripling of the data in the last 15 years or so."

What are the health benefits of spirituality and religion?

"They run across the board. Religious involvement, particularly if there is a strong spiritual component, is associated with less depression and anxiety, greater well-being, and less drug and alcohol abuse. Research using MRIs suggests that it actually alters the structure of the brain in people at high risk for depression.

It's also linked to better physical health and health behaviours — less smoking, more exercising, a better diet. Religious people have less cardiac disease and hypertension and better measurable immune function. Many studies show religious and spiritual practices delay the onset of memory loss associated with aging and slow dementia related to actual memory disorders like Alzheimer's. They also confer a longevity benefit - an extra 7 years of life among whites and 14 years for African Americans."

Are these perks a good reason to become more spiritual?

"I'd caution against doing it just for health reasons. The cake is not the health. The health benefits are unintended side benefits of being religious because it gives your life greater meaning."

Spirituality means different things to different people. What aspects of a person's spirituality or religion matter most when it comes to health outcomes?

"It turns out that belief itself doesn't mean much. It's whether the belief is carried out through some sort of action, such as gathering with others in a faith community, spending time in prayer or meditation, reading scripture, or volunteering -generally conforming your life to the teaching of your faith. That's where the biggest benefits are."

What can doctors learn about spirituality to better tend patients' health?

"Most medical schools sensitize students to the importance of spirituality in the lives of patients. But only about 10 percent of doctors address these issues in practice. I'd like to see all physicians assess their patients' spiritual needs and, if need be, refer them to someone who can address those needs. There's enormous healing potential in our spiritual practices and faith traditions."

Prayer is Popular
Prayer has been called the science of sciences and art of arts, and rightly so.

Prayer is the most widespread alternative therapy in America today.

A research study conducted by the University of Rochester at 20 sites across America and funded by the National Cancer Institute and the American Cancer Society showed that over 85 percent of people confronting a major illness pray. That is far higher than taking herbs or pursuing other non-traditional healing modalities. And increasingly the evidence is that *prayer works.*

Health Benefits of Prayer

Numerous scientific studies have evaluated the therapeutic effects of prayer. Generally, the research has shown that people who pray regularly are less likely to become ill and that when they do, they tend to recover faster. Interestingly, not only does prayer seem to have healing effects upon the people who pray, it also appears to benefit those who are prayed for by others.

Research reveals that people who pray have lower depression and suicide rates. Prayer even appears to lower blood pressure. In a study funded by the National Institutes of Health, investigators found that individuals who attended religious services at least once a week and prayed at least once a day or studied the Bible frequently, were 40% less likely to have high blood pressure than those who did so infrequently.

In other research, elderly women recovering from hip-fracture surgery who had strong religious beliefs and practices were able to walk greater distances when they left the hospital than those who were not as religious.

A 2011 study of inner city youth with asthma conducted by researchers at the *University of Cincinnati* indicates that those who practiced prayer and meditation experienced fewer and less severe symptoms than those who had not.

Other studies show that prayer boosts the immune system and helps to lessen the severity and frequency of a wide range of illnesses.

A recent survey reported in the *Journal of Gerontology* of 4,000 senior citizens in Durham, NC, found that people who prayed or meditated coped better with illness and lived longer than those who did not.

But the question remains: *By what physiological mechanisms does prayer impact our health?* Herbert Benson's most recent research suggests that long term daily spiritual practices help to deactivate genes that trigger inflammation and prompt cell death. That the mind can affect the expression of our genes is exciting evidence for how prayer may influence the functioning of the body at the most fundamental level.

Spiritual practice aims to connect the individual with God or a Higher Power, to open one to the Divinity dwelling within the self, and to make one fully present to life in the here and now.

These are not goals that lend themselves to being measured in double blind experiments. The sense of deep peace and radiant well-being that spiritual practitioners in different religious traditions report are also not testable by scientific means.

What science *can tell us* is that people who pray and meditate tend to be statistically healthier and live longer than those who do not. Whether these boons are merely unintended side effects of still deeper spiritual benefits remains a matter of faith.

Prayer as a Healing Tool

"He who is able to pray correctly, even if he is the poorest of all people, is essentially the richest. And he who does not have proper prayer, is the poorest of all, even if he sits on a royal throne"

- St John Chrysostom

Let me begin by saying that I believe in one-God for all the peoples of the world. Religion and religious denominations are man-made and we need to transcend these often-fanatical beliefs and focus on the one-God that symbolizes true, unconditional love. This is where our hearts need to be open to becoming more loving and empathic beings, so that we can help all those around us, including ourselves.

Intrinsic Characteristics of Love

In this following Scripture, Apostle Paul has given a clear description regarding the intrinsic characteristics of that love:

Love is patient, love is kind. It does not envy, it does not boast, it is not proud. It does not dishonour others, it is not self-seeking, it is not easily angered, it keeps no record of wrongs. Love does not delight in evil but rejoices with the truth. It always protects, always trusts, always hopes, always perseveres (1 Corinthians 13:4-7).

Love is the personification of the character of God.

Love is not an abstract. Love is not a feeling. Love is not really an attitude. Love is a deed. Love is an activity. In the original Greek, the word is a verb, not a noun. It describes an *action*.

Apostle Paul in Corinthians lists sixteen characteristics of love. Every time I read this list I feel deeply challenged. I know how far short of all these characteristics I often am – it is humbling:

- ✓ Love never gives up, love is patient
- ✓ Love cares more for others than for self
- ✓ Love doesn't want what it doesn't have
- ✓ Love doesn't strut

- ✓ Doesn't have a swelled head
- ✓ Doesn't force itself on others
- ✓ Isn't always "me first"
- ✓ Doesn't fly off the handle
- ✓ Doesn't keep score of the sins of others
- ✓ Doesn't revel when others grovel
- ✓ Takes pleasure in the flowering of truth
- ✓ Puts up with anything
- ✓ Trusts God always
- ✓ Always looks for the best
- ✓ Never looks back
- ✓ But keeps going to the end.

Praying to the One-God

So, irrelevant of our religious denomination, we can all pray to the one-God that should be in everyone's hearts. Prayer may be a requirement for Christians, but it is not only for Christians – God listens to all of us, no matter our colour, creed, or religion.

Years ago, I never used to pray. I thought nothing really ever came of it. However, in my later years, I began to master the art of prayer and now systematically pray daily - it is an inherent and important part of my life. I pray many times per day; for my children, for my wife, for my patients, for those that are suffering, for the politicians who wish to harm us, as well as all those that do not pray and those who have their focus on materialism and consumerism and other mundane interests.

Prayer is an *experience*. It is not a feeling, even though prayer is from the heart, not the mind. As we learn the art of prayer, we experience things happening in our lives and the lives of others that cannot be explained logically – it is like small miracles happen that are against all probabilities.

There is nothing more important or enriching than having a personal relationship with God. When you take time to walk with God each day through prayer, your relationship will grow with him – this is the goal of prayer.

Prayer is the most powerful way to experience God, but we often fall short. However, when we work at our prayer lives daily, and make it a point to be accountable with God, we begin to enter a space of full vulnerability and openness to receive God's work in our lives. Be open and allow God to guide – you will often be surprised at the positive outcome and usually what you witness is not what you planned personally. God will often nudge us to evolve Spiritually, to open our hearts, to love our family, friends and neighbours. This is what God wants from all of us – just surrender yourself to Him and let him guide.

Prayer is more personal and powerful when we accept prayer not as a daily or daunting task, but as a way of life. When we strive for closeness with Him, we grow in our intimacy with Him and can ultimately deal with the everyday challenges we face. Let go and let God in your life today.

How Should We Pray?

People often ask: how should we pray, in what words, and in what language? Some even say, *"I do not pray because I do not know how; I do not know any prayers."* You do not need any specialized skill for prayer. You can simply talk with God. We can pray to God in the language we use when speaking with people, when thinking.

Prayer should be very simple. St. Isaac the Syrian said: *"The whole fabric of your prayer should be succinct. One word saved the publican, and one word made the thief on the cross heir to the Heavenly Kingdom."*

Let us recall the parable of the Publican and the Pharisee:

Two men went up into the temple to pray; the one a Pharisee, and the other a publican. The Pharisee stood and prayed thus with himself, God, I thank thee, that I am not as other men are, extortioners, unjust, adulterers, or even as this publican. I fast twice in the week, I give tithes of all that I possess. And the publican, standing afar off, would not lift up so much as his eyes unto heaven, but smote upon his breast, saying, God be merciful to me a sinner (Luke 18:10-13).

And this short prayer saved him. Let us also remember the thief who was crucified with Jesus and who said to Him: *Lord, remember me when Thou comest into Thy kingdom* (Luke 23:42). This alone was enough for him to enter Paradise.

Prayer can be extremely brief. If you are just starting out on your path of prayer, begin with very short prayers, to allow you to focus. God does not need words; He needs hearts. Words are secondary; of paramount importance are the feeling and disposition with which we approach God.

To approach God without a feeling of reverence or with distraction is much more dangerous than saying the wrong words in prayer.

Distracted prayer has neither meaning nor value. A simple law is at work: if the words of prayer do not reach our heart, they will not reach God. Therefore, it is very important that each word of prayer should be felt deeply by us.

We do not need to say long prayers, or read from a prayer book. Perhaps the most famous and often-used prayer amongst Christians is the Jesus Prayer, it is simple and short, but very powerful and can make profound changes in our hearts when repeated many times each day.

One ascetic struggler said that if we could, with the full force of our feelings, with all our heart and soul, just say the prayer *"Lord, have mercy,"* then that would be enough for salvation. But the problem is that, as a rule, we cannot say this with all our heart; we cannot say this with our whole life. Therefore, in order to be heard by God, we tend to use many words.

The Jesus Prayer is very simple:

"Lord Jesus Christ, have mercy on me, a sinner,"

If you are including others in your prayers, then it is often enough to say: *"Lord Jesus Christ, have mercy on us"* while thinking of your children or patients or whoever – God knows who you are praying for, without even mentioning their name.

The words are really quite simple, but we need them to reverberate from the heart, and this requires us to quieten the mind, believe in the importance of prayer and make time during our day; have empathy and let the words touch your heart – after much practice this will begin happening automatically, and the changes in your life and those of others that you pray for will change for the better.

The Secrets to Maximum Prayer Power

Perhaps the most interesting and important detail of all this research is that certain factors do affect how powerful the benefits of prayer will be. Those factors are basically qualities of human consciousness, like:

- ❖ Caring
- ❖ Compassion
- ❖ Empathy
- ❖ Love

The stronger these qualities are, the greater the benefits of prayer. One thing holds true for all the studies on prayer — and that is that **it's not important** *what specifically you* **believe in. What matters is whether you believe in something, and** *how you* **put that belief into practice.**

References

Journal of Physiology and Pharmacology December 2011; 62(6):591-9.

Neurogastroenterology and Motility 2011 Dec;23(12):1132-9.

Proc Natl Acad Sci U S A. 2011 Sep 20;108(38):16050-5.

Lightning Source UK Ltd.
Milton Keynes UK
UKOW07f0225021117

312009UK00003B/20/P